15 Mansfield Street
London W1M OBE
Tel: 071-580-6523
Fax: 071-436-3951

The Royal College of Midwives

Membership gi
benefits of a
Professional Or
and a
Trade Union

GW00708163

229 Local Branches
Voting Rights in Ele

Expert Advice on Professional, Industrial Relations and Educational Matters

Representation on the Nursing and Midwifery Staffs Negotiating Council

Third Party Indemnity Insurance, Legal Representation, Personal Accident

Insurance

Involvement with the Statutory Bodies in each of the four U.K. Countries

Parliamentary and Press Advice and Contact

Educational Opportunities

Reference and Lending Library Facilities

Corporate Membership with the International Confederation of Midwives

Representation on Midwives' Liason Committee of the European Community

Representation on national bodies and committees

Free copy of the Midwives' Chronicle each month

Reduced Insurance Premiums

Further details available from
The General Secretary
Ruth Ashton, OBE SRN SCM MTD

Mayes' Midwifery 11/e

Betty R. Sweet

This classic text continues to meet the needs of students and practising midwives worldwide.

Key Features include:

* The changing role of the midwife and women in society
* AIDS, in vitro fertilization
* Applied psychology, counselling and communication skills, understanding grief and bereavement

"This edition should lead the way for a new generation of well-referenced, research-based textbooks for midwives"

Midwives Chronicle

0 7020 1236 X   638pp   217 ills   Pb
1987 Baillière Tindall   £16.95

Clear and Concise Text

Bevis
Caring for Women: Obstetric and Gynaecological Nursing (4/e) *(Nurses' Aids Series)*

To reflect the holistic concept of caring for the whole woman, the Fourth Edition of this unique title has been radically and sensitively revised to add broader women's health issues to its full coverage of obstetric and gynaecological care.

Key Features include:
- new chapters on the breast and urinary tract
- Exploration of socio-cultural and emotional influences in motherhood
- New chapter on women and sexuality
- Preparation for parenthood - including preconceptual care and counselling
- Women and HIV/AIDS

"...a useful and accessible book...helpful to those undertaking projects on women's issues"

Nursing Times

0 7020 1461 3   ELBS Edition 300pp
85 ills Pb 1991 Baillière Tindall £1.50`

NEW!

Watson's Medical - Surgical Nursing & Related Physiology 4/e

Joan Royle & Mike Walsh

Extensively revised and updated to accord with Project 2000's ethos, the fourth edition refers to health education, rehabilitation and health promotion, enhancing the text's holistic approach.

> *"...an excellent book which certainly meets the needs of today's students."*
>
> **Nursing Times**

Key features
● Socio-psychological effects and causes of illness, in addition to pathophysiology
● Care studies and care plans
● Nursing orientated presentation of care with reference to the nursing process

0 7020 1515 6   1056pp   225 ills   Hb
March 1992   Baillière Tindall   £16.95

Beischer & Mackay
Obstetrics and the Newborn
(Second British Edition)

Extensively adapted and enhanced for UK midwives, this edition includes expanded coverage of pregnancy diagnosis, nutrition, pharmacology, investigative procedures, genetics, infectious and medical disorders of pregnancy, operative obstetrics, fetal distress and labour and its conduct.

Two colour sections cover paediatric problems and psychosocial aspects of obstetrics. Each chapter is introduced by an authoritative overview which provides a rapid perspective in an easily assimilated form.

0 7020 1163 0   770pp   748 ills   Pb
1986   Baillière Tindall   £19.95

Psychology and Health Care

Oliver

A comprehensive, fully illustrated textbook of psychology applied to health care, particularly to nursing. It contains coverage of the major theories, developmental psychology, behavioural psychology, and physiological aspects of behaviour. It takes a practical approach, allowing the reader to apply its content directly, in all areas of health care.

Contents: Individual Differences: Patterns of Upbringing - Personality - Physiological Origins of Behaviour - Motivations - Communication - Cognition - The Self - Attitudes - **Reaction to Life Events:** Stressors and Coping - Personality and Life Events - Social Learning and Life Events - **Health Care Intervention:** Reactions to Illness - Reaction to Hospitalization.

0 7020 1601 2   ca 320pp   ca146ills   Pb
1992   Baillière Tindall   ca £12.95

Thorpe

A Practical Guide to Taking Blood

An introductory yet comprehensive guide to taking blood from patients. Features relevant anatomy and physiology, all blood taking procedures from thumb and heel pricking to the more recent and advanced evacuated system of venepuncture, safety aspects and first aid. It also includes features on AIDS/HIV and hepatitis, interpersonal skills with patients, an appendix of useful addresses and normal values for blood tests, and a large colour plate section.

"...highly recommend this pocket-size reference book to all budding phlebotomists."

Nursing Times

0 7020 1508 3   100pp   Ills   1991
Baillière Tindall   £6.50

Exciting New Learning Resource!

Values: A Primer for Nurses

Verena Tschudin

An exciting new training package covering health care professional values, designed for use in a workshop setting.

Workshop Guide: enables the course leader to present thought-provoking material in a flexible manner, with handouts and exercises designed to promote stimulating discussion.

Workbook: contains exercises and examples from everyday experience and societal issues for use in the workshop setting, but can also be used for independent self-learning.

Valuable for communication, ethics and personal development courses.

A discounted pack containing one Workshop Guide and ten Workbooks is also available.

Workshop Guide 0 7020 1580 6 116pp £55.00
Workbook 0 7020 1581 4 128pp £9.95
Workshop Pack 0 7020 1593 8 £150.00

Baillière Tindall
24-28 Oval Rd, London NW1 7DX
071-267-4466

Baillière's
Midwives'
Dictionary

Baillière's Midwives' Dictionary

Eighth Edition

BETTY R. SWEET BEd (Hons), RGN, RM
MTD, DN (PtA)
Senior Lecturer in Midwifery Studies
Royal College of Midwives
London, UK

Baillière Tindall
LONDON   PHILADELPHIA   TORONTO
SYDNEY   TOKYO

This book is printed on acid free paper.

Baillière Tindall
W. B. Saunders

24-28 Oval Road
London NW1 7DX

The Curtis Center
Independence Square West
Philadelphia, PA 19106-3399

55 Horner Avenue
Toronto, Ontario M8Z 4X6, Canada

Harcourt Brace & Company, Australia
30-52 Smidmore St
Marrickville, NSW 2204, Australia

Harcourt Brace & Company, Japan
Ichibancho Central Building,
22-1 Ichibancho
Chiyoda-ku, Tokyo 102, Japan

© 1992 Baillière Tindall

All rights reserved. No part of this publication may be reproduced,
stored in a retrieval system or transmitted in any form or by any
means, electronic, mechanical, photocopying or otherwise, without
the prior permission of Baillière Tindall, 24-28 Oval Road, London
NW1 7DX, UK

First published 1951
Sixth edition 1976
Seventh edition 1983
  Reprinted 1988
Eighth edition 1992
  Reprinted 1993, 1994, 1995, 1996
A catalogue record for this book is available from the British Library

ISBN 0-7020-1414-1

Typeset by Photo-graphics, Honiton, Devon
Printed and bound in Great Britain by BPC Paperbacks Ltd,
a member of the British Printing Company Ltd

CONTENTS

PREFACE

Baillière's Midwives' Dictionary is firmly established as a classic publication for midwives and other professional groups both in the UK and abroad. Over the years it has been updated by midwives well-known for their contribution to the midwifery profession and I have been challenged to uphold the high standards which they have established for the dictionary.

Changes over recent years in midwifery education and practice, in the National Health Service (NHS) and in the Statutory Bodies for Nursing, Midwifery and Health Visiting have created the need for a major revision of the dictionary.

In 1989 there was only one pre-registration midwifery programme in the UK (then called direct entry), but now there are 25 validated at diploma and in some cases degree level up and down the country. Post-registration midwifery education for registered general nurses continues, but by 1994 all these programmes will also be at diploma or degree level. The dictionary has therefore been enlarged to meet the particular needs of the large increase in number of pre-registration students and the higher academic status of all midwives. In addition, it is commonly used by student nurses during their maternity care and care of the newborn experience and will now be more relevant to their requirements.

Both the increase in midwifery research and the clearly expressed wishes of women for less intervention and more information, choice and autonomy in childbirth have led to major changes in midwifery practice in the last decade. These changes are reflected in this new edition of the dictionary. The large number of organizations concerned with maternal and child health and conditions affecting the well-being of mother and child are included in Appendix 25.

Fundamental changes in the National Health Service are in the process of being implemented according to the National Health Service and Community Care Act, 1991. An outline of these changes is included. The Nurses, Midwives and Health Visitors Act, 1992 will also lead to changes in the structure, role and function of the Statutory Bodies for Nursing, Midwifery and Health Visiting, thereby changing the way the professions regulate their own education, standards and conduct. At the time of writing the professions are being consulted about the implementation of this new Act and the main changes are included in Appendix 22.

It is my hope that this major revision of the *Midwives' Dictionary* will meet the needs of both students and practising midwives in the UK and overseas as they seek to increase their knowledge and understanding of midwifery and related issues in order to maintain high standards of care. Midwives returning to practice after a break should also find the dictionary helpful for updating practice and their knowledge of the changes being implemented in the NHS and the Statutory Bodies for Nursing, Midwifery and Health Visiting. Other professional groups concerned with maternal and child health should also find the dictionary a useful source of information. A study of the publications of current interest outlined in Appendix 23 should further aid understanding of current issues in midwifery today.

Betty R Sweet

ACKNOWLEDGEMENTS

I should like to express my thanks to family and friends for their support whilst I have been updating the dictionary, and to Sarah Smith, Senior Editor at Baillière Tindall for her patience and understanding, particularly when progress was slow.

A

A a name given to an agglutinogen in human red blood cells. Hence blood group A.

a- or **an-** prefix meaning absence of, or lacking, e.g. acardiac, lacking a heart; anoxia, lack of oxygen.

AB the blood group containing agglutinogens A and B.

abdomen the belly. The cavity between the diaphragm and the pelvis, lined by a membrane called the peritoneum and containing the stomach, intestines, liver, gallbladder, spleen and pancreas; and, lying behind the peritoneum, the kidneys, suprarenal glands and ureters. The urinary bladder and the uterus become abdominal organs when distended. For descriptive purposes, its area can be divided into ten regions (see Figure).

Pendulous a. a condition in which the anterior part of the abdominal wall hangs down over the pubis.

abdominal concerning the abdomen.

abdominal decompression a means of relaxing, by external suction, the external abdominal wall, thus allowing the uterus to come forward for its long axis to take up the optimal angle for the presenting part to enter the pelvic brim at a right angle and so descend efficiently through the pelvis. It has also been used

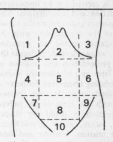

1. *Right hypochondrium*; 2. *epigastrium*; 3. *left hypochondrium*; 4. *right lumbar region*; 5. *umbilical region*; 6. *left lumbar region*; 7. *right iliac fossa*; 8. *hypogastrium*; 9. *left iliac fossa*; 10. *pubic.*
ABDOMEN

in an attempt to improve the uteroplacental circulation where there is placental insufficiency.

abdominal enlargement enlargement of the abdomen due to pregnancy can be seen from the 16th week of pregnancy; the enlargement is progressive, due to the growth of the gravid uterus. Undue enlargement of the abdomen may be caused by twins, polyhydramnios, fibroids in the wall of the uterus, or an abnormal development of the ovum (hydatidiform mole).

abdominal examination systematic examination of the abdomen. During pregnancy and labour this is carried out by inspection, palpation and auscultation. The purpose is to determine the equality of the uterine size with the calculated period of gestation and, when relevant, to decide the lie, presentation and position of the fetus and whether the widest presenting transverse diameter is engaged, that is, has passed through the brim of the pelvis. Inspection is made for shape, size, scars, striae gravidarum, skin tension, contour and fetal movements. Palpation (feeling) should be carried out gently and systematically. The uterus is palpable abdominally by the 12th week and increases in size at a regular rate. This completes the examination, except for the fetal heart sounds. Auscultation (listening) is carried out with a stethoscope (monaural or binaural) or with an electronic monitor. Its object is to hear and count the fetal heart sounds. Other sounds, such as the UTERINE SOUFFLE may be heard.

abdominal striae See STRIAE GRAVIDARUM.

abdominal swellings certain conditions, apart from pregnancy, may be responsible for swelling of the abdomen. (a) Fat may cause the abdomen to appear larger. (b) Fibroids, ovarian cysts or other tumours, if large enough, cause abdominal enlargement. (c)

The bowel (and the abdomen) may be distended with gas. (d) Fluid, as in ascites or in internal haemorrhage, causes abdominal swelling. (e) PSEUDOCYESIS also causes the abdomen to appear enlarged.

abdominal wall the structures covering the abdominal organs, namely skin, fat, fascia, muscles and peritoneum. Preparation for operation: before CAESAREAN SECTION, or any other abdominal operation, the skin must be prepared by careful cleansing. Immediately prior to operation the skin is painted with an antiseptic in spirit. See also Appendix 10.

abduct to draw away from an axis or the median plane.

abduction the act of drawing away from the centre; the state of being away from the centre.

aberrant wandering or deviating from the normal site or course.

abnormal any deviation from the normal pattern.

ABO blood groups a classification of human red blood cells according to the presence or absence of two agglutinogens, A and B. See Appendix 18.

abort to bring to a premature end, especially a pregnancy. To check the course of a disease.

abortifacient any means used to cause abortion.

abortion expulsion from the uterus of the products of conception before the 24th week of pregnancy, the fetus not being born alive. Therapeutic abortion: a term often used to describe an

induced abortion in accordance with the provisions laid down in the Abortion Act 1967. *See* Appendix 6.

abortionist one who induces abortion.

abrachia congenital absence of arms.

abreaction the reliving of an experience in such a way that previously repressed emotions associated with it are released.

abruptio tearing asunder. *A. placentae* or *placental abruption* is where the placenta is partially or completely torn from its site, usually in the upper uterine segment, after the 24th week of pregnancy. *See* Appendix 6.

abscess a localized accumulation of pus in a space or cavity. Abscesses may form in any part of the body, and those most likely to concern the midwife are: *Bartholin's a.*, in Bartholin's gland near the orifice of the vagina; *breast a.*, in the breast; and *pelvic a.*, in the pouch of Douglas.

abuse misuse, maltreatment, or excessive use. *See* CHILD ABUSE. *Drug a.*, use of illegal drugs or misuse of prescribed drugs.

accelerated labour *See* AUGMENTED LABOUR.

accessory extra or supplementary. *A. auricles* are commonly found immediately anterior to the ear.

accidental antepartum haemorrhage now more often called haemorrhage from placental abruption or ABRUPTIO PLACENTAE.

accouchement childbirth.

accoucheur a person who conducts a birth.

accountable liable to be held responsible for a course of action. In midwifery this refers to the responsibility the registered midwife takes for his/her practice. The midwife is accountable to his/her clients, peers and employing authority. *See also* Exercising Accountability, A UKCC Advisory Document, 1989.

accreta morbid attachment. *Placenta a.* a placenta attached to the uterine muscle due to a deficiency of decidua basalis.

acetabulum a cup-shaped socket in the innominate bone, into which fits the head of the femur.

acetoacetic acid a product of abnormal fat metabolism, occurring in diabetic and dehydrated patients.

acetone a by-product of acetoacetic acid. Acetone is one of the ketone bodies produced in abnormal amounts in uncontrolled diabetes and metabolic acidosis. Acetone has a characteristic smell which may be noticed in the patient's breath or urine.

acetonuria ketones in the urine. *See* Appendix 18.

achlorhydria absence of hydrochloric acid from the gastric juice; associated with conditions such as pernicious anaemia and stomach cancer.

achondroplasia failure to form cartilage. An inherited type of dwarfism characterized by marked shortening of the long bones. The achondroplastic dwarf has a large head, a normal trunk and very short limbs. Mentality is normal. The great majority of cases occur as a result of a new MUTATION and the gene is an autosomal dominant.

acid a substance which, when combined with an alkali, will form a salt. Any acid substance will turn blue litmus red. *Hydrochloric a.* a colourless compound of hydrogen and chlorine. In 0.2 per cent solution it is present in gastric juice and can cause MENDELSON'S SYNDROME if inhaled. Acids play a vital role in the chemical processes that are normally part of the functions of the cells and tissues of the body. A stable balance between acid and bases in the body is essential to life. *See also* ACID–BASE BALANCE.

acid–base balance a state of equilibrium between acidity and alkalinity of the body fluids; also called hydrogen ion (H$^+$) balance because, by definition, an acid is a substance capable of giving up a hydrogen ion during a chemical exchange, and a base is a substance that can accept it. The positively charged hydrogen ion (H$^+$) is the active constituent of all acids.

Most of the body's metabolic processes produce acids as their end products, but a somewhat alkaline body fluid is required as a medium for vital cellular activities. Therefore chemical exchanges of hydrogen ions must take place continuously in order to maintain a state of equilibrium.

An optimal pH (hydrogen ion concentration) between 7.35 and 7.45 must be maintained; otherwise, the enzyme systems and other biochemical and metabolic activities will not function normally.

Although the body can tolerate and compensate for slight deviations in acidity and alkalinity, if the pH drops below 7.30, the potentially serious condition of ACIDOSIS exists. If the pH increases to more than 7.50, the patient is in a state of ALKALOSIS. In either case the disturbance of the acid–base balance is considered serious, even though there are control mechanisms by which the body can compensate for an upward or downward change in the pH. Shifts in the pH of body fluids are controlled by three major regulatory systems which may be classified as chemical (the buffer systems), biological (blood and cellular activity), and physiological (the lungs and kidneys).

Chemical controls. The chemical buffer systems are dependent on the capability of certain substances to either combine with or release hydrogen ions. In the plasma and the intracellular and interstitial fluids there are three major buffer systems that regulate hydrogen ion activity; the carbonic acid–bicarbonate system, the protein buffer system, and the phosphate buffer system.

Of these three, the carbonic acid–bicarbonate system is the most important in fluids outside the cell. It is the most extensive and is the first to react to an acid–base imbalance.

The carbonic acid–bicarbonate buffer system is capable of either accepting or releasing hydrogen ions without forcing the pH to dangerous levels.

The protein buffer system is especially remarkable because proteins are powerful buffers that can function as either acid or base, depending on the state of the body fluids. This system is active in the plasma and in intracellular and extracellular fluids.

The phosphate buffer system operates in much the same way as the carbonic acid–bicarbonate system but is more active within the cell than in extracellular fluids. It is important in the regulation of pH in the red blood cells and kidney tubular fluids.

Biological regulators. This type of control is concerned with the shifting of excess acid or alkali in and out of the cell. The haemoglobin–oxyhaemoglobin system is another regulatory control.

Physiological regulators. The lungs begin to compensate for an acid–base imbalance within minutes of its onset. They do this by regulating the retention or the excretion of carbon dioxide. If acidosis is present, respiratory activity is increased so that CO_2 is blown off before it unites with the water in the blood to form carbonic acid. If alkalosis is present, respiratory activity is automatically decreased, CO_2 is retained, and carbonic acid is produced to neutralize the excess alkali.

The kidneys act as regulators by reabsorbing bicarbonate when it is needed to control excess acidity and by excreting it when there is a deficit of acid in the body. The kidneys also facilitate the excretion of excess hydrogen ions in combination with phosphate ions (in the form of phosphoric acid), or in combination with ammonia (excreted in the form of ammonium).

acidaemia an alteration, due to an accumulation of acids, in the reaction (pH) of the blood, which is normally slightly alkaline. It may occur in hyperemesis gravidarum and diabetes mellitus (*See* Appendix 6). If untreated, it will lead to coma and death. It can occur in labour if the woman is dehydrated and tissue perfusion is poor. The fetus or baby may suffer from acidaemia due to HYPOXIA.

acidosis a pathological condition resulting from accumulation of acid or depletion of the alkaline reserve (bicarbonate content) in the blood and body tissues, and characterized by increase in hydrogen ion concentration (decrease in pH). adj. **acidotic**. *Metabolic a.* acidosis resulting from accumulation in the blood of ketoacids (derived from fat metabolism) at the expense of bicarbonate, thus diminishing the body's ability to neutralize acids. Occurs in diabetic ketoacidosis, lactic acidosis and failure of renal tubules to reabsorb bicarbonate. *Respiratory a.* acidosis resulting from ventilatory impairment and subsequent retention of carbon dioxide. Carbon dioxide accumulats in the blood and unites with water to form carbonic acid. Occurs with severe birth asphyxia and other respiratory conditions affecting the newborn. In the mother occurs with either an acute obstruction of the airways or a chronic condition involving the organs of respiration. *See also* ACIDAEMIA.

acinus a minute hollow structure, lined by secreting cells and having a duct. The acini in the breast secrete milk. Sometimes called alveoli. pl. *acini*.

acquired immune deficiency syndrome (AIDS) part of the spectrum of disease caused by human immunodeficiency virus (HIV) infection. This virus, previously known as human T-cell lymphotrophic virus III (HTLV-III) and lymphadenopathy associated virus (LAV), causes an impairment of the body's cellular immune system which may result in infection by organisms of normally no or low pathogenicity (opportunistic infections) principally *Pneumocystis carinii* pneumonia (PCP), or the development of unusual tumours, principally KAPOSI'S SARCOMA (KS).

Infection occurs after virus in the blood, semen, vaginal secretions or breast milk of a carrier gains entry to a particular form of lymphocyte—the helper T-lymphocyte—of the host. After

a variable period, antibodies to the virus appear in the blood. This seroconversion may coincide with a transient glandular fever-like illness. These antibodies do not seem to be protective as the virus continues to be found in the helper T-lymphocytes where its continued replication destroys these cells and hence causes disordered immune function. The current experience of HIV-infected individuals is that many remain as asymptomatic infectious carriers. Some of the remainder may be asymptomatic but develop a persistent generalized lymphadenopathy. Others, in addition to the enlarged lymph nodes, develop symptoms such as night sweats, diarrhoea, weight loss and malaise; this latter condition is called AIDS-related complex. Examination of the blood may show abnormally low platelet and neutrophil counts as well as low lymphocyte counts.

Only individuals with an opportunistic infection or unusual tumour can be diagnosed as having AIDS.

During pregnancy previously asymptomatic carriers may develop symptoms and transplacental infection is likely to occur. This may cause conditions such as intrauterine growth retardation and microcephaly. There is also some evidence that the infection may be transmitted to the baby postnatally through breast milk.

acromegaly a chronic disease in which the bones and tissues of the hands, feet and face are enlarged. It results from over-function of the pituitary gland resulting in hypersecretion of growth hormone and is often caused by a pituitary tumour.

acromion a process of the scapula, which forms the point of the shoulder.

acrosome the cap-like, membrane-bounded structure covering the anterior portion of the head of the spermatozoon; it contains enzymes involved in penetration of the ovum.

Act of Parliament a law placed on the Statute Book after having passed through both Houses of Parliament and having received the assent of the monarch. The legislation relating to midwives is incorporated in the Nurses, Midwives and Health Visitors Acts, 1979 and 1992.

ACTH *See* ADRENOCORTICO-TROPHIC HORMONE.

active management of labour an active approach designed to prevent prolonged labour, so avoiding its many complications. *See* Appendix 9.

active transport the movement of ions or molecules across the cell membranes and epithelial layers, usually against a concentration gradient, resulting directly from the expenditure of metabolic energy. For example, under normal circumstances more potassium ions are present within the cell and more sodium ions extra-cellularly. The process of maintaining these normal differences in electrolytic composition between the intracellular fluids is active transport. The process differs from simple diffusion or osmosis in that it requires the expenditure of metabolic energy.

acupuncture the Chinese practice of inserting needles into specific points along the 'meridians' of the body to relieve the discomfort associated with painful disorders, to induce surgical anaesthesia, and for preventive and therapeutic purposes.

In general, acupuncture is employed to treat functional disorders rather than organic diseases that bring about severe tissue changes. It may be employed in combination with other therapies in the treatment of degenerative diseases. Acupuncture as a form of anaesthesia is considered by traditional Chinese practitioners to be a minor part of acupuncture practice.

Advocates of acupuncture base the practice on the concept of a vital energy flow or life force (*chi*) which circulates through the body along meridians similar to the blood, lymphatic and neural circuits. It is believed that there are two energy flows and that these forces are in everything in the universe. *Yang*, the positive principle, tends to stimulate and to contract; *yin*, the negative principle, tends to sedate and to expand. Health depends upon the equilibrium of *yang* and *yin*, first in the body and secondly in the universe.

The therapeutic objective of acupuncture is to rectify an imbalance in the energy flow.

This is accomplished by the insertion of needles, which are either of silver or gold, at specific points along the meridians. The needles are inserted in the skin to varying depths according to the point of insertion and the condition being treated. They may be left in place for varying lengths of time and are vibrated manually or electrically.

Traditionally an Oriental practice, acupuncture is becoming accepted in Western countries as a valid form of therapy. There is some experimental evidence that the procedure produces an analgesic effect because it causes the release of ENDORPHINS, the body's natural pain-suppressing substances. It is increasingly being used for the relief of pain in labour and for some other conditions associated with pregnancy and childbirth.

acute developing rapidly and running a short course. The reverse of chronic.

acute fatty atrophy (acute yellow atrophy) a rare complication of pregnancy characterized by rapid progressive atrophy of the liver, where there is massive fatty necrosis. The mortality rate is above 80 per cent.

acute inversion of the uterus turning inside out of the uterus. A rare, serious complication of labour. *See* Appendix 11.

acute renal failure a sudden severe interruption of kidney function. It is usually the complication of another disorder such as haemorrhage or shock and is reversible. Oliguria (diminished secretion of urine) is the hallmark of the condition and other symptoms are related to fluid and electrolyte imbalances, anaemia, hypertension and uraemia. Dialysis will be required to monitor fluid and electrolyte imbalances until kidney function improves.

acyclovir an antiviral agent used to treat *Herpes simplex*.

adactylia, adactyly congenital absence of the fingers or toes.

adaptation the ability to overcome difficulties and to adjust oneself to changing circumstances. Neuroses and psychoses are often associated with failures of adaptation.

addict a person exhibiting addiction.

addiction physiological or psychological dependence on some agent, e.g. alcohol or drug, with a tendency to increase its use.

adduct to draw towards a centre or median line.

adduction the art of adducting; the state of being adducted.

adherent placenta a placenta which is firmly attached to the wall of the uterus, and which fails to separate during the third stage of labour.

adhesion union between two surfaces normally separated: usually the result of inflammation when fibrous tissue forms; e.g. peritonitis may cause adhesions between organs; a possible cause of intestinal obstruction, or of sterility through occlusion of the lumen of the fallopian tubes.

adnexa appendages. *Uterine a.* the ovaries and fallopian tubes.

adolescence the period of development from puberty to the cessation of physical growth.

adoption the legal procedure by which a child is transferred from its natural parents to adopting parents. *See* Appendix 5.

adrenal pertaining to the adrenal or suprarenal glands, two complex endocrine glands, situated one at the upper pole of each kidney.

adrenaline one of several hormones secreted by the medulla of the adrenal or suprarenal gland. Its function is to aid in the regulation of the sympathetic branch of the autonomic nervous system. Adrenaline is a powerful vasopressor which increases blood pressure, heart rate, cardiac output and the release of glucose from the liver.

A pathological increase in adrenaline secretion is very rare and is due to a tumour of the adrenal medulla (phaeochromocytoma). It causes acute hypertension. Removal of the tumour cures the condition. In cases of severe hypertension in pregnancy a 24 hour collection of urine may be required to measure the level of vanillyl-mandelic acid (VMA), an excretory product of the catecholamines, which is raised in cases of phaeochromocytoma.

Adrenaline can also be produced synthetically.

adrenocorticotrophic hormone (ACTH) a hormone of the anterior lobe of the pituitary gland, which stimulates the adrenal cortex.

aerobe an organism requiring air or free oxygen to sustain life.

aerobic requiring air or free oxygen in order to grow and multiply.

aerosol a liquid agent dispersed in air in the form of a fine mist, possibly for therapeutic purposes, e.g. as a bactericide. Aerosol therapy is a major component of respiratory therapy in the treatment of bronchopulmonary disease.

aetiology the science of causes, e.g. of disease.

afebrile without fever.

affective pertaining to emotional tone or feeling. *A. disorder* any mental disorder characterized by a disturbance of mood accompanied by either manic or depressive symptoms or both. Major affective disorders are those in which the full syndrome of a manic or depressive episode is present: bipolar disorder (manic-depressive illness) and major depression. Other affective disorders include cyclothymic disorder and dysthymic disorder (depressive neurosis), which have less severe mood fluctuations.

afferent towards the centre. *A. nerve* a sensory nerve fibre carrying impulses from the periphery to the central nervous system.

affiliation order a court order made to compel a father to make regular payments towards his child's maintenance. *See* Appendix 5.

afibrinogenaemia absence of fibrinogen in the blood; more usually HYPOFIBRINOGENAEMIA.

Acquired hypofibrinogenaemia is usually secondary to disseminated intravascular coagulation (DIC). *See also* Appendix 11.

AFP *See* ALPHA-FETOPROTEIN.

afterbirth the placenta and membranes expelled from the uterus after the birth of the fetus.

aftercoming head the fetal head (coming after the trunk) in a breech delivery. *See* BREECH *and* Appendix 9.

afterpains painful uterine contractions occurring after labour. They are common, especially in multigravid women, in the early puerperium, are frequently felt during breast feeding and, if troublesome, are usually relieved by a mild analgesic drug. Severe and persistent afterpains would raise the suspicion that blood clot, membrane or even a fragment of placenta might be retained in the uterus.

agenesis absence of an organ due to non-appearance of its primordium in the embryo.

agglutination aggregation of separate particles into clumps or masses. 1. the clumping together of red blood corpuscles in serum. This may occur in the body if incompatible cells are transfused. Agglutination of sensitized red blood cells by urine reveals the presence of chorionic gonadotrophin in a pregnancy test. 2. the clumping together of platelets owing to the action of platelet agglutinins. 3. the clumping of bacteria when brought into contact with specific immune serum.

agglutinin a substance which reacts with an AGGLUTINOGEN and causes agglutination to occur.

agglutinogen a substance which stimulates a specific agglutinin to cause agglutination.

agnathia failure of development of the jaw.

AID artificial insemination of a woman with donor semen. The woman must be menstruating regularly and be physically fit. The donor has no responsibility or legal rights to the child. The husband may legally adopt the child.

AIDS *See* ACQUIRED IMMUNE DEFICIENCY SYNDROME.

AIH artificial insemination with semen from the husband.

AIMS Association for the Improvement of the Maternity Services. *See* useful addresses, Appendix 25.

air the atmosphere surrounding the earth, mainly composed of two gases: oxygen (approximately 21 per cent) and nitrogen (approximately 79 per cent).

air hunger deep, sighing respiration which occurs when the body's oxygen supply is deleted as in severe haemorrhage or shock.

airway 1. the passage by which air enters the lungs. 2. a mechanical device used for securing unobstructed respiration during general anaesthesia or other occasions when the patient is not ventilating or exchanging gases properly.

ala a wing, e.g. the sacral ala. pl. *alae.*

alba, albicans white.

albumin any protein that is soluble in water and moderately concentrated salt solutions and is coagulable by heat. *Serum a.* a plasma protein formed principally in the liver. Albumin is responsible for much of the colloidal osmotic pressure of the blood, and thus is a very important factor in regulating the exchange of water between the plasma and the interstitial compartment (space between the cells). A drop in the amount of albumin in the plasma leads to an increase in the flow of water from the capillaries into the interstitial department. This results in an increase in tissue fluid which, if severe, becomes apparent as oedema. Albumin also serves as a transport protein carrying substances such as fatty acids, bilirubin, many drugs and some hormones.

albuminuria the presence in the urine of albumin, usually serum albumin. It occurs in renal disease, severe cardiac disease and in some complications of pregnancy. *See* Appendix 6.

alcohol see FETAL ALCOHOL SYNDROME.

aldosterone one of the hormones of the adrenal cortex, the principal biological activity of which is the regulation of the electrolyte and water balance by promoting the retention of sodium (and, therefore, of water) and the excretion of potassium; the retention of water induces an increase in plasma volume and an increase in blood pressure. Its secretion is stimulated by angiotensin II.

alimentary pertaining to nutrition. *A. tract* the passage through which the food passes from mouth to anus.

alkalaemia increased alkalinity or pH of the blood, caused either by an overdose or accumulation of alkaline substances or by an excessive loss of acids, e.g. by vomiting.

alkali a substance capable of uniting with an acid to form a salt. Alkalis turn red litmus blue. In the body, alkalis form carbonates and combine with fatty acids to form soaps. Alkalis play a vital role in maintaining the normal functioning of the body chemistry. *See also* ACID–BASE BALANCE *and* BASE. *A. reserve* the ability of the combined buffer systems of the blood to neutralize acid. The pH of the blood is normally slightly on the alkaline side, between 7.35 and 7.45. Since the principal buffer in the blood is bicarbonate, the alkali reserve essentially is represented by the plasma bicarbonate concentration. However, haemoglobin, phosphates and other bases also act as buffers. A lowered alkali reserve means a state of acidosis; an increased reserve indicates alkalosis. Alkali reserve is measured by the combining power of carbon dioxide, which is the amount of carbon dioxide that can be bound as bicarbonate by the blood.

alkaloids organic nitrogenous substances which form the active principle of certain drugs, e.g. morphine, atropine and strychnine.

alkalosis a pathological condition

resulting from accumulation of base or from loss of acid without comparable loss of base in the body fluids, and characterized by decrease in hydrogen ion concentration (increase in pH). Alkalosis is the opposite of ACIDOSIS.

allele one of two or more alternative forms of a gene at the same site in a chromosome, which will determine alternative characters in inheritance.

alpha-fetoprotein (AFP) a plasma protein produced by the fetal liver, yolk sac and gastrointestinal tract. It is present in amniotic fluid and maternal serum and is usually measured in maternal serum prenatally between 16 and 18 weeks. A raised level at that time may be indicative of wrong gestational age, multiple pregnancy, neural tube defect, fetal death or, rarely, Turner's syndrome. A low level could be due to wrong gestational age or Down's syndrome. See Appendix 4.

alveolus any hollowed out structure, e.g. a tooth socket, an air sac in the lungs, or an acinus as in the breasts. pl. *alveoli*.

ambient surrounding or prevailing.

ambivalence the property of having equal power in two directions or on both sides at the same time. In psychiatry, having equally strong opposing emotions, such as love and hate for the same person.

ambulatory walking.

amelia a developmental anomaly with absence of the limbs.

amenorrhoea absence of menstruation. Amenorrhoea is physiological during pregnancy and lactation, and after the menopause; it often occurs following a change of climate, work or environment; or it can be a symptom of disease. Sudden and complete cessation of the menstrual flow in a woman of childbearing age whose periods have previously been regular will give rise to a strong suspicion of pregnancy.

amino acids organic substances derived from proteins, and essential to human nutrition.

aminophylline an alkaloid from camellia, which relaxes plain muscle spasm of the bronchioles and coronary arteries. It may be given by mouth, intravenously or as a suppository, and is useful in treating asthma and heart failure.

amnesia loss of memory, especially inability to recall past events or words.

Amnihook a device for performing an AMNIOTOMY. See Appendix 9.

amniocentesis puncture of the amniotic sac, usually through the abdominal wall and uterus, to obtain a sample of amniotic fluid on which the following tests may be carried out: the LECITHIN/SPHINGOMYELIN RATIO, CHROMOSOME ANALYSIS, estimation of concentrations of BILIRUBIN and ALPHA-FETOPROTEIN, and DNA analysis for fetal sexing and to detect certain gene-carrying conditions such as Duchenne muscular dystrophy, sickle cell disease and thalassaemia. It may also be carried out to relieve extreme discomfort in cases of severe polyhydramnios. *See* Appendix 4.

amnion the innermost membrane enveloping the fetus and enclosing the liquor amnii. *A. nodosum* a nodular condition of the fetal surface of the amnion, observed in oligohydramnios which may be associated with absence of kidneys in the fetus.

amnioscope an endoscope which is passed through the abdominal wall into the amniotic cavity and allows direct visualization of the fetus and amniotic fluid or is passed *per vaginam* in late pregnancy or during labour for visualization of the amniotic fluid.

amnioscopy 1. inspection of the amniotic sac, amniotic fluid and fetus by direct visualization using an endoscope passed through the abdominal wall. 2. visualization of the intact amniotic membranes and fluid *per vaginam* in late pregnancy when there is some cervical dilatation or during labour by means of an amnioscope to detect meconium-stained liquor and oligohydramnios.

amniotic fluid the fluid contained in the amniotic sac, also called liquor amnii and 'waters'. This fluid surrounds and is swallowed by the fetus. It is secreted from the cells of the amnion, transudate from fetel vessels in the cord and placenta and from maternal vessels in the decidua. The amount varies from 500 to 1500 ml at term. Amniotic fluid is normally clear and straw-coloured, and is composed of 99% water and 1% solids, which include protein, carbohydrate, lipids and phospholipids, electrolytes, urea, uric acid and creatinine, pigments, enzymes and placental hormones. In addition it contains desquamated cells, lanugo, vernix caseosa and increasing amounts of urine from the fetus. The fluid allows the fetus to move freely and equalizes pressure, acts as a shock absorber, equalizes the temperature and provides some nutritive substances for the fetus. Excess amniotic fluid is called POLYHYDRAMNIOS and an abnormally small amount is referred to as OLIGOHYDRAMNIOS.

amniotic fluid embolism the entry of liquor amnii, which contains vernix and other solids, into the maternal circulation via the sinuses of the placental site. A rare cause of collapse in labour or of HYPOFIBRINOGENAEMIA.

amniotomy surgical rupture of the amniotic sac for induction of labour. *See* Appendix 9.

amoxycillin a penicillin analogue similar in action to ampicillin but more efficiently absorbed from the gastrointestinal tract and therefore requiring less frequent dosage and not as likely to cause diarrhoea.

ampicillin a broad-spectrum penicillin of synthetic origin which is active against many of the Gram-negative pathogens, in addition to the usual Gram-positive ones that are affected by penicillin.

ampulla the dilated end of a canal, e.g. of a fallopian tube.

amyl nitrite a vasodilator given by inhalation for angina pectoris and to relieve the muscular spasm in CONSTRICTION RING.

anaemia a reduction in the number of red blood cells, or in the amount of haemoglobin present in them. Anaemia may result from haemorrhage, excessive breakdown of red blood cells or failure to manufacture them. *See* Appendix 6.

anaerobe a micro-organism which requires no free oxygen for its existence, e.g. *Clostridium welchii.*

anaesthesia a state in which the whole body (*general anaesthesia*) or part of it (*local* or *regional anaesthesia*) is insensible to pain, feeling or sensation. Anaesthesia may be produced by a number of agents. It is induced to permit the performance of surgery or other painful procedures.

anaesthetic an agent which induces anaesthesia. A general anaesthetic renders the patient unconscious; a local anaesthetic induces anaesthesia of a particular part of the body.

anal pertaining to the anus.

analgesia insensibility to pain. *See* Appendix 8.

analgesic an agent capable of inducing analgesia. A pain-relieving drug.

anaphylaxis an unusual or exaggerated allergic reaction of an organism to foreign protein or other substances. adj. *anaphylactic.* Substances most likely to produce anaphylaxis include drugs, particularly antibiotics, local anaesthetics, and codeine; drugs prepared from animals such as insulin, adrenocorticotrophic hormone, and enzymes; diagnostic agents such as iodinated X-ray contrast media; biological fluids used to provide immunity, such as vaccines, antitoxins, and gamma globulin; protein foods, the venom of bees, wasps, and hornets; and pollens, moulds and animal dander.

Anaphylaxis is the immediate reaction to allergens (often within a few seconds). The resultant release of histamines causes bronchospasm, widespread peripheral vasodilation and increased permeability of the capillaries. In addition there is increased constriction of the bronchioles and bronchi. As a result of these reactions there is a collapse of the vascular network by permitting the loss of fluid from the blood vessels into the interstitial compartment.

Immediate treatment in cases of severe anaphylaxis is the administration of adrenaline which causes bronchodilatation, reduces laryngeal spasm and elevates the blood pressure. Steroid therapy is initiated to counteract the effects of histamine by decreasing capillary permeability. Additional measures include the administration of intravenous fluids and plasma to restore intravascular fluid volume. Pressor agents, such as dopamine, noradrenaline and isoprenaline, are given to increase and maintain the blood pressure.

anastomosis a communication between two vessels or other structures, either natural or established operatively.

anatomy the science of the structure of the body.

androgens any steroid hormone that promotes male characteristics. The two main androgens are androsterone and testosterone. adj. *androgenic*. The androgenic hormones are manufactured mainly by the testes under stimulation from the PITUITARY GLAND. They are responsible for the growth of the penis and scrotum and for the secondary sexual characteristics, such as the growth of hair on the face and a deep voice. They also stimulate the growth of muscles and bones throughout the body, and thus account in part for the greater strength and size of men as compared with women.

android male-like, masculine. *A. pelvis see* PELVIS.

anencephaly a gross congenital malformation in which the cranial vault and the cerebral hemispheres fail to develop. Causes primary face presentation. *See* Appendix 9.

angiography radiography of vessels of the body after introduction into them of a suitable contrast medium.

angioma a tumour composed of blood vessels, e.g. a naevus on the skin.

angiotensin a vasoconstrictor principle formed in the blood when RENIN is released from the kidney. By its vasopressor action it raises blood pressure and diminishes fluid loss in the kidney by restricting blood flow.

angular pregnancy implantation of the fertilized ovum in the angle where the fallopian tube enters the uterus.

ankylosis abnormal fixation or union of the bones forming an articulation, resulting in a stiff joint. Ankylosis of the sacrococcygeal joint is a rare cause of difficulty during delivery.

anococcygeal pertaining to the anus and coccyx. The anococcygeal body or raphe is a mass of muscular and fibrous tissue between the anus and the coccyx; part of the insertion of the levatores ani.

anode a positive electrode to which negative ions are attracted. adj. *anodal*.

anodyne an agent which relieves pain.

anomaly marked deviation from normal.

anoxia the state of being deprived of OXYGEN. *See also* ASPHYXIA.

anoxic relating to or affected with anoxia.

antacid a substance neutralizing acid, e.g. mist. magnesium trisilicate.

ante- prefix meaning 'before'.

anteflexion bending forwards, e.g. of the body of the uterus on the cervix.

antenatal before birth. *See* Appendix 3.

antenatal bag equipment provided for community midwives to enable them to give antenatal care in the home.

antepartum before parturition.

anterior before; in front of.

anteroposterior from front to back.

anteversion turning forwards, e.g. of the uterus in relation to the vagina.

anthropoid man-like, e.g. anthropoid apes, man-like apes. *A. pelvis see* PELVIS.

anti- prefix meaning 'against', 'opposite'.

antibiotic pertaining to antibiosis, therefore destructive to life. Antibiotic drugs are drugs derived from living micro-organisms, which destroy or inhibit the growth of pathogenic bacteria.

antibodies specific substances formed in the body which counteract the effects of antigens or bacterial toxins. Antibodies, the effectors of the immune response, can be transferred passively from one individual to another as, for example, the transfer of maternal antibody across the placental barrier to the fetus, which has not yet developed a mature immune system. The developmental process of antibody production is usually completed a few months after birth.

anticoagulant an agent which prevents or delays the clotting of blood, e.g. heparin.

anticonvulsant a drug which prevents fits or convulsions, e.g. phenobarbitone. *See* Appendix 19.

anti-D gamma globulin a sterile solution of globulin derived from human blood plasma containing antibody to the erythrocyte factor Rh D. It is used to suppress formation of active Rh antibodies in Rh-negative mothers after delivery or miscarriage of a Rh-positive baby or fetus, or after invasive investigations such as amniocentesis, and thus to prevent haemolytic disease of the newborn in the next pregnancy, or later in the existing pregnancy, if the child or fetus is Rh-positive. It is given to a Rh-negative mother within 72 hours of delivery or miscarriage, or following an invasive procedure.

antidepressant effective against depressive illness. A drug used for relief of symptoms of depression.

antidiuretic 1. pertaining to or causing suppression of rate of urine formation. 2. an agent that causes suppression of urine formation. *A. hormone (ADH)* vasopressin; a hormone that suppresses the secretion of urine. It has a specific effect on the epithelial cells of the renal tubules, stimulating the reabsorption of water independently of solids, and resulting in concentration of urine. Secreted by the hypothalamus, but stored and released by the posterior lobe of the PITUITARY GLAND, it also has vasopressor activity.

antidote an agent which counteracts the effect of poison.

antigen any substance which, on introduction into the body, brings about immunity by stimulating antibody production.

antihistamine a term used to describe a group of drugs which block the tissue receptors for histamine. They are used in the treatment of various allergic conditions. They are often effective in relieving troublesome vomiting in pregnancy, the aetiology of which is not fully understood. *See* Appendix 19.

anti-hypertensive effective against hypertension. An agent that reduces high blood pressure. Anti-hypertensive drugs are used in cases of severe hypertension in pregnancy and there are many different types of drugs. Some, such as methyldopa (Aldomet), act on alpha-adrenergic mechanisms in the central or sympathetic nervous system to reduce peripheral vascular resistance. Vasodilators act directly on the arterioles to produce the same effect. Some other drugs act on adrenergic control of blood pressure. Beta-blockers, such as propranolol (Inderal), act at beta-adrenergic receptors in the heart and kidneys to reduce cardiac output and renin secretion.

antiseptics drugs employed to hinder the growth of bacteria.

antiserum a serum derived from the blood of an animal or human being with a disease and possessed of properties that are antagonistic to the bacteria producing the disease. pl. *antisera*.

antisocial against society. *A. behaviour* a term used in psychiatry to describe the refusal of an individual to accept the normal obligations and restraints imposed by the community upon its members.

antispasmodic relieving spasm. One of the actions of pethidine, hence its value in aiding relaxation of the cervix in the first stage of labour.

antistatic capable of draining away a charge of electricity.

antithrombin any naturally occurring or therapeutically administered substance that neutralizes the action of thrombin and thus limits or restricts blood coagulation.

antithromboplastin any agent or substance that prevents or interferes with the interaction of blood clotting factors as they generate prothrombinase (thromboplastin).

antitoxin an antibody produced to neutralize a bacterial toxin. Serum from immunized animals containing the specific antitoxin is used in the prevention and treatment of DIPHTHERIA and TETANUS.

anuresis retention of urine in the bladder.

anuria failure of the kidneys to secrete urine. It may complicate severe concealed haemorrhage from abruptio placentae, eclampsia and septic abortion, and lead to bilateral cortical necrosis of the kidney.

anus the extremity of the alimentary canal, through which the faeces are discharged. *Imperforate a.* one which, owing to congenital defect, is not patent.

anxiety feelings of apprehension, fear and uncertainty.

aorta the large artery proceeding from the left ventricle of the heart. *Abdominal a.* that part of the vessel in the abdomen. *Arch of the a.* the curve of the tube over the heart. *Thoracic a.* that part which passes through the chest.

aperient a drug which produces an action of the bowels.

Apert's syndrome a congenital abnormality in which there is fusion at birth of all the cranial sutures in addition to syndactyly (webbed fingers).

Apgar score a scoring system devised to assess the condition of a baby during its first few minutes of birth, so that severe asphyxia neonatorum can be diagnosed and treated at once. It is based on five criteria: heart rate, respiratory effort, muscle tone, response to stimulation and colour. *See also* ASPHYXIA NEONATORUM and Appendix 16. The infant is rated from 0 to 2 on each of the five items, the highest possible score therefore being 10. Each of the factors is rated at 1 and 5 minutes after birth and, in cases of asphyxia, subsequently at 5 minute intervals during the process of resuscitation.

aphtha the whitish spots caused by the fungus *Candida albicans.* THRUSH. pl. *aphthae.*

aphthous vulvitis infestation of the vulva with thrush (*Candida albicans*).

aplastic relating to any structure with incomplete or defective development.

APL principle the anterior pituitary-like hormone of the placenta, chorionic gonadotrophin.

apnoea absence of breathing.

Apnoeic periods occur in the respiration of newborn infants in whom the respiratory centre is immature or depressed. *A. monitors* are all designed to give an audible signal when a certain period of apnoea has occurred.

apoplexy sudden failure of cerebral function due to haemorrhage from, or thrombosis of, a cerebral vessel. It is characterized by coma, stertorous breathing and a varying degree of paralysis.

appendicitis inflammation of the vermiform appendix. Common in young people of both sexes. Uncommon and much more dangerous in pregnancy since the appendix is drawn up in the abdomen and the inflammatory process can spread more readily.

appendix vermiformis the vermiform appendix. A worm-like tube with a blind end, projecting from the caecum in the right iliac region.

apprehension fear or dread of some known or unknown factor.

aqua Latin for water.

aqueduct a canal for the passage of fluid. The *a. of Sylvius* is a canal leading from the third to the fourth ventricle of the brain. One of the causes of hydrocephalus is stenosis of this aqueduct. An obstruction of the absorption of cerebrospinal fluid occurs after meningitis or subarachnoid haemorrhage.

arachnoid the web-like membrane which is the middle covering of the brain between the dura mater and the pia mater. In the subarachnoid space beneath it, the cerebrospinal fluid circulates.

arbor vitae literally, the tree of life. 1. the tree-like appearance of white matter in the cerebellum. 2. the appearance of the folds of columnar epithelium lining the cervix uteri.

arborescent branching like a tree.

arcuate arched, bow-shaped. The arcuate ligament is a strong ligament stretching across the sub-pubic arch of the pelvis.

arcus tendineus a thickening, generally known as the 'white line' in the pelvic fascia, which gives origin to part of the levator ani.

areola the pigmented area which surrounds the nipple. It darkens during pregnancy and is termed the primary areola, with a secondary areola developing later around its perimeter. The lacteal sinuses lie under this area of the breast.

artefact an artificially produced lesion.

arteriography radiography of an artery or arterial system after injection of a contrast medium into the blood stream.

arteriole a small artery.

arteriosclerosis a hardening and thickening of the artery walls. Atheromatous plaques are deposited on the inner surface so that ischaemia of the organ or tissues occurs. It causes high blood pressure and precedes the degeneration of internal organs associated with old age or chronic disease.

artery a vessel which carries blood from the heart to some other part of the body.

arthritis inflammation affecting a joint.

artificial feeding 1. feeding via orifices other than the mouth, e.g. gastrostomy, jejunal, nasal, oesophageal and rectal feeding. In preterm or sick babies, one of these routes may be employed. 2. in reference to the feeding of infants, giving food other than human milk.

artificial respiration any method of forcing air into and out of the lungs to start breathing at birth or subsequently in cases when breathing has stopped. Artificial respiration can be given with no equipment whatsoever, so that it is an ideal emergency first-aid procedure. The mouth-to-mouth technique is commonly used in an emergency, together with cardiac massage if cardiac arrest or weakness occurs. Clear airways are essential before starting further resuscitative measures. Only the resuscitator's cheeks are filled with air when giving mouth-to-mouth resuscitation to a newborn baby and cardiac massage is carried out by either depressing the sternum with two fingers or gripping the baby around the chest with both hands with thumbs on the sternum and fingers on the thoracic spine. The chest is squeezed sharply four times between each lung inflation at a rate of 120 per minute.

artificial rupture of membranes (ARM) an aseptic procedure performed *per vaginam* by a doctor to induce labour, or carried out in labour by the doctor or midwife to accelerate the progress of labour.

A-scan ULTRASOUND display used for measuring size and thickness accurately. It is used particularly for fetal CEPHALOMETRY. *See also* ULTRASOUND *and* Appendix 4.

ascites an accumulation of free fluid in the peritoneal cavity. The condition is rarely seen in pregnancy. In the fetus or neonate, ascites is associated with HYDROPS FETALIS.

aseptic free from pathogenic bacteria.

asexual without sexual organs.

asphyxia suffocation. *A. neonatorum* is failure of the child to breathe at birth. There is a deficiency of oxygen in the blood and an increase in carbon dioxide in the blood and tissues. In mild to moderate birth asphyxia the baby makes some attempt to breathe, has fair to good muscle tone and reflex activity, a strong, fairly slow heart rate and is cyanosed. In cases of severe birth asphyxia the infant makes no attempt to breathe, is greyish white in colour, has a slow heart rate, and poor muscle tone and reflex activity. Urgent resuscitative measures are needed. *See* Appendix 16.

aspiration the withdrawing of fluid or air from a cavity by suction. *Meconium a.* fetal inhalation of meconium stained liquor. The hypoxic fetus passes meconium into the liquor. Premature inhalation prior to, or immediately following delivery draws the meconium-stained liquor into the lungs where it causes chemical pneumonitis and plugging of the airways. The obstruction produces areas of consolidation and under-aeration, as well as hyperinflation, contributing to the potentially pathological condition meconium aspiration syndrome. Preventative measures include careful suction under direct vision and intubation by an experienced paediatrician at birth, if possible before the baby breathes. *Chorionic villus a.* a sample of the chorionic villi is aspirated by a syringe or suction pump towards the end of the first trimester of pregnancy. The procedure is carried out under ultrasound guidance either *per vaginam* or transabdominally. The sample of villi obtained may be examined for DNA analysis, chromosomal analysis or for the diagnosis of some inborn errors of metabolism. *Vacuum a.* removal of the uterine contents by application of a vacuum through a hollow curet or a cannula introduced into the uterus.

aspirator any apparatus for withdrawing air or fluid from a cavity of the body.

assimilation the process whereby food is changed into body tissue.

assimilation pelvis a variation from the normal development of the sacrum. (*a*) In a high assimilation pelvis the last lumbar vertebra has become fused into the sacrum. The pelvis is deep, and there may be funnelling and associated difficulty in labour. (*b*) In a low assimilation pelvis the first sacral vertebra takes the characteristics of a lumbar vertebra. Thus the pelvis is shallow and the condition does not affect labour.

association coordination of function of similar parts. *A. fibres* nerve fibres linking different areas of the brain.

asthma a disease marked by recurrent attacks of paroxysmal dyspnoea, with wheezing, cough and sense of suffocation. Varying foreign proteins cause these spasms of the smooth muscle of the bronchioles in allergic people.

Astrup machine an apparatus for ascertaining the pH value of the blood.

asymmetry inequality in size or shape of two normally similar structures, or of two halves of a structure normally the same. An asymmetrical pelvis is a pelvis in which one side is distorted as a result of disease, injury or congenital maldevelopment.

asynclitism a parietal presentation of the fetal head in which the transversely placed sagittal suture lies close to the symphysis pubis or sacrum; the sideways rocking mechanism of fetal descent during labour, in a flat pelvis. In anterior asynclitism the anterior parietal bone moves down behind the symphysis pubis until the parietal eminence enters the brim. The movement is then reversed and the head rocks back until the posterior parietal bone passes the sacral promontory. In posterior asynclitism the movements are reversed, the posterior parietal bone negotiating the sacral promontory before the anterior parietal bone passes behind the symphysis pubis. *See* SYNCLITISM.

'at risk' register a register of children considered to be at risk of NON-ACCIDENTAL INJURY (NAI) or abuse. *See also* OBSERVATION REGISTER.

atelectasis incomplete expansion of the lung. *Primary a.* present from the moment of birth. *Secondary a.* this may occur owing to aspiration of meconium, infected liquor, vaginal discharge or, more rarely, maternal blood. The failure of all or part of the lungs to expand; it results from respiratory obstruction or weakness of the respiratory muscles at birth especially in the preterm baby.

athetosis a condition marked by involuntary movements of the limbs. Seen in children who have suffered intracranial birth trauma or kernicterus.

atlas the 1st cervical vertebra, articulating with the occipital bone of the skull.

atony lack of muscle tone.

atresia absence of the opening of a natural canal, e.g. of the oesophagus or vagina; usually a congenital malformation.

atrial pertaining to the atrium. *A. fibrillation* a cardiac arrhythmia marked by rapid randomized contractions of the atrial myocardium, causing a totally irregular, often rapid, ventricular rate. *A. septal defect* a congenital heart defect in which there is persistent patency of the atrial septum, owing to failure of closure of the foramen ovale.

atrium a chamber of the heart, formerly called 'auricle'. pl. *atria*.

atrophy wasting of any part of the body, due to degeneration of the cells from disuse, lack of nourishment or of nerve supply.

atropine the active principle of belladonna. An alkaloid which depresses salivation and the secretions of the respiratory tract, relaxes muscular spasm, accelerates the heart rate and dilates the pupil. It is employed before the administration of general anaesthesia.

attitude the relation of the fetal parts—head, spine and limbs—to each other.

atypical varying from the normal pattern.

auditory concerning the hearing sense. *A. response cradle* a device used to screen infants for impairment of hearing. A set of headphones is used to play noises to the baby and a computer analyses the baby's movements in response to the sounds.

augment to increase, as in *augmented labour* when progress in labour is slow and oxytocin is used to speed it up. *See* Appendix 9.

aura the premonition which often precedes an epileptic fit but not an eclamptic fit. See ECLAMPSIA.

aural pertaining to the ear.

auricle 1. the external portion of the ear. 2. former term for either of the two atria or upper chambers of the heart.

auricular fibrillation *See* ATRIAL FIBRILLATION.

auscultation a method of examining the internal organs by listening to the sounds which they give out. Auscultation of the FETAL HEART SOUNDS is an important part of abdominal examination in pregnancy and labour.

autistic withdrawn. A term describing a child who has great difficulty in making personal relationships.

autoclave a strongly built and hermetically sealed apparatus for raising the temperature of steam for the purpose of sterilization by maintaining the steam at a high pressure. This produces a much higher temperature and allows greater penetration by the steam.

autogenous generated within the body and not acquired from external sources.

autoimmune disease disease due to immunological action of an individual's own cells or antibodies on components of the body.

autoinfection self-infection, i.e. transferred from one part of the body to another by fingers, towels, etc.

autolysis self-digestion. The breakdown of tissue in the involution of the uterus which occurs in the puerperium. The surplus muscle is broken down into simple substances which are absorbed by the blood stream and excreted in the urine.

autonomic self-governing. *A. nervous system* the sympathetic and parasympathetic systems which control involuntary muscle.

autopsy post-mortem examination.

autosome any chromosome other than the X or Y sex chromosomes.

avitaminosis a state due to vitamin deficiency.

Avomine a proprietary preparation of promethazine, ANTIHISTAMINE type, used in the treatment of vomiting in pregnancy.

axilla the armpit.

axillary pertaining to the axilla. *A. tail of Spence* a process of mammary tissue extending to the axilla.

axis 1. an imaginary line passing through the centre of a body. 2. the second cervical vertebra.

axis of the birth canal an imaginary line representing the course taken by the fetus in its passage through the birth canal, downwards and backwards through the pelvic brim and the major part of the cavity; then, at the level of the ischial spines, turning through a right angle to proceed downwards and forwards. *See also* PELVIS.

axis of the pelvis an imaginary line passing at right angles through the centres of all the planes of the bony pelvis.

axis traction forceps obstetric forceps designed to allow traction to be applied in the line of the pelvic axis when the head is above the level of the pelvic outlet. Axis traction is rarely used now. *See* Appendix 10.

B

B an antigen present on the red blood cells in human blood groups AB and B.

bacille Calmette–Guérin (BCG) a vaccine used for inoculation against tuberculosis. It should be given during the first week of life to the infants of tuberculous mothers.

bacilluria the presence of bacilli in the urine.

bacillus a general term for any rod-shaped organism, e.g. *Koch's b.* instead of *Mycobacterium tuberculosis*. They are mostly Gram-negative except for *Koch's b.* and *Döderlein's b.* which are Gram-positive (*see* GRAM STAIN). pl. *bacilli*.

backache pain in the lumbar or sacral region. In pregnancy it is common and usually results from faulty posture. It may be a symptom of disease, such as pyelonephritis, or of the onset of abortion or labour. In the puerperium it occurs associated with poor muscle tone and the relaxation of the sacroiliac joints which persists after pregnancy and labour. If it is not relieved by rest the patient should have a full medical examination as the backache may be a symptom of pelvic disease. Other causes of persistent or severe backache are sacro-iliac strain and a prolapsed invertebral disc.

backward displacement of the uterus RETROVERSION of the uterus.

bacteraemia the presence of bacteria in the blood.

bacteraemic shock *see* ENDOTOXIC SHOCK.

bacteria microscopic unicellular organisms, universally distributed. When a part of the normal flora (commensals) they may be beneficial to health, e.g. DÖDERLEIN'S BACILLUS. Pathogenic bacteria are those which, on entering tissues, can cause disease. Bacteria are classified into two major groups, Gram-positive and Gram-negative, based on their reaction to the Gram stain. Other important characteristics used in the classification of bacteria are their form and structure and metabolic reactions (1) *cocci* are spherical; (a) diplococci are found in pairs, e.g. gonococcus; (b) streptococci are found in chains; (c) staphylococci are found in clumps; (2) *bacilli* are rod-shaped; (3) *vibrios* are curved rods; (4) *spirochaetes* are thin spiral filaments. Further classification depends on their requirements for atmospheric oxygen, aerobes require oxygen and anaerobes only grow in the absence of oxygen. Facultative anaerobes adapt to either environment. Bacteria can cause disease by produc-

ing *toxins*, by causing inflammation or the formation of granulomas, or by inducing a hypersensitivity reaction. *Exotoxins* are extremely potent poisons produced by some Gram-positive bacteria. *Endotoxins* cause hypotension, fever, DIC and shock. Other toxins include haemolysins and leukocidins which destroy red and white blood cells, kinases which lyse blood clots and enzymes that attack tissue.

bacteriological examination microscopic examination of body fluids or tissue to identify bacteria. In all cases of pyrexia in the puerperium it is desirable that a swab for bacteriological culture be taken from the cervix or upper part of the vagina. A mid-stream specimen of urine and, possibly, a throat swab should also be examined.

bacteriology the science of the study of bacteria.

bacteriophage a virus which infects bacteria.

bacteriostatic able to prevent the multiplication of bacteria.

bacteriuria bacteria in the urine, usually only considered of significance if there are 100 000 organisms per ml. Five per cent of all pregnant women have asymptomatic bacteriuria, some of whom will develop pyelonephritis in pregnancy if untreated.

bag of membranes the amnion and chorion which contain the liquor amnii surrounding the fetus; sometimes called the bag of waters.

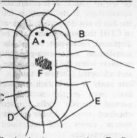

A. *Inclusion granules*; B. *flagellum*; C. *cell wall*; D. *capsule*; E. *frimbriae*; F. *nuclear material*.

TYPICAL BACTERIAL CELL

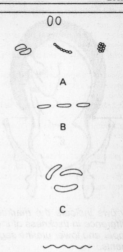

A. *Cocci*; left to right: *diplococci*, e.g. *gonococcus*, *streptococci and staphylococci*; B. *bacilli*; C. *vibrios*; D. *spirochaetes*, e.g. *Treponema*.

BACTERIAL SHAPES

ballottement bouncing. Tapping a structure which lies in fluid, such as the fetus in the amniotic sac, in such a way that it rebounds against the examining fingers. *Internal b.* is elicited by inserting two fingers into the vagina at about 16 to 18 weeks of pregnancy and tapping the fetus, causing it to float away and quickly return to the examining fingers. External ballottement can be elicited when making an examination per abdomen when the head is not engaged; the fetal head is given a sharp tap on one side, floats away and is then felt to return against the examining fingers.

Bandl's ring the extreme thickening of the RETRACTION RING of normal labour, which occurs when labour is obstructed. A

Bandl's ring is palpable as a transverse ridge across the abdomen, and is a sign of imminent rupture of the uterus.

barbiturates a large group of hypnotic drugs which are derivatives of barbituric acid.

Barlow's test a test to diagnose

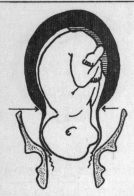

Arrows indicate the marked difference in thickness of the upper and lower uterine segments.

BANDL'S RING

congenital dislocation of the hip (CDH) in the newborn. It is a modification of Ortolani's test. The baby lies on his back with his feet pointing towards the examiner. The examiner grasps each leg with knees and hips flexed, placing middle fingers of each hand over the greater trochanter and the thumb of each hand on the inner aspect of the thigh. The thighs are then abducted and the middle finger of each hand pushes the greater trochanter forward. If the hip is dislocated the femoral head will be felt to 'clunk' as it enters the acetabulum. If no 'clunk' is felt the hip is not dislocated. In cases of CDH the femoral head can be displaced backwards out of the acetabulum by exerting slight pressure when the hips are flexed and adducted (Barlow's sign).

Barr body A small dark-staining body seen in the nucleus of normal female cells, often obtained from a smear of the buccal cavity and examined microscopically.

barrier nursing precautions taken by staff to prevent infection from one patient spreading to other patients and/or staff. This normally involves nursing the mother and/or baby in a separate room or cubicle. Staff wear gowns, and frequently gloves, masks, goggles and overshoes when carrying out care. All items used by the patient such as crockery, toilet requisites, etc. are sterilized after use. Excreta are disinfected prior to disposal; laundry is collected separately and either washed in a special container or disinfected prior to joining the main wash. Articles that cannot be disinfected or sterilized are burnt after use. In midwifery practice it is rare to have to carry out full barrier precautions, as described above, but modified precautions are sometimes required.

bartholinitis inflammation of one or both of BARTHOLIN'S GLANDS producing an abscess or cyst.

Bartholin's glands two glands situated in the labia majora, with ducts opening in the vagina, just external to the hymen; they produce the secretion which lubricates the vulva.

basal metabolic rate this is the minimum heat produced by a person who is resting, and who has fasted 18 hours. The method used enables the amount of oxygen consumed to be measured, and the result obtained is expressed as a percentage above or below what is normal for anyone of the patient's age, height and weight. In pregnancy the rate is increased by about 30 per cent. The basal metabolic test was a test of thyroid gland function but has now largely been replaced by tests to determine the levels of thyroid hormones in the blood and the radioactive iodine uptake test.

base 1. the lowest part or foundation of anything. 2. the main ingredient of a compound. 3. the non-acid part of a salt; a substance that combines with acids to form salts. In the chemical processes of the body, bases are essential to the maintenance of the normal ACID–BASE BALANCE. Excessive concentration of bases in the body fluids leads to ALKALOSIS, therefore the pH rises.

basophil a leucocyte which has an affinity for basic dyes.

battledore placenta a placenta in which the umbilical cord is attached to the margin instead of the centre. *See also* PLACENTA.

BCG *See* BACILLE CALMETTE–GUÉRIN.

bearing down the expulsive contractions in the second stage of

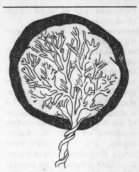

BATTLEDORE PLACENTA

labour. The mother uses her respiratory and abdominal muscles to help expulsion. During a contraction the face is congested, the pulse quickens, the blood pressure rises and the intrauterine pressure is markedly raised.

Benedict's qualitative reagent a solution containing sodium carbonate, sodium citrate and copper sulphate, used as a test for the detection of glucose and other reducing substances in urine or stools.

benzodiazepine any of a group of drugs having similar molecular structure. The group includes the sedative-hypnotics chlordiazepoxide, diazepam, oxazepam, flurazepam, and clorazepate, which are anti-anxiety agents; and the anticonvulsant clonazepam.

Prolonged use of these drugs often causes dependence.

bereavement loss, often associated with death.

beta- second letter in the Greek alphabet, B; used to denote the second position in a classification system. *B. adrenergic receptors* specific sites effector cells that respond to adrenaline. *B. blocker* a drug that blocks the action of adrenaline at beta-adrenergic receptors on cells of effector organs, e.g. anti-hypertensive drugs. *B. haemolytic streptococcus* a virulent streptococcus capable of haemolysing erythrocytes. The beta haemolytic streptococci are divided into serotype groups designated by letters, e.g. Group A. Cause of serious infections in the neonate.

betamethasone a synthetic glucocorticosteroid, the most active of the anti-inflammatory steroids. It may be administered to a mother who is likely to deliver a baby under 34 weeks' gestation. It decreases the risk of respiratory distress syndrome (RDS) by inducing an increase in the lecithin level in the infant. *See* Appendix 17.

bi- prefix meaning 'two'.

bicarbonate a salt of carbonic acid (H_2CO_3) in which one hydrogen atom has been replaced by a base, e.g. sodium bicarbonate, $NaHCO_3$. It is usually used to correct ACIDAEMIA.

bicornuate having two horns. *B. uterus* a congenital malformation in which there is a partial or complete vertical division of the body of the uterus. Normal pregnancy and labour is possible but it may be associated with persistent malpresentation and retained placenta.

bidet a low narrow basin on a stand with running water used for washing the perineum and external genitalia. Now commonly used in the postnatal period.

bifid cleft into two parts or branches. In SPINA BIFIDA the spinous processes of one or more vertebrae fail to unite and remain divided, or cleft.

bile a dark green substance secreted by the liver cells, stored in the gallbladder and passed into the intestine, where it assists digestion by emulsifying fats, and activating lipase. *B. ducts* the ducts through which the bile passes from the liver and gallbladder to the intestine. *B. pigments* BILIRUBIN and biliverdin.

bilirubin a bright yellow-orange bile pigment, resulting from the breakdown of haemoglobin. It is fat-soluble and unconjugated until it is rendered water-soluble, i.e. conjugated by the liver, when it is excreted as stercobilin in the faeces. If this process fails at any point, bilirubin passes into the skin and sclera, and JAUNDICE or ICTERUS results. See Appendix 17.

bilirubinometer an instrument for measuring the serum bilirubin concentration.

Billings' method a method of family planning. The woman and her partner are taught to recognize the changes in the cervical mucus which occur 3 to 4 days before ovulation in order that they may avoid intercourse around that time. The mucus increases in amount and becomes thinner in consistency to facilitate the passage of the spermatozoa through the cervix. This method of family planning when used in conjunction with other natural methods such as monitoring the body temperature is known as the sympto-thermal method. *See* Appendix 12.

bimanual using both hands. *B. examination* examination, usually of some part of the pelvic cavity, in which both hands are used. One hand is on the abdomen, the other with one finger in the rectum, or one or two fingers in the vagina.

bimanual compression of the uterus a manoeuvre to arrest severe postpartum haemorrhage after the third stage of labour when the uterus is atonic. The right hand is introduced into the vagina and closed to form a fist, which is pressed into the anterior vaginal fornix. The left hand, on the abdominal wall, pulls the uterus forwards, so that the anterior and posterior walls are pressed firmly together. This enables direct pressure to be applied to the placental site to stop the bleeding. It is exhausting, but should be maintained until the uterus recovers its tone and remains contracted. In an emergency, a midwife should her-

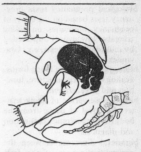

BIMANUAL COMPRESSION OF THE UTERUS

self carry out this manoeuvre. *See also* Appendix 11.

binovular developing from two ova. In binovular twin pregnancy two complete gestation sacs, each with fetus, placenta, chorion and amnion, develop in the uterus together. Also termed *dizygotic*, *dichorionic* or *fraternal* twins. The infants may be of the same or different sexes and like or unlike each other in appearance, in the same way as any siblings who are not twins. About five times as common as uniovular twins. *See also* TWINS.

biochemistry chemistry of living matter. With increased knowledge of blood chemistry, many diseases can now be treated much more successfully.

biological pregnancy tests pregnancy tests based on the effect of pregnancy hormones on living animals; now mainly superseded by immunological tests, e.g. Gravindex.

biology the science of living forms, dealing with their structure, function and organization.

biopsy observation of living matter. Removal of tissue from the body for microscopic examination and diagnosis.

biparietal diameter between the parietal eminences of the fetal skull; traditional measurement is 9.5 cm (3¾ in), in a normal baby at term. It may be determined by ultrasonic cephalometry from 9 weeks' gestation using an A-scan. Serial measurement of the biparietal diameter in pregnancy is used to assess fetal maturity and growth. The fetal head is said to be engaged when the biparietal diameter, which is the widest transverse diameter of the skull, has passed through the brim of the maternal pelvis; this indicates that delivery by the vaginal route should be possible. Crowning occurs when the biparietal diameter distends the vulva during delivery and the head no longer recedes during contractions.

bipolar relating to two poles or ends, and used in reference to the fetus and the parturient uterus.

birth the act or process of being born.

birth canal the bony and soft tissue structures through which the fetus must pass in order to be born. *See* PELVIS.

birth certificate a statement issued by the registrar for births, marriages and deaths for the district in which the child was born. It certifies details of parentage, name and sex of child, and date and place of birth. This certificate must be obtained by the parents, or failing them, anyone present at the delivery, within 42 days of birth in England (21 days in Scotland). It gives legal status to the child and is necessary before the child can receive Child Benefit. A birth certificate is issued to any child born alive, irrespective of the period of gestation. A stillbirth certificate is issued for babies of 24 weeks maturity or longer who did not breathe or show other signs of life after complete expulsion from the mother.

birth control the prevention or avoidance of conception. *See* Appendix 12.

birth injury trauma to the child, sustained during birth. *See* HAEMORRHAGE, CEPHALHAEMATOMA *and* ERB'S PARALYSIS.

birth mark a congenital blemish or spot on the skin, usually visible at birth or soon after. See also NAEVUS.

birth, notification of a person present, or in attendance, at the birth or within 6 hours afterwards, must notify the Director of Public Health within 36 hours (Public Health Act, 1936). This responsibility is accepted by the midwife when in attendance.

birth plan a plan prepared by the expectant mother, usually in conjunction with her partner and midwife, which records her preferences for care during and after labour.

birth rate the number of births during one year per 1000 total estimated mid-year population (crude birth rate), per 1000 estimated mid-year female population (refined birth rate), or per 1000 estimated mid-year female population of child-bearing age (true birth rate), that is between the ages of 15 and 45.

birth, registration of either parent must register the birth within 42 days at the registrar's office in the district in which the birth took place (21 days in Scotland). Failure to do so incurs a fine. The responsibility rests with the midwife if the parents default.

birth stool a stool on which a mother sits to give birth.

birth weight the weight of a baby immediately following delivery. Accuracy is important because it forms a baseline for assessing future development and is also used for national statistics. The average birth weight in the UK for a healthy baby born at term is currently 3.5 kg.

birthing chair a chair on which a woman gives birth. Some are electronically operated, thus can be tilted back quickly and easily as required. They combine the advantages of the upright position with good visibility and access for the midwife during delivery. Disadvantages are a higher mean blood loss and an increased incidence of postpartum haemorrhage. To reduce these problems it is recommended that the chair be tilted to 40° to the vertical immediately before delivery and throughout the third stage of labour. Some delivery beds can now be converted into a chair.

birthing room usually refers to a room for normal labour and delivery which is furnished in a comfortable and home-like fashion.

bisacromial diameter a diameter measured between the acromion processes on the shoulder blades. The fetal measurement is about 12 cm (4½ in).

bisexual hermaphrodite. Having gonads of both sexes.

Bishop's score a method of assessing the favourability of the cervix, prior to induction of labour. *See* Appendix 9.

bitemporal a diameter measured between the most distant points of the coronal suture; on the fetal skull it measures 8.2 cm (3¼ in).

bitrochanteric diameter a diameter measured between the greater trochanters of the femora; it measures 10 cm (4 in) on the fetus, and is the diameter to engage in breech presentation.

bladder the reservoir for urine, of obstetrical importance owing to its position in front of the uterus and vagina. The enlarging uterus during the first 12 weeks of pregnancy may press on the bladder and cause increased frequency of micturition. Towards term pressure from the fetal head, if engaged, has a similar effect. Incarceration by the retroverted gravid uterus may cause retention of urine between the 12th and 16th weeks of pregnancy. During labour a distended bladder may inhibit uterine contractions with the risk of prolongation of the first and second stages and of postpartum haemorrhage complicating the third stage.

blastocyst a very early pregnancy about a week after conception. The outer layer, the trophoblast, develops into the placenta and the chorion, and the inner cell mass, a mass of cells projecting into the cavity, develops into the fetus and the amnion.

bleeding time the time required for a small inflicted wound to cease bleeding. The normal time is 3–4 minutes.

blighted ovum abnormal ovum.

BLISS (Baby Life Support Systems) a charitable organization which raises money for equipment for babies requiring special and intensive care in neonatal units.

blister a bleb. A collection of serum between the epidermis and the true skin. The appearance of watery blisters on the body of an infant within the first 3 weeks of life may be a sign of PEMPHIGUS NEONATORUM.

block 1. an obstruction or stoppage. 2. regional anaesthesia. *Epidural b.* anaesthesia produced by injection of local anaesthetic between the vertebral spines and beneath the ligamentum flavum into the extradural space. It is widely used for the relief of pain in labour. *Paracervical b.* anaesthesia of the inferior hypogastric plexus and ganglia produced by injection of the local anaesthetic into the lateral fornices of the vagina. *Pudendal b.* anaesthesia produced by blocking the pudendal nerves, accomplished by injection of local anaesthetic into the tuberosity of the ischium.

blood the fluid that circulates through the heart and blood vessels, supplying oxygen and nutritive material to all parts of the body, and carrying off waste products, etc. It has an essential role in the maintenance of fluid balance. Blood is composed of two parts: 1. plasma, the fluid portion, and 2. formed elements, the blood cells and platelets suspended in the fluid. *Plasma* accounts for about 55% of the total volume of the blood. It consists of about 92% water, 7% proteins and less than 1% inorganic salts, organic substances other than proteins, dissolved gases, hormones, antibodies and enzymes. Plasma from which fibrinogen has been removed is called serum. *Blood cells and platelets* comprise the other 45% of the total volume of blood. They include erythrocytes (red blood cells), leukocytes (white blood cells) and platelets (thrombocytes). There are 35×10^{12} red blood cells in the average adult and they carry oxygen from the lungs to the tissues via the haemoglobin. Leukocytes are the body's primary defence against infections. They are longer than red blood cells and normally the blood has about 8×10^9 white blood cells per litre. When infection is present their numbers are greatly increased. Platelets initiate blood clotting and are concerned in contraction of a clot. When they encounter a leak in a blood vessel, they adhere to the edges of the injured tissue and create a matrix on which the clot forms. There are about $350–500 \times 10^9$ platelets in the blood. See Appendix 18.

blood clotting coagulation. See CLOTTING.

blood count see Appendix 18.

blood gas analysis laboratory studies of arterial and venous blood for the purpose of measuring oxygen and carbon dioxide levels and pressure or tension, and hydrogen ion concentration (pH). Analyses of blood gases provide the following information: PaO_2—partial pressure (P) of oxygen (O_2) in the arterial blood (a); SaO_2—percentage of available haemoglobin that is saturated (Sa) with oxygen (O_2); $PaCO_2$—partial pressure (P) of carbon dioxide (CO_2) in arterial blood (a); pH—an expression of the extent to which the blood is alkaline or acidic; HCO_3—the level of plasma bicarbonate; an indicator of the metabolic acid–base status.

blood grouping See Appendix 18.

blood pressure the pressure or force which the blood exerts against the walls of the blood vessels. Though there is some pressure in all blood vessels, the term is generally used in reference to the arterial blood pressure. This pressure is determined by several interrelated factors, including the pumping action of the heart, the resistance to the flow of blood in the arterioles, the elasticity of the walls of the main arteries, the blood volume and extracellular fluid volume, and the blood's viscosity, or thickness. The blood pressure is measured in the brachial artery by means of a sphygmomanometer. Two levels are recorded: a systolic pressure, which is the maximum pressure during contraction of the ventricles; and a diastolic pressure, which is the pressure in the vessel when the ventricles are at rest. It is the midwife's duty to check carefully the blood pressure of all women attending the antenatal clinic, at every visit. The midwife should consult a doctor about any woman in whom the systolic pressure rises to more than 130 mmHg or the diastolic pressure to more than 90 mmHg, or where there is an increase of 15 mmHg in diastolic pressure over the previous reading. See also Appendix 3 and Appendix 6.

blood products a group of products derived from blood. Most units of blood are issued for transfusion to patients as packed red cells; the supernatant fluid (plasma) contains platelets, white cells, coagulation factors and plasma proteins, including immunoglobulin. Blood products may be issued for immediate use, e.g. red cells, platelets, frozen down in their natural state for later use, e.g. fresh frozen plasma (FFP), or pooled and concentrated to achieve therapeutic levels, e.g. factor VIII concentrate for the treatment of haemophilia.

blood sugar the concentration of sugar in the blood. The commonest measurement is for glucose and this is recorded in millimoles per litre (mmol/l). Adult nonpregnant values are between 3.3 and 5.3 mmol/l, and pregnant values between 3.3 and 6.1 mmol/l. Neonatal concentrations may be much lower: 2.2–5.3 mmol/l. *See also* HYPOGLYCAEMIA.

blood transfusion the introduction of blood from a donor to the circulation of a recipient. *See* Appendix 11.

blood urea the proportion of urea in the blood. Normally it is between 2.5 and 5.8 mmol/l (15–35 mg/100 ml). In pregnancy the level is lowered to between 2.3 and 5.0 mmol/l (14–30 mg/100 ml).

blood volume the total quantity of blood in the body. The regulation of blood volume in the circulatory system is affected by the intrinsic mechanism for fluid exchange at the capillary membranes and by hormonal influences and nervous reflexes that affect the excretion of fluids by the kidneys. A rapid decrease in the blood volume, as in haemorrhage, greatly reduces the cardiac output and creates a condition called SHOCK or circulatory shock. Conversely, an increase in blood volume, as when there is retention of water and salt in the body because of renal failure, results in an increase in cardiac output. The eventual outcome of this situation is increased arterial blood pressure. Assessment of blood volume can be done through the use of intravascular catheters such as the CENTRAL VENOUS PRESSURE catheter, which measures pressure in the right atrium, and the Swan–Ganz catheter, which measures pressure on both sides of the heart.

bonding the development of a close emotional tie to a newborn infant, or to another person. It is now thought that optimal bonding of the parents to a newborn infant requires a period of close contact with the infant in the first few hours after birth. The infant's responses to the mother, such as body and eye movements, are a necessary part of the process, and the presence of the father during the birth increases his bonding to the infant.

bone marrow a substance found in the hollow cavities of bones. *Red b. m.*, in trunk and skull bones only, forms all red and white cells except some lymphocytes. *Yellow fatty b. m.* is present in the long bones of adults and is not normally concerned with blood formation.

borborygmus the rumbling sound produced by flatus in the intestine.

bougie a flexible instrument made of plastic or gum-elastic and used to dilate a stricture, as in the oesophagus or urethra or vagina.

bowel the intestine. *B. sounds* sounds caused by the propulsion of the intestinal contents through the lower alimentary tract. The absence of bowel sounds is symptomatic of greatly decreased or totally absent peristaltic movement. This can occur in such conditions as paralytic ileus and advanced intestinal obstruction which may occur following abdominal surgery such as caesarean section.

Bowman's capsule the commencement of the kidney nephron, which surrounds a tuft of renal capillaries—the *glomerulus*. Filtration takes place from the blood into the TUBULE; called also glomerular capsule.

Boyle's anaesthetic machine a continuous-flow anaesthetic machine which supplies oxygen and nitrous oxide together with cyclopropane, halothane and other anaesthetic agents as required.

brachial relating to the arm. *B. artery* the continuation of the axial artery along the inner side of the upper arm. *B. plexus* a nerve plexus situated just above the clavicle and in the root of the neck. It is formed by anterior primary rami of the Vth, VIth, VIIth and VIIIth cervical spinal and 1st thoracic nerves. The plexus may be damaged during birth by forcible widening of the angle between the head and shoulders during a breech delivery or a vertex presentation wih shoulder dystocia. ERB'S PARALYSIS or KLUMPKE'S PARALYSIS may result.

brachydactylia abnormally short fingers.

bradycardia an abnormally slow heart beat as shown by slowing of the pulse rate to less than 60 per minute or, in the case of the fetus, to a heart rate of less than 100 beats per minute.

brain the highly specialized area of the central nervous system contained within the cranium. The *forebrain* is expanded into the cerebral hemispheres (A), separated by the fissure of Rolando and containing the lateral ventricles which communicate with the third ventricle, inferior to which are the HYPOTHALAMUS and PITUITARY GLAND. The *mid-*

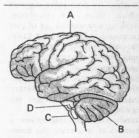

A. *Cerebral hemispheres*;
B. *cerebellum*; C. *medulla oblongata*; D. *pons varolii*.
BRAIN

brain, carries a canal, the aqueduct of Sylvius, connecting the third ventricle to the fourth ventricle in the hindbrain. The *hindbrain* consists of the pons (D), cerebellum (B) and medulla oblongata (C). The medulla is a continuation of the spinal cord. The brain and spinal cord are covered by three membranes, the MENINGES. The brain is made up of millions of nerve cells, intricately connected with each other. It contains centres (groups of neurons and their connections) which control many involuntary functions, such as circulation, temperature regulation, and respiration, and interpret sensory impressions received from the eyes, ears and other sense organs. Consciousness, emotion, thought and reasoning are functions of the brain. It also contains centres or areas for associative memory which allow for recording, recalling and making use of past experiences. *See also* FALX CEREBRI *and* TENTORIUM CEREBELLI.

brain death irreversible coma.

brain scanning an imaging technique used to detect abnormalities of the brain, e.g. intraventricular haemorrhage in the newborn.

Brandt–Andrews manoeuvre a method of delivering the membranes and placenta after their descent into the vagina. One hand lifts the contracted uterus away from the placenta, while the other hand applies counter-tension on the cord. This method has now been superseded by controlled cord traction.

Braxton Hicks contractions painless, irregular uterine contractions occurring during pregnancy, so called after the obstetrician of that name who first described them. As pregnancy advances they gradually increase in intensity and frequency and become more rhythmic during the third trimester; are often mistaken for true labour, and sometimes referred to as 'false labour'.

breast the mammary gland. The female breasts, two in number, are situated superficially on the anterior aspect of the thorax, separated from the chest wall by a layer of loose connective tissue. The nipple is composed of erectile tissue and should stand out from the breast. Surrounding each nipple is a circle of pigmented skin, the areola. Upon the surface of the areola open about 12–16 sebaceous glands, which enlarge during pregnancy and are known as Montgomery's tubules. They secrete a fatty substance which renders the skin supple. The breast is composed of glandular and connective tissue (fat and fibrous tissue) and is richly supplied with blood vessels. The glandular tissue of the breast is divided up into lobes, each surrounded by a fibrous capsule. There are about 16 lobes in each breast, and each lobe consists of lactiferous tubules held together by connective tissue. The tubules end in minute spaces called

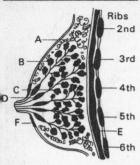

A. *Fat*; B. *alveoli*; C. *lactiferous duct*; D. *lacteal sinus or ampulla*; E. *pectoralis major*; F. *areola*.

BREAST

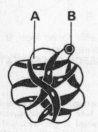

A. *Muscle fibres*; B. *Milk duct*.
ALVEOLUS SHOWING THE MYOEPITHELIAL CELLS (MICROSCOPIC)

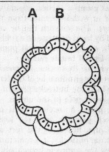

A. *Acini cells*; B. *Cavity*.
CROSS-SECTION OF AN ALVEOLUS (MICROSCOPIC)

alveoli or acini, each surrounded by contractile myoepithelial cells. Secreting cells form the lining of the alveoli, and it is here that milk is secreted during lactation. The alveoli unite with small branches of lactiferous tubules and eventually form the main tubules or lactiferous ducts; these converge towards the areola, beneath which they are dilated. The dilatations, known as ampullae or lacteal sinuses, lie under the areola and act as reservoirs for the milk. The lactiferous tubules are straight and narrow in the nipple, eventually opening onto its surface by minute apertures. *See also* LACTATION. For breast feeding and difficulties associated with feeding, *see* Appendix 14.

breast pump a suction apparatus, used to withdraw milk from the breast. The vacuum can be created by hand pressure on a rubber bulb, or by an electrical pump, e.g. Egnell breast pump.

breech the buttocks. *B. presentation* a longitudinal lie of the fetus in which the buttocks present in the lower pole of the uterus. (*a*) *The flexed b.* occurs when the breech presents with the knees and hips flexed so the feet are near the buttocks; it is sometimes called the complete breech and is more common in multigravidae. A *footling presentation* is one in which one or both feet lie below the buttocks. Similarly one or both knees may be lowermost in a *knee presentation*. (*b*) *The b. with extended legs*, sometimes known as the incomplete or frank breech, occurs when the hips are flexed but the knees are extended so that the feet lie near the child's head. This is the most common type to occur in primigravidae. *See* Appendix 9.

bregma the anterior fontanelle, a kite-shaped membranous area in the head of the fetus and infant at the junction of the frontal, coronal and sagittal sutures.

Briggs report the report of a committee commissioned in 1970 to review the roles of the nurse and midwife. *See* Appendix 23.

brim of the pelvis the pelvic inlet. *See* PELVIS.

British Pharmacopoeia (BP) the official publication containing the list of drugs and other medicinal substances in use in the United

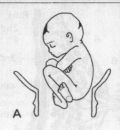

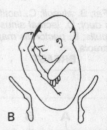

A. *with flexed legs*; B. *with extended legs.*
BREECH PRESENTATION

Kingdom. The book gives details of how these substances are obtained or prepared, and their dosages and methods of administration. It is compiled under the auspices of the General Medical Council and is regularly revised and brought up to date.

broad ligaments two folds of peritoneum, continuous with that of the uterus, and extending to the sides of the pelvis. They contain the fallopian tubes, the parametrium, the ovarian blood and lymph vessels and the nerves of the uterus and, in their bases, the ureters.

bromethol a basal anaesthetic.

bromocriptine a dopamine agonist, a derivative of ergot alkaloids used to inhibit prolactin secretion. It may be used to suppress lactation.

bronchopulmonary dysplasia a chronic respiratory condition occurring in babies who have been ventilated for long periods or have needed prolonged oxygen therapy. It results in serious disruption of lung growth. Examination of radiographs and lung specimens reveals patches of collapse and fibrosis. Following ventilation these babies usually require supplementary oxygen for several weeks or even months to keep the arterial oxygen tension above 55 kPa.

bronchus one of the main branches of the trachea. pl. *bronchi*.

brow presentation a cephalic presentation in which the attitude of the head is midway between flexion and extension. Since the mentovertical diameter of 13.0–13.75 cm (5¼–5½ in) presents, and this diameter is greater than any of those of the average pelvis, brow presentation is a possible cause of obstructed labour. *See* Appendix 9.

B-scan ULTRASOUND display which

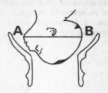

A–B *Mentovertical diameter 13.5 cm.*
BROW PRESENTATION

produces a two-dimensional cross-sectioned picture of internal anatomy. Used to locate the position of the fetal skull prior to cephalometry, for placentography and diagnosis of abnormal conditions, e.g. hydatidiform mole, pelvic tumours and intrauterine death. *See also* Appendix 4.

buccal smear scrapings from the buccal mucosa which are examined microscopically to study BARR BODIES.

buffer a chemical substance which, when present in a solution, helps to resist a change in pH. *Bicarbonate b.* this is the principal buffering system in the blood and involves the bicarbonate ions and carbon dioxide.

bulbocavernosus muscles two of the perineal muscles which surround the vaginal introitus and have a weak sphincter-like action.

bulla a blister. pl. *bullae*.

bupivacaine (Marcain) a local

analgesic drug used for epidural and paracervical analgesia. Duration of action 2–4 hours. *See* Appendix 19.

Burns–Marshall technique one method for delivering the head during a breech delivery. *See* Appendix 9.

C

C chemical symbol, carbon; cathode (cathodal); Celsius or centigrade (scale); cervical.

Ca chemical symbol, calcium; cathode.

C, c symbols used with D, d, E and e in defining Rhesus blood groups.

caecum 1. the first or proximal part of the large intestine, forming a dilated pouch distal to the ileum and proximal to the colon, and giving off the vermiform appendix. 2. any blind pouch.

caesarean section an obstetric operation whereby the fetus is extracted from the uterus through an incision made in the abdominal and uterine walls following the 24th week of pregnancy. A lower segment caesarean section (LSCS) involves a horizontal incision in the lower uterine segment. The possibility of rupture of the uterus during a subsequent labour is greatly reduced when a LSCS is performed. Classical caesarean section involves a vertical incision in the body of the uterus, the scar of which is more likely to rupture in subsequent pregnancies. *See* Appendix 10.

caffeine an alkaloid present in tea and coffee. It is used as a mild stimulant to the central nervous system.

calcaneum, calcaneus the bone of the foot which forms the heel.

calcification the deposit of lime in any tissue. Calcification is seen in the mature and postmature placenta.

calcium a chemical element. Symbol Ca. It is the most abundant mineral in the body. In combination with phosphorus it forms calcium phosphate, the dense, hard material of the bones and teeth. It is an important cation (a positively charged ion) in intra- and extracellular fluid and is essential to the normal clotting of the blood, the maintenance of a normal heartbeat, and the initiation of neuromuscular and metabolic activities. In pregnancy, a diet rich in calcium is required and can be obtained from milk, cheese and green vegetables; it may be given in vitamin form. Vitamin D is essential for its absorption. Tetany resulting from hypocalcaemia, may occur in newborn babies.

calculus a stone which may be formed in the gallbladder, bile duct, kidney or ureter. *Renal c.* a stone in the kidney.

Caldwell–Molloy classification the classification of female pelves as gynaecoid, android, anthropoid and platypelloid.

calipers compasses for measuring diameters and curved surfaces, e.g. the fetal skull.

callus 1. the tissue which grows round fractured ends of bone and develops into new bone to repair the injury. 2. localized hyperplasia of the horny layer of the epidermis due to pressure or friction.

calorie a unit of heat, the amount needed to raise 1 g of water through 1°C. A Calorie (kilocalorie) equals 1000 cal and is the amount of heat needed to raise 1 kg of water through 1°C. This unit is used to measure body heat and energy needs in food; 1 g of carbohydrate or protein gives 4 cal and 1 g of fat gives 9 cal. During pregnancy and lactation the mother needs about 2500 cal/day. A full-term infant needs 110 cal/kg body weight/day after the fourth day of life. The SI counterpart of this unit is the JOULE (J) which equals 4.2 cal.

cancer a general term to describe malignant growths. *See* CARCINOMA. It encompasses a group of neoplastic diseases in which there is a transformation of normal body cells into malignant ones. The altered cells pass on inappropriate genetic information to their offspring and begin to proliferate in an abnormal and destructive way. As the cancer cells continue to proliferate, the mass of abnormal tissue that they form enlarges, penetrating neighbouring tissues, destroying normal cells and taking their place. Cells are spread from this primary site via lymphatic or blood vessels to distant sites. This migration is called metastasis. Another way of spread is by entering a body cavity and coming into contact with a healthy organ by diffusion.

Candida a genus of yeast-like fungi that are commonly part of the normal flora of the mouth, skin, intestinal tract and vagina, but can cause a variety of infections. *See also* CANDIDIASIS. *C. albicans* the usual pathogen in human infection.

candidiasis infection by fungi of the genus *Candida*, generally *C. albicans*, most commonly involving the skin, oral mucosa (thrush), respiratory tract and vagina; rarely there is systemic infection or endocarditis.

cannula a tube for insertion into a cavity or blood vessel; during insertion its lumen is usually occupied by a trocar.

capillary hair-like. 1. minute vessels connecting arterioles and venules, the walls of which act as a semipermeable membrane for interchange of various substances between the blood and tissue fluid. 2. minute vessels of the lymphatic system.

caput head. *C. succedaneum* an oedematous swelling formed on the presenting part of the fetus, by pressure from the dilating cervical os which, after rupture of the forewaters, restricts the venous return in the superficial tissues. It is present before delivery but disperses within a few hours. Other characteristic features are that it pits on pressure, can cross suture lines when present on the scalp and is found over the face or buttocks if these are the presenting parts. Bruising may also be a feature. *See also* CHIGNON.

carbimazole an antithyroid drug used in the treatment of thyrotoxicosis.

carbohydrate that food composed of carbon, hydrogen and oxygen (CHO). The sugar, starch and cellulose foods which provide heat and energy; 1 g of carbohydrate yields 17 kJ (4 kcal). Carbohydrates may be stored in the body as glycogen for future use. If they are eaten in excessive amounts, however, the body changes them into fats and stores them in that form.

carbon dioxide (CO₂) a gas present in minute quantities in the atmosphere and formed in the body tissues by the oxidation of carbon and excreted by the lungs; used with oxygen to stimulate respiration. It is usually measured as PCO₂.

carbon monoxide (CO) a colourless, odourless, tasteless gas, formed by burning carbon or organic fuels with a scant supply of oxygen; inhalation causes central nervous system damage and asphyxiation.

carbonate a salt of carbonic acid.

carcinogenic causing carcinoma.

carcinoma cancer. A malignant epithelial tumour which may develop in any part of the body. *C. of the uterus* and of the breast are the most common in women. *C. of the uterus* may be of the body or of the cervix. *C. of the cervix* occurs most commonly, but not exclusively, in parous women between the ages of 40 and 55. The first symptom is irregular bleeding *per vaginam* and pain is present only when the condition is advanced. It is treated by radiotherapy, either alone or combined with WERTHEIM'S HYSTERECTOMY. *C. of the body of the uterus* occurs usually after the menopause and more often in nulliparous women. The first symptom is postmenopausal bleeding. Treatment is usually hysterectomy plus excision of a 3-cm cuff of vagina and bilateral salpingo-oophorectomy. The midwife should never ignore a report of bleeding *per vaginam* during or after the menopause, and should strongly recommend the patient to see a doctor without delay.

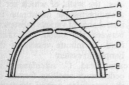

A. *Skin*; B. *subcutaneous tissue*; C. *aponeurosis*; D. *periosteum*; E. *bone*.

CAPUT SUCCEDANEUM

By means of CERVICAL CYTOLOGY much earlier diagnosis is possible. *C. of the breast* occurs in women of all ages. It is manifested first by a painless lump in the breast. The treatment used to be radical mastectomy, but now is more often a lumpectomy or a simple mastectomy and radiotherapy. A midwife who is consulted about a lump or swelling in the breast should immediately refer the patient to a doctor.

cardia 1. the cardiac opening. 2. the cardiac part of the stomach; that part of the stomach surrounding the oesophagogastric junction, distinguished by the presence of cardiac glands.

cardiac 1. pertaining to the heart. 2. pertaining to the stomach. *C. arrest* sudden and often unexpected stoppage of effective heart action. Either the periodic impulses which trigger the coordinated heart muscle contractions cease, or ventricular fibrillation or flutter occurs in which individual muscle fibres have a rapid irregular twitching. The majority of victims of cardiac disease arrest suffer from ventricular fibrillation and most of them have severe coronary artery disease. The only chance of survival for many of those who experience unexpected cardiac arrest is successful implementation of emergency cardiac care and cardiopulmonary resuscitation (CPR).

cardinal of first importance.

cardinal ligaments also known as the transverse cervical or Mackenrodt's ligaments. Two thickened bands of parametrium which stretch from the cervix uteri to the lateral walls of the pelvis, and help to support the uterus.

cardiogram a graphic representation of the heart's action made by the electrocardiograph.

cardiotocography a graphical correlation between fetal heart rate patterns and uterine contractions in labour. Also a non-stress test for fetal well-being in pregnancy.

cardiovascular relating to the heart and blood vessels.

caries decay or necrosis of bone. *Dental c.* decay of teeth.

carneous mole a mass of blood clot surrounding a dead embryo, and retained by the uterus. Also termed blood mole, fleshy mole, missed abortion. *See* Appendix 6. *See also* TUBAL MOLE.

carotene a deep yellow pigment which is converted into vitamin A by the liver.

carotid bodies small neuro-vascular structures lying in the bifurcation of the right and left carotid arteries, containing chemoreceptors that monitor oxygen content in blood and help to regulate respiration.

carpal tunnel syndrome tingling and numbness in the hand resulting from pressure on the median nerve as it passes through the carpal tunnel at the wrist. This condition may occur in pregnancy, since local oedema increases the pressure. Typically, the patient finds activities such as knitting difficult or impossible. It improves spontaneously after delivery.

carpopedal spasm muscular spasm of the hands and feet in TETANY.

carrier a person who carries in the body pathogenic organisms, but has no symptoms of disease. Such a person may transmit poliomyelitis or typhoid fever. Haemolytic streptococci from the throat of a carrier could be transmitted to the genital tract of a recently delivered woman. In genetics it is an apparently normal individual who carries a RECESSIVE or SEX-LINKED gene.

cartilage a specialized, fibrous connective tissue present in adults, and forming most of the temporary skeleton in the embryo, providing a model in which most of the bones develop, and constituting an important part of the organism's growth mechanism.

caruncle a small fleshy eminence, often abnormal. *Hymenal c's* small elevations of mucous membrane around the vaginal orifice, being relics of the ruptured hymen (also called *carunculae myrtiformes*). *Urethral c.* a small, polypoid, red growth on the mucous membrane of the female urinary meatus, sometimes causing difficulty in voiding. It may be painful, and is treated by surgical removal or cauterization.

carunculae myrtiformes *see* CARUNCLE.

case conference a meeting of professionals involved in the care of a particular person (often a child), to agree patterns of action and to monitor progress.

casein one of the proteins of milk. The casein of cows' milk is less digestible, and present in larger quantities, than that of human milk.

caseinogen the precursor of casein. Caseinogen is converted into casein by the renin of the gastric juice in babies.

cast a structure moulded in a hollow organ and retaining the shape of the cavity of the organ, when shed, e.g. a decidual cast shed from the uterus in tubal pregnancy, or casts from the renal tubules found in the urine in kidney disease.

castor oil a purgative formerly used in the medical induction of labour. By stimulating peristalsis it could reflexly stimulate uterine contractions.

castration the removal of the male testicles or the female ovaries.

CAT *See* COMPUTED AXIAL TOMOGRAPHY.

catamenia menstruation.

cataract an opacity of the crystalline lens or its capsule which impairs vision. Congenital cataract is sometimes seen in newborn babies. It may be a familial condition or it may occur in babies of women who have contracted RUBELLA in early pregnancy. It also may be associated with GALACTOSAEMIA.

catecholamine any of a group of sympathomimetic amines (including dopamine, adrenaline, and noradrenaline), the aromatic portion of whose molecule is catechol. The catecholamines play an important role in the body's physiological response to stress. Their release at the sympathetic nerve endings increases the rate and force of muscular contractions of the heart, thereby increasing cardiac output, constricts peripheral blood vessels, resulting in elevated blood pressure; elevates blood glucose levels by hepatic and skeletal muscle glycogenesis; and promotes an increase in blood lipids by increasing the catabolism of fats.

catgut a substance prepared from the gut of sheep and used, since it is absorbed, mainly for buried sutures.

catheter a tube made of polythene, rubber, gum-elastic or silver, and perforated near its blind end. Introduced into various hollow organs, vessels or canals for the purpose of CATHETERIZATION.

catheterization the introduction of a catheter to introduce or withdraw fluid or to measure fluid pressure, e.g. bladder, cardiac or umbilical catheterization.

cathode a negative electrode.

cation an ion carrying a positive electric charge. Examples are sodium (Na), copper (Cu).

cauda equina literally, horse's tail. The nerves into which the spinal cord divides at its termination in the lumbar region.

caudal block regional analgesia achieved by the introduction of the agent through the sacral hiatus. It is less reliable than entering the epidural space by the lumbar route. See EPIDURAL ANALGESIA.

caul the amnion, which occasionally does not rupture, but envelops the infant's head at birth. It should be ruptured as quickly as possible to establish a clear airway.

cautery a hot instrument or a chemical agent used to destroy tissue by burning it. Sometimes used in the treatment of cervical erosion.

cavity of the pelvis the hollow within the pelvic walls, bounded by the pelvic brim (or inlet) above and the outlet below.

CDH See CONGENITAL DISLOCATION OF THE HIP.

-cele suffix meaning 'a tumour', e.g. meningocele, a swelling consisting of a protrusion of meninges.

cell the structural unit of which all multi-celled organisms are made. It consists of a nucleus with central nucleolus, and CHROMOSOMES. The surrounding cytoplasm is semifluid and contains mitochondria, RIBOSOMES and other bodies. The whole is contained within the cell membrane. All living cells arise from other cells, either by division of one cell or to make two, as in MITOSIS and MEIOSIS, or by fusion of two cells to make one, as in the union of the sperm and ovum to make the zygote in sexual reproduction. The cells of the body differentiate during development into many specialized types with specific tasks to perform. Cells are organized into tissues and tissues into organs.

cellulitis a diffuse inflammatory process within solid tissues, characterized by oedema, redness, pain and interference with function. It may be caused by infection with streptococci, staphylococci, or other organisms. Cellulitis usually occurs in the loose tissues beneath the skin, but may also occur in tissues beneath mucous membranes, or around muscle bundles or surrounding organs. Pelvic cellulitis involves tissues surrounding the uterus and is called parametritis. It may occur as a complication of septic abortion or following labour, if infection has been introduced into the genital tract.

cellulose a carbohydrate; the outer covering of vegetable cells, i.e. vegetable fibres. Not digestible in the alimentary tract of man, but gives bulk, and as 'roughage' stimulates peristalsis.

Celsius an internationally recognized unit of temperature. Water freezes at 0° and boils at 100°. These units were called 'Centigrade' in the UK but this is not used in SYSTÈME INTERNATIONAL D'UNITES (SI units), as in some countries it is a measurement of angle.

census enumeration of a population. The national census was first introduced in England and Wales in 1801 and has since been repeated every 10 years (except 1941). It usually records name, address, sex, occupation, marital status and other social information.

Centigrade See CELSIUS.

centile See PERCENTILE.

centimetre the one-hundredth part of a metre. See Appendix 20.

Central Midwives Board (CMB) a statutory body set up under the Midwives Act, 1902, to lay down regulations for the training of midwives, for their admission to a register and for the framing of rules governing their practice. There was a separate Central Midwives Board for Scotland and a Northern Ireland Council for Nurses and Midwives. These bodies were dissolved in July 1983 when the United Kingdom Central Council for Nursing, Midwifery and Health Visiting (UKCC) and National Boards took over their functions.

central nervous system the brain and spinal cord.

central venous pressure (CVP) the pressure of blood in the right atrium. It indicates the balance between the cardiac output and the venous return. Measurement of central venous pressure is made possible by the insertion of a catheter through the median cubital vein to the superior vena cava. The distal end of the catheter is attached to a manometer on which can be read the amount of pressure being exerted by the blood inside the right atrium. The manometer is positioned at the bedside so that the zero point is at the level of the right atrium. Each time the patient's position is changed the zero point on the manometer must be reset. It is invaluable to ensure adequate fluid replacement without overloading the circulation when the amount of blood lost cannot be accurately estimated, e.g. in concealed ABRUPTIO PLACENTAE. The normal range is +5 to +10 cm of saline when the zero point of the scale corresponds to the mid-axillary line.

centrifuge an apparatus which rotates at great speed. It will hold test tubes of blood, urine, etc., and such rotation will precipitate bacteria, cells and other substances.

cephalhaematoma an effusion of blood beneath the periosteum of one of the cranial bones. It causes a fluctuant swelling which develops on the head of the newborn child within 48 hours of birth. It is seen following both easy and difficult delivery. Very occasionally the cranial bone beneath is found to be fractured. A cephalhaematoma is distinguished from a CAPUT SUCCEDANEUM by the fact that it develops after birth, and is a

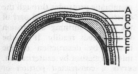

A. *Skin*; B. *subcutaneous tissue*; c. *aponeurosis*; D. *periosteum*; E. *blood under periosteum*; F. *bone*.
CEPHALHAEMATOMA

fluctuant swelling limited to the area of one bone. It takes several weeks to subside, and the mother should be told to expect this. No treatment is necessary unless severe jaundice occurs.

cephalic version conversion to a head presentation. *See* VERSION.

cephalometry measurement of the head. Antenatally this is usually the measurement of the biparietal diameter. The most accurate is by means of ULTRASOUND. It is used to assess fetal maturity and growth. *See also* BIPARIETAL DIAMETER. After birth the head is measured with a tape measure.

cephalopelvic pertaining to the relationship of the fetal head to the maternal pelvis. *C. disproportion* a misfit between the fetal head and the maternal pelvis. This may be due to a small pelvis or, more often, the attitude of the fetal head causing larger diameters to present at the pelvic brim. It is diagnosed when the fetal head will not engage in the pelvis after 36 weeks of pregnancy.

cephaloridine an antibiotic derived from CEPHALOSPORIN. It can cross into the fetal circulation via the placenta.

cephalosporin a naturally occurring antibiotic similar chemically to PENICILLIN.

cerclage encircling of a part with a ring or loop, as for correction of an incompetent cervix uteri or fixation of the adjacent ends of a fractured bone.

cerebellum the hindbrain, below

the cerebrum and behind the medulla oblongata.

cerebral pertaining to the cerebral hemispheres.

cerebral dysrhythmia a condition in which the brain shows an abnormal pattern of electrical waves on an electroencephalograph (ECG) tracing. It occurs in epilepsy and has been noted in eclampsia, such patients tending to have convulsions.

cerebral haemorrhage bleeding from or into one of the cerebral hemispheres.

cerebral palsy a persisting motor disorder which may result from hypoxia *in utero*, asphyxia neonatorum, and periods of apnoea and cyanosis, as may occur in RESPIRATORY DISTRESS SYNDROME, HYPOGLYCAEMIA and other conditions.

cerebrospinal relating to the brain and spinal cord. *C. fluid* the fluid in the ventricles of the brain, secreted by the choroid plexuses and circulating in the subarachnoid space covering the brain, and in the membranes surrounding the spinal cord. It protects the nerves in the brain and spinal cord from jar and injury. An excessive quantity of this fluid is found in HYDROCEPHALUS.

cerebrum the largest part of the brain, occupying the greater portion of the cranium and consisting of the right and left cerebral hemispheres. The centre of the higher functions of the brain.

cervical pertaining to the neck. In obstetrics, pertaining to the cervix uteri or neck of the uterus.

C. cerclage see SHIRODKAR OPERATION. *C. cytology* the examination of cells from the cervix to detect abnormal changes. *C. incompetence* failure of an injured cervix to hold the pregnancy in the uterus: a cause of abortion after the 12th week of pregnancy, characterized by premature rupture of the membranes and painless expulsion of the fetus. The incidence appears to be increasing following the Abortion Act. *C. cap* a contraceptive device worn over the vaginal portion of the cervix. *C. suture* a suture placed around the region of the internal os in patients with a history of, or clinical signs indicating, cervical incompetence. The more complex operation described by Shirodkar has now been mostly replaced by the more simple purse-string suture of McDonald.

cervicitis infection of the mucous membrane lining the cervix uteri. *Acute c.* occurs in GONORRHOEA. *Chronic c.* usually results from a low-grade infection following slight tearing of the cervix during delivery. The inflamed mucous membrane protrudes through the external os to the vaginal part of the cervix, forming an erosion which bleeds readily. It can be treated by destruction of the infected tissues by cauterization.

cervix a constricted portion or neck, e.g. *c. uteri*, the neck of the uterus; it is about 2.5 cm (1 in) long and opens into the vagina. The cervical canal starts at the internal os, which communicates with the body of the uterus, and ends at the external os, which opens into the vagina. The portion of the cervix protruding into the vagina is spoken of as the *portio vaginalis*, or vaginal portion, and the portion above the vagina as the *supravaginal c.*

Chamberlen the name of a family of Huguenot refugees, who settled in England after the persecution. This family included several generations of surgeons and physicians, and the name is now chiefly remembered because one of the Chamberlens invented and used midwifery forceps. The family managed to preserve the secret of this instrument for more than a hundred years.

chancre the initial lesion of SYPHILIS developing at the site of inoculation.

change of life the period when menstruation ceases; the menopause. Climacteric.

chemical change this differs from physical change in that a profound alteration in properties results, usually permanently and usually accompanied by use of energy in a new substance, e.g. hydrogen (2 atoms) plus oxygen produces water.

chemical compound any substance produced by chemical change which may then be broken up into its components only by chemical means, unlike a mixture, which can usually be separated mechanically.

chemoreceptor a collection of cells sensitive to alterations in chemicals contacting them. They are found in the carotid body and

aortic body. These receptors are responsive to changes in the oxygen, carbon dioxide and hydrogen ion concentration in the blood. When oxygen concentration falls below normal in the arterial blood, the chemoreceptors send impulses to stimulate tne respiratory centre so that there will be an increase in alveolar ventilation and consequently, an increase in the intake of oxygen by the lungs.

chemotherapy the treatment of illness by chemical means; that is, by medication. adj. *chemotherapeutic*. The term was first applied to the treatment of infectious diseases, but is now used to include the treatment of mental illness and CANCER with drugs.

chest the thoracic cavity containing the lungs, heart, trachea, bronchi, oesophagus and large blood vessels and nerves.

chi-squared test a statistical test to determine whether two or more groups of observations differ significantly from one another, i.e. more than would be expected by chance.

chignon the large caput succedaneum seen on the head of an infant delivered by ventouse vacuum extraction. *See* VACUUM EXTRACTOR.

child abuse abnormal and detrimental behaviour towards a child, often by one or other parent or by a custodian responsible for the care of the child. Child abuse encompasses malnutrition and other kinds of neglect through ignorance, as well as deliberate withholding from the child the necessary and basic physical care. Examples of physical abuse range from burns and exposure to extreme cold to beating, poisoning, strangulation, sexual interference and withholding food and water. *See also* NON-ACCIDENTAL INJURY (NAI).

child health clinic a centre for well children to attend on a regular basis to ensure normal progress and development. A medical officer and a health visitor are in attendance.

child minder one who is registered with the local authority social services department and who is approved by the department to mind a few children aged from birth to 5 years during the day.

childbearing pregnancy. The normal childbearing period is between the ages of 15 and 45 years, though pregnancy may occur earlier or later.

childbirth the act or process of giving birth to a child. Called also parturition. *Natural c.* a term used to describe an approach to labour and delivery whereby the mother and her partner are well prepared and remain in control of events which are allowed to progress naturally, and without intervention. Medical interference, drugs and other stimuli to labour are therefore avoided.

Children Act, 1989 this Act was implemented in October 1991 and gives new rights to children, enabling them to have more say in decisions affecting their future. The concept of parental right has been replaced by parental responsibility which is defined as 'all rights, duties, powers, responsibility and authority.' Three new public law orders have been introduced: 1. the emergency protection order replaces the place of safety order and lasts for up to 8 days, with the possibility of extension for a further 7 days; 2. the child assessment order obtained by the Social Services Department or NSPCC, if the applicant has good cause to suspect the child is suffering significant harm but is not at immediate risk; 3. the recovery order for older children. Supervision and care orders have been retained.

Chlamydia a bacterium which is grown only with difficulty. One species causes trachoma in tropical climates. *C. trachomatis* is responsible for at least half the cases of non-specific urethritis (NSU) in males, and is now more likely than the gonococcus to cause OPHTHALMIA NEONATORUM. It is acquired from the birth canal but the mucopurulent discharge is not seen until 5–10 days after birth.

chloasma mask. The 'pregnancy mask', or pigmentation of the skin of the forehead, nose and cheeks seen quite commonly in pregnancy.

chloral elixir a hypnotic for babies contains 200 mg in 5 ml of solution. Dose: 30 mg/kg body weight for the first 2 weeks of life.

chloral hydrate a hypnotic and sedative with mild action as a pain reliever but used more commonly to induce sleep. It is now rarely used.

chloramphenicol a broad-spectrum antibiotic with specific therapeutic activity against rickettsiae and many different bacteria. Side-effects include serious, even fatal, blood dyscrasias in certain patients. Frequent blood tests are recommended during therapy. Chloromyecetin is a proprietary preparation of chloramphenicol.

chlorhexidine a coal-tar derivative which has a wide antibacterial action. It is especially effective against coagulase-positive staphylococci and is extensively used in antibiotic skin cleansers for surgical scrub, pre-operative skin preparation and cleansing skin wounds. Hibitane is the proprietary preparation of chlorhexidine.

chloride a salt of chlorine. One of the electrolytes important in helping to maintain the normal balance of the blood necessary to health.

chlormethiazole (Heminevrin) a hypnotic, sedative and anticonvulsant drug with a depressant action on the central nervous system. It is used to treat insomnia, agitation and confusion. It is also used to treat acute withdrawal symptoms in alcoholism and drug addiction, and for the control of sustained epileptic fits.

chloroform a colourless liquid, the vapour of which when inhaled induces general anaesthesia. It was also one of the first drugs used to relieve pain in labour but has now been superseded by safer inhalation agents for analgesia, e.g. ENTONOX.

chlorothiazide (Saluric) a diuretic drug that also has an antihypertensive effect. It is used in the treatment of the oedema of congestive heart failure, and in hypertension.

chlorpromazine a phenothiazine used as an antipsychotic agent and antiemetic. Side-effects include drowsiness and slight hypotension. Largactil is the widely used proprietary preparation.

choanal atresia a membranous or bony obstruction of the posterior nares. As a neonate breathes mainly through the nose, considerable respiratory difficulty occurs at or shortly after birth, leading to cyanosis.

cholecystitis inflammation of the gallbladder.

chorea St Vitus' dance. A disease, related to rheumatism and probably of bacterial origin, affecting the nervous system. It is characterized by irregular involuntary muscular movements, and can prove very exhausting to the patient. This condition occurring during pregnancy has sometimes been termed chorea gravidarum. It may also be called Sydenham's chorea. It is occasionally seen in young primigravid women with or sometimes without a history of rheumatism and/or chorea in childhood. It is dangerous in so far as the pregnancy throws an additional strain on the already impaired heart.

chorioangioma a collection of fetal blood vessels in WHARTON'S JELLY, forming a tumour on the placenta. It is of little clinical significance, but is, rarely, associated with POLYHYDRAMNIOS.

choriocarcinoma formerly known as chorioepithelioma. A highly malignant NEOPLASM, usually arising from the trophoblast of a HYDATIDIFORM MOLE. It develops in about 3 per cent of hydatidiform moles and is detected by raised levels of chorionic gonadotrophin in serum or urine and by radioimmunoassay. It is treated by cytotoxic chemotherapy and, if necessary, hysterectomy.

chorioepithelioma see CHORIOCARCINOMA.

chorion the outer of the two membranes enclosing the fetus *in utero*. It is derived with the PLACENTA from the trophoblast. It is opaque and friable in nature and may sometimes be retained after delivery. *C. biopsy* tissue removed from the gestational sac early in pregnancy so that chromosome and other inherited disorders can be identified. Because this can be done as early as 8 weeks gestation, termination (where recommended and agreed) can be undertaken before 12 weeks, which is not possible with amniocentesis. *C. frondosum* the part of the chorion covered by villi in the early weeks of embryonic development before the placenta is formed. *C. laeve* the nonvillous, membranous part of the

trophoblast which develops into the chorion.

chorionic gonadotrophin a substance produced from the BLASTOCYST, stimulating the CORPUS LUTEUM to produce oestrogen and progesterone as the pituitary GONADOTROPHINS are decreasing, so ensuring the continuation of the pregnancy. The presence of the human chorionic gonadotrophins (HCG) in a woman's urine is diagnostic of pregnancy. *See also* PREGNANCY TESTS.

chorionic villi minute fingerlike projections arising from the TROPHOBLAST and persisting in the chorion frondosum. These have an outer SYNCYTIOTROPHOBLASTIC layer with multiple nuclei and without cell walls, and an inner CYTOTROPHOBLASTIC layer with cell walls containing single nuclei. Within are fetal capillaries embedded in mesoderm. Oxygenated maternal blood spurts in cascades over the villi in the intervillous spaces, so that oxygen, nutrients, etc., may pass into the fetal circulation and carbon dioxide, etc., may pass out. This exchange becomes easier after 24 weeks of gestation when the cytotrophoblastic cell layer remains only in isolated areas.

choroid plexus vascular fringeline folds in the pia mater in the third, fourth and lateral ventricles of the brain; concerned with formation of cerebrospinal fluid.

Christmas disease a hereditary haemorrhagic diathesis clinically similar to haemophilia A (classic haemophilia) but due to deficiency of clotting factor IX; called also haemophilia B.

chromatin the substance of the chromosomes, composed of DNA and basic proteins (histones), the material in the nucleus that stains with basic dyes. *Sex c.* Barr body; the persistent mass of the material of the inactivated X chromosome in cells of normal females.

chromatography a technique for analysis of chemical substances. The term literally means colour writing and the technique is used for some investigations, for example, to detect and identify in body fluids certain sugars and amino acids associated with inborn errors of metabolism.

chromosome one of a number of minute thread-like structures contained in the cell nucleus, composed of DEOXYRIBONUCLEIC ACID (DNA) and protein and carrying the genes, which transmit the inherited characteristics. In the human body the cells carry 46 chromosomes, 22 pairs of autosomes, and the two sex chromosomes (XX or XY), which determine the sex of the organism. *C. analysis* fetal cells obtained by AMNIOCENTESIS or by lymphocytes from a blood sample can be cultured in the laboratory until they divide. Cell division is arrested in mid-metaphase by the drug colchicine. The chromosomes can be stained by one of several techniques that produce a distinct pattern of light and dark bands along the chromosome, and each chromosome can be recognized by its size and banding pattern. The chromosomal characteristics of an individual are referred to as his/her karyotype. *See also* GENE.

chronic prolonged or permanent, e.g. chronic disease.

cilia fine hair-like processes which grow on the free border of certain epithelial cells. The lining of the fallopian tubes is ciliated epithelium, and the cilia, waving to and fro, produce a current which carries the ovum from the ovarian end of the fallopian tube to the uterus. sing. *cilium.*

ciliated having cilia.

CIP *see* CONTINUOUS INFLATING PRESSURE.

circulation movement in a circular course, as of the blood. *Coronary c.* the system of vessels which supplies the heart muscle itself. *Fetal c.* the circulation of blood in the fetus. Before birth the foramen ovale and the ductus arteriosus bypass the lungs, and blood is carried to and from the

ONE PAIR OF CHROMOSOMES SHOWING GENE BANDING

placenta by the umbilical vessels and the ductus venosus. *Lymph c.* the flow of lymph through lymph vessels and glands. *Placental c.* the exchange of substances between the maternal blood, brought to the placenta by the uterine vessels, and the fetal blood in the CHORIONIC VILLI of the placenta. *Portal c.* the blood flow from the gastric, splenic and superior mesenteric veins to the portal vein, which enters the liver. *Pulmonary c.* that of the blood from the right ventricle via the pulmonary artery through the lungs and back to the heart by the pulmonary veins. *Systemic c.* that of the blood throughout the body. The direction of flow is from the left atrium to the left ventricle and through the aorta and its branches; then through arterioles, capillaries and venules to veins, which carry it back to the right atrium, and so into the right ventricle. *Uterine c.* the blood supply to the uterus. The uterus is supplied with oxygenated blood by the two uterine arteries which enter near the cervix, and the two ovarian arteries which enter near the fallopian tubes. The deoxygenated blood is returned by corresponding veins.

circumcision excision of the prepuce. It is performed on healthy Jewish male children on the eighth day of life as a religious ceremony. Medically, it is considered necessary if the urinary meatus of the prepuce is obstructed. The PLASTIBELL is commonly used for circumcision in many hospitals.

circumference of fetal skull measurements taken round the skull at various points. *See* FETAL SKULL.

circumvallate literally, surrounded by a wall. A *c. placenta* has a distinct ridge on the fetal surface, caused by a double fold of chorion near its periphery. This is slightly more likely to partially separate, causing antepartum haemorrhage.

clamp a surgical instrument used to compress any part of the body, e.g. to prevent or arrest haemorrhage. *Hollister'c.* a plastic device for occluding the vessels of the umbilical cord. It is applied at birth, almost flush with the umbilicus, for about 48 hours, after which it is removed.

clavicle the collar bone, articulating with the sternum and the acromion process of the scapula. Fracture of the fetal clavicle is an uncommon birth injury. It may be due to a traumatic breech delivery or in shoulder dystocia, as with an undetected large baby of a mother with gestational diabetes. Alternatively, it may occur spontaneously during easy birth in the rare condition of congenital OSTEOGENESIS IMPERFACTA. *See also* CLEIDOTOMY.

cleft lip a congenital defect resulting from the failure of fusion, in the embryo, of the median nasal and maxillary processes. It may be unilateral or bilateral. It is usually repairable

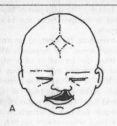

A

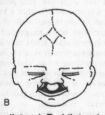

B

A. *unilateral*; B. *bilateral*.
CLEFT LIP

during the first few weeks or months of life.

cleft palate a congenital defect which is often associated with CLEFT LIP. The cleft may be central or on one side of the palate only. The most severe variety is a complete cleft of the palate accompanied by a bilateral cleft lip, in which case there is an unsightly fleshy projection below the nose. Cleft palate interferes with the child's ability to suck, and, later, with speech.

Modern operative treatment is very successful. Considerable responsibility rests on the midwife who should: (*a*) by careful routine inspection of the child's mouth at birth, detect the condition and consult a doctor immediately, who should inform the parents; (b) explain if necessary, and support the parents during their initial distress; (*c*) give the mother careful advice and instruction about feeding, which may be achieved by using a dropper, a cup, a spoon, or an obturator, a device inserted in the mouth to close the cleft while the baby is sucking. Cleft palate allows the food to get in the nose, and it causes difficulty in chewing and swallowing. Later it will hinder speech. Treatment of cleft palate and lip is by surgery, often in several stages, dental plates being used temporarily prior to surgery. Speech therapy may then be required.

cleidotomy division, with scissors, of the fetal clavicles, in very rare cases, to facilitate delivery where there is obstruction due to excessive breadth of the shoulders, e.g. in a large ANENCEPHALIC fetus.

climacteric the changes in the body occurring at the time of the MENOPAUSE.

clinic a place where patients or clients receive advice and treatment. Teaching given in the presence of a patient.

clinical pertaining to or founded on actual observation and treatment of patients, as distinguished from theoretical or experimental.

C. trial assessment of the effectiveness of modes of treatment by carefully following response to therapy in defined patient groups. A controlled clinical trial is one where a comparison is made of one or more active treatments against each other and against placebo. *Double-blind c. trial* comparison of different treatments (active and placebo) in which neither patients nor observers know which patient is receiving treatment until a trial code is decoded after completion of the study.

clinical thermometer an instrument for taking the body temperature. The temperature should be taken in the mouth if possible, but can also be taken in the axilla or in the rectum. A note should be made as to where the temperature was taken, if not in the mouth.

clitoris a small sensitive organ, consisting of erectile tissue, situated at the anterior junction of the labia minora. It is the homologue of the male penis.

clomiphene citrate a GONADO-TROPHIC drug used to stimulate ovulation. A proprietary preparation is Clomid.

clonic of the nature of a jerk. The convulsive stage of a fit is called the clonic stage.

Clostridium an anaerobic Gram-positive spore-bearing bacillus, e.g. that of tetanus or gas gangrene.

clot usually blood cells forming a partially solidified mass in a matrix of fibrin. It may also occur in lymph. The solid part of blood after it escapes from the blood vessels.

clotrimazole (Canesten) an antifungal agent. *See* Appendix 19.

clotting the formation of a jelly-like substance over the ends or within the walls of a blood vessel, with resultant stoppage of the blood flow. Clotting is one of the natural defence mechanisms of the body when injury occurs. A clot will usually form within 5 minutes after a blood vessel wall has been damaged. It is possible for a clot to form within a blood vessel if the inner wall of the vessel has been roughened by injury or disease. Clots may form in conditions such as arteriosclerosis, varicose veins, and thrombophlebitis. An internal clot that remains at the place where it forms is called a thrombus; the general condition is called THROMBOSIS. If the clot (or pieces of it) breaks loose and flows through the blood vessels, it is called an embolus, and the condition is called EMBOLISM. *C. time* the time taken for shed blood to clot, usually within 5 minutes.

cloxacillin a semi-synthetic penicillin; its sodium salt is used in treating staphylococcal infections due to penicillinase-producing organisms.

clubfoot *see* TALIPES.

CNP *see* CONTINUOUS NEGATIVE PRESSURE.

coagulase a substance formed by certain strains of staphylococci (thus termed *coagulase-positive*) causing clotting in plasma.

Coagulase-positive staphylococci (e.g. *Staphylococcus aureus*) are considerably more dangerous, especially to newborn babies, than those which are coagulase-negative (e.g. *Staphylococcus albus*).

coagulation formation of a clot. *Disseminated intravascular c. (DIC)* a disorder characterized by reduction in the elements involved in blood coagulation due to their utilization in widespread blood clotting within the vessels; the activation of the clotting mechanism may arise from disorders such as abruptio placentae and prolonged intrauterine death. In the late stages it is marked by profuse haemorrhage.

coarctation of the aorta stricture of the aorta at, or just below, the position of the ductus arteriosus; often diagnosed by absence of femoral pulses.

coccus a spherical microorganism. *See* BACTERIA.

coccygeus one of two muscles arising from the ischial spines and inserted into the lateral borders of the sacrum and coccyx, and forming part of the PELVIC FLOOR. Also called ischiococcygeus.

coccyx the terminal bone of the spinal column, in which four rudimentary vertebrae are fused together.

coitus sexual intercourse. Copulation. *C. interruptus* an unsatisfactory method of contraception where the penis is withdrawn from the vagina before ejaculation of semen.

colic severe spasmodic pain in the abdomen; most common during the first 3 months of life. The infant may pull up his legs, cry loudly, turn red-faced, and expel gas from the anus or belch it up from the stomach. *Biliary c.* colic due to the passage of a gallstone through the bile ducts. *Renal c.* colic caused by the passage of a stone along the ureter. Painful, ineffective, irregular contractions of the uterus are sometimes termed colicky.

coliform resembling *E. coli. See* BACTERIA.

collapse a state of prostration due to circulatory failure. SHOCK. *C. therapy* operative collapse and immobilization of the lung in treatment of pulmonary disease; artificial pneumothorax.

colloidal solution a suspension in water or other fluid, of molecules of a type which do not readily pass through animal membrane. Examples are blood, plasma, and the various plasma substitutes, which are valuable in the treatment of shock, because they are retained in the circulation.

colon the section of the large intestine extending from the caecum to the rectum.

colostrum the thin, yellow, milky fluid secreted by the breasts from 16 weeks of pregnancy and for 3 to 4 days after birth until lactation is initiated. Colostrum is high in protein, and initially low in lactose; its fat content is equivalent to breast milk. It is an important source of passive antibody.

colour index a measurement of

the proportion of haemoglobin in the red blood cells. In normal blood the figure is 1, in iron deficiency anaemia it is less than 1 and in megaloblastic anaemia it is more than 1.

colpoperineorrhaphy repair of the pelvic floor, vagina and perineal body, usually undertaken for PROLAPSE.

colporrhaphy repair of the vagina. *Anterior c.* for CYSTOCELE. *Posterior c.* for RECTOCELE.

colposcope a speculum for examining the vagina and cervix by means of a magnifying lens; used for the early detection of malignant changes.

colpotomy incision of the vaginal wall. *Posterior c.* incision through the posterior vaginal fornix to the pouch of Douglas to drain a pelvic abscess.

coma a condition of deep unconsciousness from which it is not possible to rouse the patient. It may have various causes including cerebrovascular accident, diabetes mellitus, alcoholism, eclampsia and uraemia.

comatose in a condition of coma.

commensal an organism which lives on another without harming it. *See also* LACTOBACILLUS ACIDOPHILUS.

commissure a connection. *Posterior c.* a fold of skin connecting the labia minora posteriorly.

Committee on Nursing set up in June 1970 to review the midwife's and nurse's roles both in the hospital and in the community and their education. A report (the Briggs Report) was published in 1972.

Committee on Safety of Medicines (CSM) an organization responsible for controlling the release of new drugs in the UK. Also collects data on adverse reactions to drugs via the yellow card system. This data enables the CSM to issue warnings about serious adverse effects.

Community Health Council an organization which enables the consumer's interests to be represented to those responsible at district level for the National Health Service. Apart from a paid secretary, the members are drawn from local organizations, whose representatives work on a voluntary basis.

community midwife a midwife who normally works in the community rather than the hospital, although many midwives now work in both areas. Previously called domiciliary midwife.

compatibility mixing together of two substances without chemical change or loss of power.

compensation in heart disease, the ability of the weakened heart nevertheless to function adequately.

complement that which makes up a deficiency. A non-specific complex group of serum proteins which have the ability with antibody, to LYSE red blood cells, destroy certain bacteria and facilitate PHAGOCYTOSIS. *C.-fixation tests* immunological tests utilizing complement to detect antigens and antibodies, e.g. Wassermann's test to detect antibodies to SYPHILIS.

complementary making up a deficiency. A complementary feed is an artificial feed given to an infant to make up the deficient amount of a breast-feed. Not now recommended for normal healthy babies. cf. Supplementary.

compound presentation presentation of more than one part of the fetus, e.g. head and hand; head and foot; breech, hand and cord. A rare complication of labour.

computed tomography (CT) a radiological imaging technique that produces images of 'slices' 1–10 mm thick through a patient's body.

computed axial tomography (CAT) computed tomography; used to diagnose such conditions as subdural haemorrhage, excess fluid or intraventricular haemorrhage in preterm infants.

conception 1. the formation of an idea. 2. the fusion of spermatozoon and ovum to form a viable zygote. The onset of pregnancy.

condom a contraceptive device, a sheath covering the penis, worn during coitus.

confinement childbirth, or more broadly childbearing, i.e. pregnancy, labour and puerperium.

congenital born with. Used to describe a condition, generally a malformation, present at birth. Also includes an infection which takes place *in utero*.

Congenital Disabilities (Civil Liabilities) Act, 1976 this act is applicable in England, Wales and Northern Ireland and provides for a child to be entitled to recover damages where the child has suffered as result of a breach in a duty of care owed to the mother or the father unless that breach of duty of care occurred before the child was conceived and either or both parents knew of the occurrence. In Scottish law the same provisions are made. The accuracy and preservation of records is therefore essential (UKCC, 1991).

congenital dislocation of the hip (CDH) the hip should be examined neonatally as a routine. The thigh is abducted with the hip at an angle of 90° to the spine. The examining thumb is placed in front of the femoral head and the fingers over the greater trochanter. An attempt is then made to dislocate the hip by pressing backwards with the thumb. A distinct judder will be felt if the hip is dislocated; a click may also be significant. Early splinting avoids complicated treatment later.

congestion abnormal accumulation of blood in a part of the body.

congestive pertaining to or associated with congestion. *C. heart failure* a broad term denoting conditions in which the heart's pumping capability is impaired.

conjoined twins *see* TWINS.

conjugate 1. to join or yoke together as, in the liver, bilirubin is combined with albumin by the activity of GLUCURONYL TRANSFERASE to render it water-soluble so that it may be excreted via the gut. *See also* ICTERUS GRAVIS *and* JAUNDICE. 2. a conjugate diameter of the pelvis. *See also* PELVIS.

conjunctiva the mucous membrane lining the inner surface of the eyelids and covering the anterior aspect of the eye.

conjunctivitis inflammation of the conjunctiva. *See* OPHTHALMIA NEONATORUM.

connective tissue tissue which binds together or supports the structures of the body. Adipose tissue, areolar tissue, bone, cartilage, fat, blood and fibrous tissue are all connective tissues.

consent in law, voluntary agreement with an action proposed by another. Consent is an act of reason; the person giving consent must be of sufficient mental capacity and be in possession of all essential information in order to give valid consent. Written informed consent is generally required before many invasive clinical procedures, such as investigations, including amniocentesis and surgery.

constipation delay in the passage of food through the bowel, characterized by infrequent bowel actions and the passage of hard stools. In pregnancy it appears to be common, and probably due to the increased progesterone in the blood, which inhibits the tone of plain muscle. The woman is advised to take extra water, fruit, vegetables, bran cereals and, if necessary, mild aperients. Breast-fed babies have soft stools, but those artificially fed have harder stools, usually causing no trouble. Any really constipated baby should be carefully examined to exclude HIRSCHSPRUNG'S DISEASE.

constriction ring a localized annular spasm of the uterine muscle at any level but often near the junction of the upper and lower uterine segments. In the first and second stages of labour it may form round the neck of the fetus and in the third stage forms an HOURGLASS CONSTRICTION of the uterus, causing a retained placenta. It may result from the use of oxytocic drugs in a uterus with incoordinated function, following early rupture of the membranes, and especially if intrauterine manipulation is carried out. Relaxation may occur with inhalation of amyl nitrite but often deep anaesthesia is required.

Consultant in Public Health Medicine following recent changes in the NHS the Consultant in Public Health Medicine has replaced the community physician and is now responsible for functions such as promoting health, preventing disease and fostering cooperation between the health and social services.

contagion communication of disease from one person to another by direct contact.

continuing education further study after the attainment of basic qualifications. This is vital for all midwives so that they keep up to date, and is accomplished by reading appropriate professional journals and research reports and by attending a variety of courses, including statutory refresher courses which practising midwives are required to attend every 5 years. A variety of patterns and types of refresher courses for midwives are now available.

continuous inflating pressure (CIP) pressure of water used against a baby's spontaneous breathing in respiratory distress syndrome (RDS). Its purpose is to prevent HYPOXAEMIA, apnoeic attacks or rising levels of carbon dioxide in the blood ($P\text{CO}_2$). *See* Appendix 17.

continuous negative pressure (CNP) a rarely used method of treating a neonate with the RESPIRATORY DISTRESS SYNDROME. Subatmospheric pressure is applied to the baby's thorax in a body box.

continuous positive airways pressure (CPAP) a technique used to prevent total alveolar collapse on expiration in a baby with RESPIRATORY DISTRESS SYNDROME. Positive pressure of 2–5 cmH_2O is applied into the respiratory tract by the nasal or endotracheal route or by face mask. CPAP is used with patients who are breathing spontaneously. When the same principle is used in mechanical ventilation, it is called positive end-expiratory pressure (PEEP).

contraception the prevention of conception. *See* Appendix 12.

contraceptive pertaining to contraception. Any means used to prevent conception.

contracted pelvis a pelvis in which

any diameter of the brim, cavity or outlet is so shortened as to interfere with the progress of labour.

contraction a temporary shortening of muscle fibre, which returns to its original length during relaxation. Contractions of the uterus during pregnancy are painless and are termed Braxton Hicks contractions, after the obstetrician of that name. During labour they may and generally do, become painful and are accompanied by RETRACTION.

controlled drugs preparation subject to the Misuse of Drugs Act, 1971, Misuse of Drugs (Notification of and Supply to Addicts) Regulations, 1973, and the Misuse of Drugs Regulations, 1985, which regulate the prescribing and dispensing of psychoactive drugs, including narcotics, hallucinogens, depressants and stimulants.

convulsions violent involuntary contractions of voluntary muscle. In a newborn baby the commonest causes are HYPOXIA, cerebral birth injury and HYPOGLYCAEMIA. In a pregnant woman they may be due to eclampsia, epilepsy or hysteria. Convulsions may also occur during labour or after delivery.

Cooley's anaemia an uncommon, severe type of anaemia found mainly in the Mediterranea races. Thalassaemia. *See also* Appendix 6, *under anaemia.*

Coombs' test a test for detecting antibody in blood. *Indirect C.t.* to detect free antibody in maternal blood. *Direct C.t.* to detect antibody on red cell surfaces in umbilical cord blood.

copper cuprum. Symbol Cu. An element, minute quantities of which are essential to health.

Copper-7 an INTRAUTERINE CONTRACEPTIVE DEVICE containing copper wire embedded within the plastic shape.

copulation sexual intercourse. Coitus.

Coramine see NIKETHAMIDE.

cord in midwifery, the UMBILICAL CORD which connects the fetus and placenta, and contains the umbilical vein carrying oxygen and nutrients to the fetus and the two umbilical arteries carrying CO_2 and waste products from the fetus to the placenta.

cornea the transparent anterior part of the eyeball situated in front of the lens. It is covered by conjunctiva, and severe conjunctivitis may be associated with a spread of infection to the cornea, causing ulceration, scarring and impairment of vision. *See also* OPHTHALMIA NEONATORUM.

cornu a horn. The junction of uterus and fallopian tube. pl. *cornua*.

coronal suture the suture between the two frontal and the two parietal bones. *See* FETAL SKULL.

coronary encircling. *C. arteries* those which supply the heart. *C. thrombosis* see THROMBOSIS.

corpus body. *C. albicans* white body. The white scar left on the surface of the ovary following the retrogression of a corpus luteum. *C. luteum* literally, yellow body.

The structure, first greyish and later yellow, which develops from the graafian follicle after ovulation. In the menstrual cycle it lasts 12 days before degenerating. If pregnancy occurs it lasts about 14–16 weeks, i.e. until the placenta is formed and fully functioning. *C. uteri* the body of the uterus.

corpuscle a small body or cell, e.g. the blood cell.

corrosive an agent which destroys or eats into other substances.

cortex the outer layers of an organ, e.g. the cerebral hemispheres, kidney, suprarenal gland or ovary.

cortical necrosis irreparable damage to the renal cortex due to severe vasospasm of the arteries supplying the cortex, which can occur following any severe shock, especially after abruptio placentae. *See* Appendix 6.

corticoids the name given to a group of hormones secreted by the adrenal cortex.

corticosteroid any of the hormones produced by the ADRENAL CORTEX; also their synthetic equivalents. Called also adrenocortical hormone and adrenocorticosteroid. All the hormones are steroids having similar chemical structures, but quite different physiological effects. Generally they are divided into *glucocorticoids* (cortisol, or hydrocortisone; and cortisone and corticosterone), *mineralocorticoids* (aldosterone and desoxycorticosterone, and also corticosterone) and androgens.

cortisone one of several hormones known as CORTICOSTEROIDS or STEROIDS, produced from the adrenal cortex. It is an anti-allergic and anti-inflammatory agent, among many other beneficial effects. It is widely used in allergic states, e.g. asthma, rheumatoid arthritis, severe skin conditions and ulcerative colitis. Hydrocortisone has a similar action. Prednisone and prednisolone are synthetic forms of cortisone and hydrocortisone respectively. Sudden withdrawal of these drugs is dangerous.

coryza a cold in the head, with headache, watery discharge from the eyes and nasal catarrh.

costal pertaining to the ribs.

cot death *see* SUDDEN INFANT DEATH SYNDROME.

cotyledon a division or lobe. A lobe of the placenta.

counselling a generic term used to describe a process of consultation and discussion in which one individual, the counsellor, listens and enables the other, the client, to make appropriate decisions. The general aim is to help the client solve problems, increase awareness and promote constructive exploration of difficulties so that the future may be approached more confidently and more constructively.

Couvelaire uterus the appearance of the uterus in severe concealed abruptio placentae (accidental haemorrhage), where the high tension in the uterus forces blood between the fibres of the myometrium, giving it a deep purplish-blue bruised appearance.

CPAP *see* CONTINUOUS POSITIVE AIRWAYS PRESSURE.

cracked nipple a fissure on the skin of the nipple, which causes much pain during suckling, and exposes the breast tissue to bacterial infection causing MASTITIS or an abscess. It is usually preventable by good management of breast feeding, which ensures that the baby is correctly latched on to the breast. If possible the mother should continue breast feeding, ensuring that the baby is correctly fixed. After feeding exposure of the nipple to the air promotes healing. If the nipple is too painful to continue feeding, the mother should gently express the milk and give it to the baby by bottle or spoon. When the crack has healed sufficiently breast feeding can gradually be resumed. *See* Appendix 14.

cramp painful spasmodic muscular contraction, common in pregnancy. *See* Appendix 3.

cranioclast an instrument rarely used now for crushing the fetal skull.

craniotomy the almost obsolete operation of perforation and extraction of the crushed fetal skull to allow vaginal delivery.

cranium the skull.

creatine a non-protein substance synthesized in the body from three amino acids; arginine, glycine (aminoacetic acid), and methionine. Creatine readily combines with phosphate, which is present in muscle, where it serves as the storage form of high-energy phosphate necessary for muscle contraction.

creatinine a nitrogenous compound formed as the end-product of creatine metabolism. It is formed in the muscle in relatively small amounts, passes into the blood and is excreted in the urine. A laboratory test for the creatinine level in the blood may be used as a measurement of kidney function. Since creatinine is normally produced in fairly constant amounts as a result of the breakdown of phosphocreatine and is excreted in the urine, an elevation in the creatinine level in the blood indicates a disturbance in kidney function or an abnormal muscle-wasting process. To determine the creatinine clearance, urine is collected for 24 hours and the serum creatinine is measured by a venous blood sample. Thus the rate of creatinine excretion per minute can be calculated. This test may be carried out in cases of severe hypertension in pregnancy.

crèche a DAY NURSERY.

Credé's expression a manoeuvre to complete the separation of, and to expel, a partially separated placenta when severe postpartum haemorrhage occurs. It consists in massaging the uterus to make it contract, the squeezing it behind and in front of the fundus in an attempt to force the placenta down into the vagina, from which it is expelled. It is rarely performed, since it is intensely painful and shock-producing.

cretinism congenital thyroid deficiency. It causes arrested physical and mental development with dystrophy of bones and soft tissues. The child has a large head, short limbs, puffy eyes, a thick and protruding tongue, excessively dry skin, lack of coordination and mental handicap. The acquired or adult form of thyroid deficiency is MYXOEDEMA. Administration of thyroid extract, which must be administered for life, can result in normal growth and mental development.

cri du chat syndrome a hereditary congenital syndrome characterized by hypertelorism, microcephaly, severe mental deficiency, and a plaintive cat-like cry; due to the deletion of part of the short arm of chromosome 5.

cricoid 1. ring-shaped. 2. the cricoid cartilage. *C. cartilage* a ring-like cartilage forming the lower and back part of the larynx. Pressure on the cricoid cartilage during the induction of general anaesthesia occludes the oesophagus, thereby preventing acid reflux from the stomach. Cricoid pressure is maintained until the endotracheal tube is in position and the anaesthetist has checked that the seal provided by the cuff is effective.

criminal abortion *see* Appendix 6.

cross-matching a procedure vital in blood transfusions and organ transplantation. The donor's erythrocytes or leukocytes are placed in the recipient's serum and vice versa. Absence of agglutination, haemolysis and cytotoxicity indicates that the donor and recipient are blood group compatible or histocompatible.

crown-rump length (CRL) this is measured in the first trimester to assess accurately the age of a fetus by a REAL-TIME SCANNER. *See* Appendix 4.

crowning the moment during birth when the suboccipitobregmatic and biparietal diameters of the fetal head are distending the vulval ring, and the head no longer recedes between contractions.

cryosurgery the use of a refrigerated probe to remove abnormal tissue such as a cervical erosion.

cryptomenorrhea subjective symptoms of menstruation without flow of blood.

culture 1. the propagation of micro-organisms or of living tissue cells in special media conductive to their growth. 2. to induce such propagation. 3. the product of such propagation. 4. a collective norm for the symbolic and acquired aspects of human society, including convention, custom and language. 5. a singular noun for the customs and features of an ethnic (racial, religious or social) group.

curette a metal loop, which may be blunt or sharp, used for the removal of unhealthy tissues by scraping, or to obtain biopsy material. This operation of *curett-*

age is commonly performed to remove the uterine endometrium.

Cushing's syndrome overactivity of the adrenal cortex resulting in excess glucocorticoids governing carbohydrate metabolism, leading to obesity especially of the face ('moon face') and trunk. Amenorrhoea, hirsutism (*see* HIRSUTE) and weakness also occur.

cutaneous concerning the skin.

cyanosis blueness of the skin and mucous membranes due to a deficiency of oxygen.

cyclopropane a gas used for general anaesthesia.

cyesis pregnancy.

cyst a tumour with a membranous capsule and containing fluid. *Chocalate c.* of the ovary is associated with endometriosis. *Corpus luteum* or *luteal c.* is one which develops from the corpus luteum. It occurs in HYDATIDIFORM MOLE. *Dermoid c.* contains skin, hair, teeth, etc., and is due to abnormal development of embryonic tissue. *Multilocular c.* of the ovary is divided into compartments. *Papilliferous c.* of the ovary is lined with papillae which may grow through the cyst wall into the peritoneal cavity, and give rise to ascites. *Pseudomucinous c.* of the ovary contains fluid similar to mucin. In pregnancy the presence of an ovarian cyst should be diagnosed early. It is generally removed about the middle of pregnancy. It might otherwise interfere with the normal course of labour or become malignant.

cystic fibrosis also known as

mucoviscidosis or fibrocystic disease of the pancreas. A disease with an autosomal recessive inheritance, in which the mucus-secreting glands of the body secrete an unusually thick tenacious mucus. This causes fibrosis in the pancreas and MECONIUM ILEUS in the newborn. Later complications are repeated chest infections. The diagnosis is made by the serum immune-reactive trypsin (IRT) test. A sweat test, if carried out, shows a raised level of sodium chloride. A raised ALBUMIN level in the meconium may also be significant. One individual in 25 is a genetic CARRIER of the disease and in Britain one individual in 2000 is affected.

cystitis inflammation of the bladder.

cysto- a prefix relating to the bladder.

cystocele a hernia of the bladder into the vagina, as a result of damage to the pelvic floor during childbirth. *See* COLPORRHAPHY.

cystoscope an instrument for inspecting the interior of the bladder.

cystoscopy inspection of the interior of the bladder with a cystoscope.

cystotomy incision of the bladder, e.g. for the removal of calculi.

cytogenetics a branch of GENETICS mainly concerned with the study of CHROMOSOMES.

cytology the science of the structure and functions of cells. Vaginal and cervical cytology are being applied increasingly in the early detection of abnormalities.

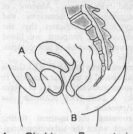

A.   Bladder;   B.   anterior vaginal wall.
CYSTOCELE

In pregnancy, desquamated cells from the vaginal wall suggest hormone changes which reveal placental insufficiency and danger to the fetus. It is possible by cervical cytology to detect very early malignant disease in the genital tract, and, although this is not common in women of childbearing age, routine examination in antenatal, postnatal and family planning clinics has been recommended. Similar routine checks are advisable in gynaecological clinics, especially for women over 35.

cytomegalic inclusion disease an infection due to cytomegalovirus and marked by nuclear inclusion bodies in large infected cells. In the congenital form, there is hepatosplenomegaly with cirrhosis and microcephaly with mental or motor handicap.

Acquired infection may cause a clinical state similar to infectious mononucleosis.

cytomegalovirus a virus found in the human salivary gland. Infection *in utero* may, rarely, cause cytomegalic inclusion disease in the newborn. The baby may be small for gestational age, and suffer from JAUNDICE with liver and spleen enlargement and THROMBOCYTOPENIA. MICROCEPHALY may also follow this disease.

cytoplasm all the protoplasm of a cell, excluding the nucleus.

cytotrophoblast the cellular layer of the trophoblast. Langhans' cell layer. It becomes much less obvious after 19–20 weeks of gestation. *See also* CHORIONIC VILLI.

D

D, d symbols used with C, c, E and e in defining Rhesus blood groups. The simplest typing, Rhesus positive and Rhesus negative, refers to blood with or without the substance D.

dactyl a finger or toe.

Danol trademark for a preparation of danazol, an anterior pituitary suppressant.

day nursery a centre for the care, during the daytime, of children up to the age of 5 years. Provided by the Social Services Department or by voluntary agencies. Priority is given to children from 'at risk' families and to those with a handicap.

deadbirth a STILLBIRTH.

deafness lack or loss, complete or partial, of the sense of hearing. Total deafness is quite rare but partial deafness is common. A great many cases of congenital deafness are caused by infectious diseases, especially viral infections, contracted by the mother during pregnancy. Of these, rubella is the most common.

death the cessation of all physical and chemical processes that occurs in all living organisms or their cellular components. *Brain d.* the diagnosis of clinical brain stem death is governed, in the UK, by a set of guidelines ratified by the Medical Royal Colleges and their Faculties. *Cot d.* sudden infant death syndrome (SIDS). *D. certificate* a certificate issued by the registrar for deaths after receipt of a preliminary certificate completed and signed by an attending doctor, indicating the date and probable cause of death. Only after issue of this certificate, indicating that the death has been registered, can burial or cremation take place. *D. grant* a payment made by social security from the social fund which is payable to low income families only. This payment is recoverable from the estate of the deceased.

D. intrauterine death of the fetus *in utero. See* INTRAUTERINE. *D. rate* the number of deaths per stated number of persons (100 or 10 000 or 100 000) in a certain region in a certain time period.

decapitation severing the head from the body. A destructive operation occasionally employed in obstructed labour in a neglected shoulder presentation.

decentralized clinics clinics held locally to reduce the distances travelled; they include antenatal clinics, attended by midwives and general practitioners, and sometimes by consultant obstetricians.

decidua the name given to the endometrium of the uterus during pregnancy. It is thickened and more vascular, to receive and provide for the nutrition of the fertilized ovum. It is shed when pregnancy terminates. *D. basalis* the part on which the ovum rests and which covers the maternal surface of the placenta. *D. capsularis* that part covering the ovum as it projects into the uterine cavity. *D. vera* the true lining of the uterus, which for the first 12 weeks of pregnancy is not in contact with the ovum.

decidual cast the expulsion of the decidua intact, in the shape of the uterine cavity, following the death of the ovum in an ectopic pregnancy. *See* ECTOPIC GESTATION.

decompensation inability of the heart to maintain adequate circulation; it is marked by dyspnoea,

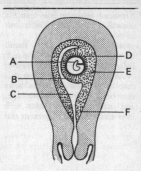

Sixth week of pregnancy.
A. *Embryo*; B. *capsular decidua*; C. *uterine cavity*; D. *chorionic villi*; E. *basal decidua*; F. *true decidua*.
DECIDUA

venous engorgement, cyanosis and oedema.

defaecation evacuation of the bowels.

defibrillation termination of atrial or ventricular fibrillation, usually by electric shock.

deflexion a fetal attitude in which the head is not flexed, or only partially flexed, as may occur in occipitoposterior positions of the vertex.

degeneration a structural change which lowers the vitality of the tissue in which it takes place. *Fatty d.* fat is deposited in tissues. *Red d. See* NECROBIOSIS.

dehydration excessive loss of fluid

from the body or failure to take sufficient fluid to balance loss. The term usually means actual dehydration together with the ketoacidosis which often accompanies it. It occurs in severe vomiting in pregnancy and in prolonged labour. The skin is dry and inelastic, the tongue is dry and the eyes are sunken. The breath may smell of acetone, and the urine is scanty and contains ketone bodies. The electrolyte balance and the reaction of the blood are disturbed. Dehydration with ketoacidosis in the mother is dangerous to the fetus. It is treated by giving intravenous dextrose, with saline if the urinary chlorides are much diminished. In babies, dehydration fever may occur if insufficient fluid is taken. Severe dehydration is usually caused by diarrhoea; the fontanelle is depressed, skin turgor poor and weight loss occurs. This condition can be corrected orally if mild, or intravenously if severe.

delay in labour unusual prolongation of any one of the three stages of labour, especially of the first stage. *See* Appendix 9.

deletion in genetics, loss from a chromosome of genetic material.

Delfen foam an aerosol SPERMICIDE.

delirium a mental disturbance of relatively short duration usually reflecting a toxic state, marked by illusions, hallucinations, delusions, excitement, restlessness and incoherence. Almost any acute illness accompanied by a very high fever can bring on delirium.

delivery natural expulsion or extraction of the child, placenta and fetal membranes at birth. *Abdominal d.* delivery of an infant through an incision made into the uterus through the abdominal wall (CAESAREAN SECTION). *Instrumental d.* delivery facilitated by the use of instruments, particularly forceps. *Spontaneous d.* delivery occurring without assistance of forceps or other mechanical aid. *Vaginal d.* complete expulsion of the baby, placenta and membranes via the birth canal. Normally the head comes first presenting by the vertex. Breech delivery is also possible.

delivery bag equipment provided to enable a community midwife to conduct a delivery in the home.

demand feeding feeding when the baby appears hungry and not according to a fixed timetable. Sometimes called 'on demand' feeding or baby-led feeding.

Demerol an American proprietary form of PETHIDINE.

demography the statistical science dealing with populations, including matters of health, disease, births, and mortality.

denaturation test Singer's test; a blood test to distinguish fetal from maternal blood.

denidation the degeneration and expulsion during menstruation, of certain epithelial elements, potentially the nidus of an embryo. The term used to describe the intended shedding of uterine lining when postcoital contraceptive pills are used.

Denis Browne splint a special boot designed for the correction of TALIPES.

denominator in obstetrics, a particular point on the presenting part of the fetus used to indicate its position in relation to a particular part of the mother's pelvis. In a vertex presentation the denominator is the occiput, in a breech presentation it is the sacrum, and in a face presentation the mentum or chin.

dental caries decay of teeth.

dentition teething. *Primay d.* cutting of the temporary or milk teeth, beginning at the age of 6 or 7 months and continuing until the end of the second year. A full set consists of 8 incisors, 4 canines and 8 premolars; 20 in all. *Secondary d.* appearance of the permanent teeth, beginning at 6 or 7 years and complete by 12 to 15 years, except for the posterior molars or 'wisdom teeth' which appear between the ages of 17 and 25. There are 32 permanent teeth: 8 incisors, 4 canines, 8 premolars or bicuspids, and 12 molars.

deoxyribonucleic acid (DNA) a nucleic acid of complex molecular structure occurring in cell nuclei as the basic structure of the GENES. DNA is present in all body cells of every species, including unicellular organisms and DNA viruses. DNA is the molecule that directs all the activities of living cells, including its own reproduction and perpetuation in generation after generation.

Department of the Environment (DoE) a State department set up in 1970 to combine the previous ministries of Housing and of Local Government and of Public Building and Works.

Department of Health (DH) the body responsible for administering the National Health Service.

depression a lowering of the spirits. A mood change experienced as sadness or melancholy. *Endogenous d.* occurs in the course of the manic-depressive psychosis. The mood change is associated with slowing of thought and action and feelings of guilt. *Reactive d.* depression occurring as a result of some event which influences the person

Age of appearance of teeth

Tooth	Age
Milk teeth	
Incisors	6 months
1st molars	12 months
Canines	18 months
2nd molars	24 months
Permanent teeth	
1st molars	6 years
Incisors	7–8 years
Premolars	9–10 years
Canines	11 years
2nd molars	12 years
3rd molars	17–25 years

unfavourably. Either type may occur in the puerperium and usually starts in the first 2 weeks after delivery, but develops gradually. Early recognition and treatment with support, psychotherapy and often anti-depressant drugs are required for those less severely disturbed. Mothers with severe depressive illness are treated in a psychiatric hospital, preferably a mother and baby unit where anti-depressant drugs and sometimes ECT are necessary. About 60% of postnatal women experience the 'blues' on or around the fifth day after delivery. This normally lasts only a day or so, the mother quickly responding to emotional support and reassurance.

dermoid cyst a tumour consisting of a fibrous wall lined with stratified epithelium containing pulpy material in which epithelial elements such as hair are found.

descent a downward movement, e.g. of the fetus. During labour the fetus must descend through the brim, cavity and outlet of the pelvis in order to be born. The descent may be measured in fifths. *See* Appendix 7.

desquamation the shedding of the superficial cells from the epithelium of any part of the body.

detergent a cleansing agent. Detergents are commonly used as soap substitutes, both in domestic and in professional practice. An example is Cetavlon, a proprietary preparation of cetrimide.

detoxication the process of neutralizing toxic substances. A function of the liver.

detrusor a general term for a body part, e.g. a muscle, that pushes down.

development the process of growth and differentiation.

developmental pertaining to development. *D. anomaly* absence, deformity, or excess of body parts as a result of faulty development of the embryo. *D. milestones* significant behaviours which are used to mark the process of development, e.g. sitting, walking, talking, etc. *D. tests* a standard series of tests performed on children to assess their development.

dexamethasone a synthetic glucocorticoid used primarily as an anti-inflammatory agent in various conditions, including diseases and allergic states; it is also used in a screening test for the diagnosis of CUSHING'S SYNDROME. Dexamethasone is given to some women prior to preterm delivery because of the suggestion that it accelerates the maturation of the fetal lungs and therefore reduces the incidence of respiratory distress syndrome.

dextran a polysaccharide preparation used as a plasma substitute in the treatment of shock. Its disadvantages are: (*a*) that it restores the circulatory volume; (*b*) it does not leak out of the blood vessels in the same way as physiological saline; (*c*) it can be used when blood grouping is not possible; and (*d*) it carries no risk, as does genuine plasma, of viral infections. *See* Appendix 11.

dextrose glucose. A monosaccharide. The simplest form of carbohydrate.

diabetes insipidus a rare disease of deficiency in secretion of the antidiuretic hormone of the posterior lobe of the pituitary gland. It is characterized by polyuria and consequent dehydration and thirst. Treated by the administration of vasopressin.

diabetes mellitus a familial disease of deficient secretion of insulin from the islet cells of the pancreas or increased resistance to the action of insulin, possibly caused by anterior pituitary growth hormone. Insulin resistance increases during pregnancy and gestational diabetes may develop. Pregnancy has a diabetogenic influence because of the increased metabolic workload and insulin resistance. However, this occurs only in women who have a genetic predisposition to the disease. The symptoms are polyuria, weight loss, thirst and lassitude. There is hyperglycaemia and later ketosis which may be severe enough to cause coma. Treatment is by the administration of insulin and a carefully regulated diet. For diabetes mellitus in pregnancy, *see* Appendix 6.

diabetic pertaining to diabetes. *D. coma* loss of consciousness occurring as a result of severe ketosis.

diacetic acid acetoacetic acid, a colourless compound found in minute quantities in normal urine and in abnormal amounts in the urine and in abnormal amounts in the urine of diabetic patients and of those who have excessive vomiting.

diagnosis determination of the nature of a disease. *Clinical d.* is made by study of actual signs and symptoms. *Differential d.* the patient's symptoms are compared and contrasted with those of other diseases. *Tentative d.* a provisional one judged by apparent facts and observations.

diagonal conjugate an internal measurement of the pelvis, taken from the promontory of the sacrum to the lower border of the symphysis pubis; it should measure 12.5 cm (5 in) in a normal pelvis. By subtracting 1.3 cm (0.5 in) from the measurement, the true conjugate can be estimated. In practice, the examining finger cannot as a rule reach the sacral promontory unless the pelvis is unusually small, and in normal cases the true conjugate is inferred to be of average size because the promontory is not felt, i.e. is out of reach.

dialysis the passage of salts, water and metabolites through a semipermeable membrane. *Renal d.* the use of an artificial kidney. The patient's blood is separated from the dialysing fluid by the membrane, retaining blood cells and plasma proteins and losing the toxic substances normally excreted by the kidney.

diameter a straight line passing through the centre of a circle or sphere. The pelvic girdle is nearly

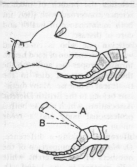

A. *True conjugate*; B. *diagonal conjugate*.

MEASUREMENT OF THE DIAGONAL CONJUGATE

circular at certain levels and the fetal skull is nearly spherical, hence a number of diameters are described in both. *See* FETAL SKULL *and* PELVIS.

diamorphine hydrochloride heroin. A powerful analgesic and drug of addiction. *See* Appendix 19.

diaphragm the muscular dome-shaped partition separating the thorax from the abdomen. It is an important muscle of respiration, and, as such, it is one of the secondary forces in labour. When relaxed, the diaphragm is convex but it flattens as it contracts during inhalation, thereby enlarging the chest cavity and allowing for expansion of the lungs. In the second stage of labour the contraction of the diaphragm and abdominal muscles aids the expulsive force of the uterine contractions. *Contraceptive d.* a device of moulded rubber or other soft plastic material, fitted over the cervix uteri to prevent entrance of spermatozoa.

diarrhoea the frequent passage of loose stools. It is usually caused by infection. In the neonate it is dangerous, as the baby may become rapidly dehydrated, with a disturbed electrolyte balance. If caused by infection it is very dangerous in a maternity unit, as it is rapidly transmitted. *See also* ESCHERICHIA COLI.

diastole the resting stage of the cardiac cycle. Following atrial and ventricular SYSTOLE the cardiac muscle is now in a state of relaxation.

diastolic murmur an abnormal sound produced during diastole, and occurring in valvular disease of the heart.

diastolic pressure the pressure of blood in the arteries during the resting stage of the heart. *See* BLOOD PRESSURE.

diathermy the use of high-frequency electrical currents as a form of physiotherapy and as a coagulative, cutting and haemostatic agent in surgical procedures. The term diathermy is derived from the Greek words dia and therma, and literally means 'heating through'. Surgically it is commonly used to treat neoplasms, warts, infected tissues and to cauterize blood vessels to prevent excessive bleeding. In obstetrics and gynaecology it is often used to treat cervical lesions. *See also* CRYOSURGERY.

diazepam a benzodiazepine tranquillizer used primarily as an anti-anxiety agent, and also used as a skeletal muscle relaxant, as an anticonvulsant, as preoperative medication to relieve anxiety and tension, and in the management of alcohol withdrawal symptoms.

DIC *see* DISSEMINATED INTRAVASCULAR COAGULATION.

dicephalus a fetus or infant with two heads.

dichorial, dichorionic having two distinct chorions, said of dizygotic twins.

dichotomy a division into two parts.

didactylism the presence of only two digits on a hand or foot.

didelphia the condition of having a double uterus.

didymitis inflammation of the testicle. Also called orchitis.

didymus a testis; also used as a word termination designating a fetus with a duplication of parts or one consisting of conjoined symmetrical twins.

diembryony the production of two embryos from a single egg.

dienoestrol a synthetic oestrogen used in the treatment of atrophic vaginitis and kraurosis vulvae.

diet the customary amount of food and drink taken by a person from day to day; more narrowly, a diet planned to meet specific requirements of the individual, including or excluding certain foods.

dietetics the branch of medical science concerned with diet, for both maintenance of health and cure of disease.

dietician one who is concerned with the promotion of good health through proper diet and with the therapeutic use of diet in the treatment of disease. Many dieticians belong to the British Dietetic Association, which acts as both a professional body and a trade union.

differential making a difference. *D. blood count* comparison of the numbers of the different white cells present in the blood. *D. diagnosis see* DIAGNOSIS.

difficult labour DYSTOCIA. A term sometimes used to describe a labour which is prolonged or complicated by mechanical difficulty. Prolonged labour should not occur now that PARTOGRAMS and active management are used more commonly. *See* Appendix 9.

diffusion the passage of substances in solution into an area of weaker concentration through a semipermeable membrane. Oxygen, carbon dioxide, some minerals and urea diffuse across the CHORIONIC VILLI of the placenta. More complex substances such as protein, lipids and carbohydrates are conveyed by active transport.

digestion the process by which food taken into the body is changed and rendered suitable for absorption into the blood.

digit a finger or toe.

digital pertaining to the finger or toe, usually the former, e.g.

...igital examination. An examination carried out with one or more fingers.

...gitalis the active principle of the ...oxglove plant, *Digitalis purpurea*. ...t is used in congestive heart ...ailure and atrial fibrillation to ...low and strengthen the heart ...eat.

...goxin a drug obtained from the ...eaves of *Digitalis lanata*; used in ...he treatment of congestive heart ...ailure.

...latation stretching of either an ...rifice or, rarely, a hollow organ. ...t may be natural, as in the cervix ...uring the first stage of labour, ...or artificial, as in that of the ...ervix preceding curettage of the ...terine cavity.

...lator an instrument used to ...ffect dilatation, e.g. HEGAR'S D.

...metria a condition characterized ...y a double uterus.

...morphism the quality of existing ...n two distinct forms. *Sexual* ...*. 1. physical or behavioural ...lifferences associated with sex. ...*. having some properties of both ...exes, as in the early embryo and ...n some hermaphrodites.

...indevan a proprietary preparation of phenindione, a synthetic anticoagulant.

...noprost trometamol a PROSTA-...LANDIN (PGF$_2$a) administered ...ntra-amniotically and intra-...enously to induce abortion.

...iodone a contrast medium similar ...o iodoxyl, used in radiography.

...phtheria an acute, specific infec-...ious disease caused by infection ...with *Corynebacterium diphtheriae* ...Klebs–Loeffler bacillus). Highly dangerous prior to the introduction of diphtheria immunization. In the UK diphtheria toxoid is given in combination with tetanus toxoid and pertussis vaccine as 'triple-antigen' at 3 months, 4½–5 months and 8½–11 months of age. A booster dose of triple vaccine against diphtheria, tetanus and whooping cough is given just before the child starts school at the age of 5 years.

diphtheroids   non-pathogenic corynebacteria resembling the bacilli of diphtheria, common COMMENSALS of the throat, nose, ear, conjunctiva and skin.

diplococci cocci found always in pairs. They may be encapsulated, e.g. pneumococci, or intracellular, e.g. gonococci. *See* GONOCOCCUS.

diploid the condition in which the cell contains two sets of CHROMOSOMES. In man the diploid number is 46, i.e. 23 pairs.

diplosomatia a condition in which complete twins are joined at some of their body parts.

disability any restriction or lack (resulting from an impairment) of ability to perform an activity in the manner or within the range considered normal for a human being. *Developmental d.* a substantial handicap of indefinite duration, with onset before the age of 18 years, and attributable to mental handicap, autism, cerebral palsy, epilepsy, or other neuropathy.

disabled living allowance provides a weekly sum for the disabled to help with costs of care and mobility. From April 1992 this benefit replaces attendance and mobility allowances for people disabled before the age of 65. Attendance allowance continues for those disabled after the age of 65.

disabled working allowance provides a weekly payment for disabled people on a low income.

disaccharide a carbohydrate formed of two simple sugar units. Examples are lactose in milk, sucrose and maltose. These may readily be broken down into MONOSACCHARIDES.

disc a circular or rounded flat plate. *Embryonic d.* a flattish area in a cleaved ovum in which the first traces of the embryo are seen. *Intervertebral d.* the layer of fibrocartilage between the bodies of adjoining vertebrae. *Prolapsed intervertebral d.* rupture of an intervertebral disc. Most commonly occurs in the lower back and occasionally in the neck.

discharge the flow of substances from the body. The term is more commonly used in reference to abnormal conditions, e.g. discharge from the child's eyes in ophthalmia neonatorum, or vaginal discharge resulting from infection.

discoloration an alteration in the colour of the skin or mucous membranes. A bluish discoloration of the cervix and vagina is seen in early pregnancy and is known as Jacquemier's sign.

discus proligerus the compact mass of follicular cells surrounding the ovum before it is expelled from the graafian follicle.

disease any abnormal condition which causes a local or general disturbance in the structure or function of the body.

disinfect to destroy micro-organisms but not usually bacterial spores, reducing the number of micro-organisms to a level which is not harmful to health.

dislocation the displacement of a bone from its natural position. Some dislocations, especially of the hip, are congenital, usually resulting from a faulty construction of the joint. Such a condition is best treated with a splint fitted after birth to prevent the need for surgery later.

displacement a movement to an unusual position. The non-gravid uterus normally lies in the centre of the pelvic cavity, anteverted and anteflexed. Retroversion and PROLAPSE may therefore be termed displacements.

disproportion lack of harmony or lack of a proper relationship between one object and another. In obstetrics, this refers to disparity between the fetal head and the particular pelvis through which it is to pass. The fault lies either in the maternal pelvis, which is too small or abnormally shaped, or in the child's head, which is presenting by an unfavourable diameter, or unusually large. It is recognized in the last 3 weeks of pregnancy by failure of the fetal head to engage, either spontaneously or on pressure. The degree of disproportion may be assessed accurately by means of X-rays or ultrasound. In minor degrees the action of the uterus in labour is sufficient to mould the fetal head through the pelvis, often with increased flexion, and labour may proceed without complication to mother or child. This is anticipated in TRIAL OF LABOUR. In moderate and severe degrees, delivery is by caesarean section.

disseminated intravascular coagulation (DIC) widespread formation of thromboses in the microcirculation, mainly within the capillaries. It is a secondary complication of conditions which introduce coagulation-promoting factors into the circulation, such as abruptio placentae, retained dead fetus, amniotic fluid embolism and various types of infections and bacteraemias. Paradoxically, the intravascular clotting ultimately produces haemorrhage because of rapid consumption of fibrinogen, platelets, prothrombin and clotting factors, V, VIII and X. Treatment of DIC consists of replacement of the inadequate blood products and correction, when possible, of the underlying cause. When the primary condition cannot be treated, intravenous injections of heparin may inhibit the clotting process and raise the level of the depleted clotting factors.

distress *see* fetal hypoxia, Appendices 7 *and* 16.

district general hospital a hospital equipped to provide a full range of specialist services to a natural catchment area.

district health authority (DHA) *See* Appendix 1.

diuresis increased secretion of urine.

diuretic a drug which increases the excretion of urine, e.g. Frusemide. Many diuretics, especially the thiazides, are used in the management of hypertension, particularly when used in conjunction with other kinds of antihypertensive agents. *See* Appendix 19.

diurnal pertaining to or occurring during the daytime, or period of light.

dizygotic pertaining to or derived from two separate zygotes (fertilized ova); said of twins.

DNA *See* DEOXYRIBONUCLEIC ACID.

Döderlein's bacillus a non-pathogenic lactobacillus occurring normally in vaginal secretions. Metabolism of glycogen within the squamous epithelium lining the vagina produces lactic acid. The resulting pH of 4.5 effectively counteracts the alkalinity of cervical mucus and proves hostile to pathogenic organisms.

dolichocephalic having a long head, where the anteroposterior diameter is increased.

domiciliary midwifery the confinement of a woman in her own home, where she is attended by a midwife and, probably, by her family doctor. For selection of place of confinement, *see* Appendix 3.

dominant inheritance the mode of inheritance by which one parent passes on a characteristic to the offspring. One of the pair of GENES carries the characteristic and is dominant over, or rules over, the other gene. There is a 1 in 2 chance of the offspring being affected, as in ACHRONDO-PLASIA. cf. RECESSIVE inheritance.

'domino' booking a plan of maternity care whereby a mother has her baby in a consultant unit, cared for by the community midwife. They return home any time after 6 hours following delivery. The name derives from *domi-ciliary midwife in and out*.

donor one who gives. A blood donor is a person who gives blood for transfusion. A milk donor is one whose abundant lactation enables her to supply milk for a human milk bank.

dopamine an intermediate product in the synthesis of noradrenaline. It is a neurotransmitter in the central nervous system. Dopamine is administered intravenously to correct haemodynamic imbalance in shock syndrome.

Doppler ultrasound that in which measurement and a visual record are made of the shift in frequency of a continuous or pulsed ultrasonic wave proportional to the blood flow velocity in underlying vessels; used in diagnosis of occlusive vascular disease. It is also used in detection of the fetal heart beat and the velocity of blood across a stenotic heart valve.

dorsal concerning the back. *D. position* the patient lies on her back with her head and shoulders slightly elevated.

dorso- a prefix meaning related to the position of the back of the fetus, in cases of shoulder presentation.

double uterus abnormal development of the uterus resulting from failure of fusion of the Müllerian ducts. There are two uterine bodies with or without duplication of the cervix and of the vagina.

douche 1. a stream or jet of water or other fluid applied to some part of the body. A vaginal douche of up to 5 litres of warm saline is occasionally used to provide hydrostatic pressure to distend the vagina and thus cause INVERSION OF THE UTERUS to revert to its normal position. 2. the apparatus used for a douche.

Douglas' pouch a pouch of peritoneum between the upper third of the vagina in front and the anterior wall of the rectum behind.

Down's syndrome a chromosome abnormality, the commonest type having 47 instead of 46 chromosomes. The extra one is attached to the 21st pair, so that the condition is also called *trisomy 21*. This condition is associated with increasing maternal age. In the other form of Down's syndrome a translocation occurs, usually between chromosomes 14 and 21, as a *de novo* structural arrangement in the child, although the parents have normal chromosomes. Alternatively the translocations may occur as a result of a similar translocated chromosome in the parents, in which case there is a 10% chance of the condition recurring in a further pregnancy. The child exhibits certain characteristics and is always mentally handicapped. The slanting eyes and broad flat nose suggest the common name of mongolism. The child also has brachycephaly, with a short neck with loose skin, and HYPOTONIA. The hands are broad, with a single palmar crease. A third fontanelle is often present, as well as Brushfield's spots in the iris. Many of these individuals have other congenital abnormalities, i.e. congenital heart disease, and may not survive infancy. These children are often friendly and affectionate and benefit from special education.

drain 1. to withdraw liquid gradually. 2. any device by which a channel or open area may be established for exit of fluids or purulent material from a cavity, wound or infected area.

dram a unit of weight in the avoirdupois (27 344 grains, 1/16 ounce) or apothecaries' (60 grains, 1/8 ounce) system; symbol 3. Sometimes also spelled drachm. *Fluid d.* a unit of liquid measure of the apothecaries' system, containing 60 minims, and equivalent to 3.697 ml. Abbreviated fl. dr.

Dramamine a proprietary preparation of dimenhydrinate, an anti-emetic drug.

draught reflex *see* MILK FLOW MECHANISM.

drepanocyte sickle cell.

drepanocytosis occurrence of drepanocytes (sickle cells) in the blood.

dressing the covering applied to a wound surface.

Drew–Smythe cannula an S-shaped metal CATHETER designed for introduction into the birth canal to pass into the cervical os past the fetal head. The purpose is to puncture the hindwaters when the head is not engaged. It is rarely used now, as it can cause placental separation.

drip the introduction into the body of fluid run through tubing and a 'drip' connection so slowly that the drops can be counted and regulated by hand or by a pump. *Intravenous d.* usually dextrose solution or blood introduced into a vein. *Intragastric* or *gastric d.* milk or other fluid run slowly into the stomach.

droplet infection the passage of pathogenic bacteria, conveyed during talking, coughing, sneezing, etc., in minute droplets, from the respiratory tract of an infected person.

drug 1. any medicinal substance. 2. a narcotic. 3. to administer a drug. *D. abuse* the use of one or more drugs for purposes other than those for which they are prescribed or recommended. *D. addiction* a state of periodic or chronic intoxication produced by the repeated consumption of a drug characterized by: (*a*) an overwhelming desire or need (compulsion) to continue use of the drug and to obtain it by any means; (*b*) a tendency to increase the dosage; (*c*) a psychological and usually a physical dependence on its effects; and (d) a detrimental effect on the individual and on society. *D. interaction* modification of the potency of one drug by another (or others) taken concurrently or sequentially. Some drug interactions are harmful and some may have therapeutic effects.

drugs in midwifery *see* Appendix 19.

Dubowitz score a method used to assess gestational age in a low-birth-weight infant.

Duchenne's muscular dystrophy the childhood type of muscular dystrophy. 1. spinal muscular atrophy. 2. bulbar paralysis. 3. tabes doralis.

Ducrey's bacillus the organism which causes soft chancre (*Haemophilus ducreyi*).

duct (ductus) a tube or channel for conveying away the secretion of a gland.

ductus arteriosus a fetal blood vessel which bypasses the pulmonary circulation by connecting the pulmonary artery and the descending aorta, and which normally closes at birth. *ductus venosus* the umbilical vein travels in the cord to the fetus and divides into two branches, one of which is the ductus venosus and this joins the inferior vena cava.

Duffy blood group a type of blood containing a rare antigen.

Dulcolax a proprietary form of bisacodyl given orally as an aperient and also used as suppository.

duodenum the first part of small intestine, from the pylorus to the jejunum. It is about 25–27 cm (10–11 in) in length. *duodenal atresia* incomplete canalisation of the duodenum. Projectile vomiting will occur as soon as the infant begins to be fed. Characteristically the vomitus contains bile.

dura mater the tough fibrous membrane lining the skull and forming the outermost covering of the brain and spinal cord. A double fold of the inner layer of dura mater, the falx cerebri, dips down between the cerebral hemispheres, and a horizontal fold, the tentorium cerebelli, separates the cerebellum from the cerebral hemispheres above. These two membranes carry the large venous sinuses which drain blood from the skull. They may be stretched and are sometimes torn during delivery, causing serious INTRACRANIAL HAEMORRHAGE.

dural tap puncture of the dura mater causing a leakage of cerebrospinal fluid. This causes a headache which may persist for about a week. Undue exertion and straining may cause further loss of cerebrospinal fluid so should be avoided.

duration of pregnancy duration averages 266 days from conception to delivery and 280 days (40 weeks or 9 months and 1 week) from the date of the last menstrual period to the date of delivery. If the woman knows the date of the first day of her last menstrual period, a useful calculation of the estimated date of delivery (EDD) can be obtained by adding 40 weeks. If the cycle is x days less than 28, the EDD will be x days earlier. Similarly, it will be 28 days plus x if the cycle is longer. About 67 per cent of women may be expected to begin labour within a period of 7 days before or 7 days after the calculated date. Other symptoms of pregnancy, such as quickening, the size of the uterus and liquor studies, may be of value in determining the duration of a pregnancy. However, the most accurate method is by ultrasound. At 7–14 weeks the CROWN–RUMP LENGTH (CRL) is very accurate. A biparietal measurement between 13 and 20 weeks is as accurate as the CRL in the first trimester of pregnancy.

Dutch cap a contraceptive device. See DIAPHRAGM.

Duvadilan trademark for preparations of isoxsuprine, a vasodilator.

dydrogesterone an orally effective, synthetic progestin used mainly in the diagnosis and treatment of primary amenorrhoea and severe dysmenorrhoea, and in combination with oestrogen in dysfunctional menorrhagia.

dys- prefix meaning 'difficult', 'disordered' or 'painful'.

dysentery a notifiable intestinal infection characterized by severe diarrhoea, with the passage of blood or mucus and pus usually caused by a *Shigella* species or *Entamoeba histolytica*.

dyslexia impairment of ability to comprehend written language, due to a central lesion. adj. *dyslexic*.

dysmature a vague term commonly used to describe a baby who is small for gestational age. See also Appendix 17.

dysmenorrhoea difficult or painful menstruation. It is characterized by cramp-like pains in the lower abdomen, and sometimes by headache, irritability, mental depression, malaise and fatigue.

dyspareunia difficult or painful coitus.

dyspepsia indigestion.

dyspnoea difficult or laboured breathing.

dystocia difficult or abnormal labour.

dystrophia literally, difficult or abnormal growth. *Dystocia d. syndrome* a rare unfortunate obstetric sequence to which a certain type of woman is said to be prone. She is short, heavily built, subfertile, hirsute and often has pre-eclampsia. She has an android pelvis, an occipito-posterior position of the fetus with its many possible complications. See Appendix 9.

dysuria difficult or painful micturition.

E

E, e symbols used in conjunction with C, c, D, d to denote Rhesus types.

early transfer the transfer home of mother and baby from a maternity unit within the early POSTNATAL PERIOD.

ecbolic oxytocic, i.e. makes uterine muscles contract.

ecchymosis effusion of blood beneath the skin, causing discoloration. Bruising.

ECG electrocardiogram.

echovirus a group of viruses (enteroviruses) isolated from man which produce many different types of human disease, especially aseptic meningitis, diarrhoea and various respiratory diseases.

eclampsia a serious complication of pregnancy characterized by fits and accompanied by severe hypertension, oedema and proteinuria. adj. *eclamptic. See* Appendix 6.

econazole an anti-fungal agent similar to clotrimazole or miconazole.

ECT electroconvulsive therapy; electroplexy.

ecto- a prefix meaning 'outside'.

ectoblast the ectoderm.

ectocervix portio vaginalis.

ectoderm the outer germinal layer of the developing embryo from which the skin, external sense organs, mucous membrane of the mouth and anus and nervous system are derived.

-ectomy a suffix meaning 'cutting out', e.g. appendicectomy, hysterectomy.

ectopia abnormal position of any structure. *E. vesicae* an uncommon congenital defect of the abdominal wall in which the interior of the bladder is exposed.

ectopic gestation the embedding of a fertilized ovum, usually in the fallopian tube, but occasionally in the ovary or abdominal cavity. Such a pregnancy is unlikely to continue for more than 6 or 7 weeks, and there is a considerable risk of haemorrhage. *See* Appendix 6.

ectro- a prefix meaning miscarriage, congenital absence.

ectrodactyly congenital absence of all or part of a digit.

ectromelia gross hypoplasia or

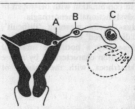

A. *Interstitial (angular).* B. *isthmic;* C. *ampullar.*
ECTOPIC GESTATION

aplasia of one or more long bones of one or more limbs. adj. *ectromelic*.

ctrosyndactyly a condition in which some digits are absent and those that remain are webbed.

czema a serious allergic skin condition. There are hereditary traits, and infantile eczema can be precipitated by giving cows' milk feeds. A mother with a family history of eczema, hay fever or asthma should be encouraged to breast feed her baby totally, as even one complementary feed can induce these conditions.

EDD expected date of delivery. It is calculated by counting forwards 9 months and adding 7 days from the first day of the last normal menstrual period or counting back 3 months and adding 7 days. Adjustments have to be made for a regular long cycle by adding days in excess of 28 days and in a regular short cycle by subtracting days less than 28.

Edward's syndrome trisomy 18 syndrome. The baby is small for gestational age and has typical facies, hands and feet and a shield-shaped chest. Most of these children have severe congenital heart disease and all are mentally retarded.

effacement 'taking up' of the cervix. The process by which the internal os dilates, so opening out the cervical canal and leaving only a circular orifice, the external os. This process precedes cervical dilatation, particularly in a primigravida, whilst both occur simul-

taneously in a multigravida during labour.

efferent carrying outward, i.e. from the centre to the periphery. The *e. nerves*, also called motor nerves, obey impulses from the nerve centres of the brain.

effleurage stroking movement in massage. In natural childbirth, a light circular stroke of the lower abdomen, done in rhythm to control breathing, to aid in relaxation of the abdominal muscles, and to increase concentration during a uterine contraction. The stroking is accomplished by moving the wrist only. Concentrating on the coordination of stroking and breathing is believed to block out some of the sensations created by the contracting uterus.

effusion the escape of blood or serum into surrounding tissues or cavities.

egg 1. an ovum; a female gamete. 2. an oocyte. 3. a female reproductive cell at any stage before fertilization and in derivatives after fertilization, and even after some development. *E. donation* the donor takes drugs to induce multiple ovulation; the ova are removed by laparoscopy, fertilized *in vitro* and then placed in the recipient's uterus.

ego in psychoanalytic theory, one of the three major parts of the personality, the others being the ID and the SUPEREGO. The word ego is Latin for 'I'. The ego may be considered the psychological aspect of one's personality, the id comprising the physiological

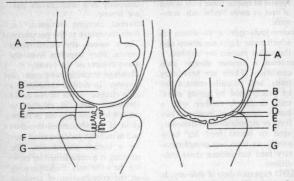

A. *Upper uterine segment*; B. *lower uterine segment*; C. *uterine contents*; D. *internal cervical os*; E. *columnar epithelium lining cervical canal*; F. *external cervical os*; G. *vagina.*

CERVIX BEFORE (left) AND AFTER (right) EFFACEMENT

aspects and the superego the social aspects.

Eisenmenger's syndrome large ventricular septal defect, overriding of the aorta and right ventricular hypertrophy. It is associated with a high maternal mortality.

ejaculation forcible, sudden expulsion; especially expulsion of semen from the male urethra, a reflex action that occurs as a result of sexual stimulation.

electrocardiogram (ECG) a tracing of the heart's action shown by electrical waves, used in the diagnosis of heart disease.

electrode a conductor through

which electricity leaves its source to enter another medium. *Fetal scalp e.* an electrode applied to the fetal scalp to record the ECG. *See* Appendices 7 *and* 16.

electroencephalogram (EEG) a tracing of electrical waves from the brain. Epileptic patients show a characteristic abnormal pattern which has also been noted in some patients with eclampsia.

electrolyte a substance which in solution dissociates into electrically charged particles (IONS), e.g. sodium bicarbonate, potassium chloride. Imbalance, e.g. from severe vomiting or renal failure, is diagnosed by examination of the serum.

electrophoresis the movement of charged particles suspended in a liquid or various media under the influence of an applied electric field. The various charged particles of a particular substance migrate in a definite and characteristic direction—toward either the anode or the cathode—and at a characteristic speed. This principle has been widely used in the separation of proteins and is therefore valuable in the study of diseases in which the serum and plasma proteins are altered. The principle has also been applied in the separation and identification of various types of human haemoglobin.

eliminate to expel waste substances of the body; e.g. the kidney eliminates urea, the bowel eliminates the unabsorbed food products, the lungs eliminate carbon dioxide.

embolism the blocking of a blood vessel by a solid or foreign substance introduced into the circulation. *Air e.* air bubbles entering the circulation, possibly in vaginal or intrauterine douching in pregnancy. *Amniotic fluid e.* amniotic fluid with the substances it may contain entering the circulation; an occasional complication of labour. *Pulmonary e.* following labour in the event of pelvic or leg vein thrombosis, part of the clot is detached and travels in the blood stream until it is arrested in a branch of the pulmonary artery. Any large embolus will cause immediate death. A smaller embolus will cause the patient to collapse with pain in the chest, dyspnoea and cyanosis. Oestrogens appear to increase the risk of venous thrombosis, so that most authorities have abandoned their use to suppress lactation.

embolus a foreign particle or substance circulating in the blood, e.g. a detached portion of thrombus, a mass of bacteria, an air bubble or amniotic fluid.

embryo the developing offspring of viviparous animals before birth. The human embryo is usually so called for the first 8 weeks after conception, the term fetus being employed subsequently.

embryology the science of the development of the embryo.

embryonic plate that portion of the inner cell mass of the blastocyst from which the embryo itself is formed.

embryotomy cutting up the fetus to make delivery possible, occasionally necessary in neglected obstructed labour where there are no facilities for operative procedures. Extremely rare in modern obstetrics.

emergency a condition requiring immediate attention. The UKCC Handbook of Midwives' Rules 1991, 40(2) states: 'A practising midwife shall not, except in an emergency, undertake any treatment which she has not been trained to give, either before or after registration as a midwife, and which is outside her sphere of practice'. *E. obstetric unit* an emergency team from a consultant obstetric unit who go out to obstetric emergencies in the community or, in general practitioner units, taking the appropriate equipment, including O-negative blood for transfusion.

E. protection order a court order whereby a child is arbitrarily removed from the care of its parents in the interests of his/her safety.

emetic a substance which induces vomiting. Examples are common salt in water, and apomorphine.

Emotril apparatus an apparatus for administering trichloroethylene (Trilene) and air to patients in labour. It is no longer to be used by midwives in the UK.

empathy the recognition of and entering into another's feelings. adj. **empathic**.

Employment Protection Act, 1975 an act to protect employees' security. After childbirth, provided a woman has been employed for 2 years, she is entitled to 6 weeks' pay when her absence is due to pregnancy or childbirth. If she also works up to 29 weeks' gestation, she is entitled to reinstatement in her old job or similar, provided she informs her employer of her wish to return and if she returns to work within 29 weeks following delivery. If any employee is suspended on medical grounds, she (or he) must be offered suitable alternative employment or receive 26 weeks' full pay.

Employment Protection Act, 1980 entitles employees to minimum dismissal notice. It must be 1 week where an employee has

given at least 4 weeks' service, and 2 weeks after 2 years' service. An additional 1 week's notice must be given for each subsequent year, to a maximum of 12 weeks.

Employment rights for the expectant mother an employee who is expecting a baby has the following rights, subject to various conditions: 1. paid time off work to receive antenatal care. 2. the right to complain of unfair dismissal because of pregnancy. 3. the right to statutory maternity pay is granted in certain conditions under the Social Security Act, 1986. 4. the right to return to work with her employer after a period of absence due to pregnancy or confinement within 29 weeks of the week in which the child was born, providing the woman has been continuously employed for 2 years, generally with the same employer.

emulsion a mixture of minute particles of a fatty or oily substance suspended in fluid.

encephalitis inflammation of the brain. Viral encephalitis may be caused by such conditions as *Herpes simplex*; it may also be caused by bacterial infections such as tuberculosis or syphilis, by fungal infections such as histoplasmosis and protozoal infections such as toxoplasmosis.

encephalocele hernia of the brain through a congenital or traumatic opening of the skull.

encephalopathy a non-specific term meaning diffuse disease or damage of the brain. *Wernicke's* *e.* an inflammatory haemorrhagic encephalopathy due to thiamine deficiency. It may be a complication of hyperemesis gravidarum.

endemic pertaining to an infectious disease which, to a greater or lesser degree, is always present in the locality.

endo- a prefix meaning 'inside' or 'within'.

endocarditis inflammation of the endocardium or lining of the heart.

endocervicitis inflammation of the lining membrane of the cervix uteri, more commonly termed CERVICITIS.

endocervix the mucous membrane lining the cervical canal.

endocrine secreting within. Applied to those glands whose secretions (hormones) pass directly into the blood stream.

endoderm entoderm.

endogenous originating inside the body. In puerperal sepsis, inside the birth canal.

endometriosis tissue resembling endometrium, and functioning similarly, developing outside the uterus. Chocolate cyst of the ovary contains some endometrial material.

endometritis inflammation of the endometrium, or lining of the uterus.

endometrium the mucous membrane lining the body of the uterus.

endorphins one of a group of opiate-like peptides produced naturally by the body at neural synapses at various points in the central nervous system pathways where they modulate the transmission of pain perceptions. Endorphins raise the pain threshold and produce sedation and euphoria; the effects are blocked by naloxone, a narcotic antagonist.

endoscope an instrument, fitted with a light, used to inspect hollow organs and structures. CYSTOSCOPES and LAPAROSCOPES are examples.

endotoxic shock a rare condition associated with septicaemia caused by Gram-negative organisms, especially *Escherichia coli* and *Clostridium welchii* and, more recently, *beta-haemolytic streptococcus*. The endotoxins released from the bacteria are thought to cause widespread dilatation of arterioles in liver, lungs and other organs, so that diminished venous return causes profound shock.

endotracheal within the tracheal. *E. tube* an airway catheter inserted in the trachea during endotracheal intubation to assure patency of the upper airway and enable removal of secretions. Endotracheal intubation is carried out for resuscitation purposes, when it may be accompanied by cardiac massage, and also during general anaesthesia. In the latter case a 'cuffed' tube is used which protects the lungs because, when inflated, it prevents any regurgitated gastric fluid from passing the 'cuffed' area and entering the lungs.

enema an injection of fluid into the rectum. In midwifery, the following types are occasionally used: (a) simple enema, 0.5–1 litre (1–2 pt) of water, during the first stage of labour, before induction of labour or before operation, now often replaced by suppositories. (b) pre-packed enema (c) 120–180 ml of olive oil, to be retained for an hour, followed by a simple enema, to soften the faeces and secure an easy motion following repair of a third-degree PERINEAL LACERATION when conservatively treated.

energy (calorie) requirement every bodily process—the building up of cells, motion of the muscles, the maintenance of body temperature—requires energy, and the body derives this energy from the food it consumes. Digestive processes reduce food to usable 'fuel', which the body 'burns' in the complex chemical reactions that sustain life. The amount of energy required for these chemical processes vary. A woman during pregnancy requires about 2500 Cal (625 kJ) per day. Excess energy foods are stored as fat. This fat provides a supplementary source of energy if the diet is inadequate.

engagement the entry of the presenting part of the fetus, generally the head, into the true pelvis. A head is said to be engaged when its greatest presenting transverse diameter, the BIPARIETAL, has passed the plane of the pelvic brim. In a primigravida the fetal head usually becomes engaged after the 36th week of pregnancy; in a multigravida it is usually later and may not occur until after the onset of labour.

engorgement of the breasts painful accumulation of secretion in the breasts, often accompanied by lymphatic and venous stasis and oedema at the onset of lactation. If breast feeding, the milk may need to be expressed, either manually or by machine, until the AREOLA is softer and the baby may fix correctly onto it.

enkephalin either of two naturally occurring pentapeptides isolated from the brain, which have potent opiate-like effects and probably serve as neurotransmitters. They are classified as ENDORPHINS.

enteritis intestinal infection. See DYSENTERY.

entoderm those cells in the inner cell mass which line the yolk sac and which later develop into the epithelium of the alimentary tract, trachea, bronchi, bladder and urethra.

Entonox nitrous oxide and oxygen, 50 per cent of each, premixed in one cylinder and used as an analgesic. See Appendix 8.

environmental health the concept that the health of any individual can be affected by his or her environment. Levels of pollution and poor housing are two instances of factors which can affect health.

environmental health officer the person employed by the local authority to improve and regulate environment and to enforce statutory regulations. Responsibilities include housing, food hygiene and refuse collection, and also infestation, air pollutants and noise. Some authorities employ several officers, each specializing and responsible to a chief officer.

enzyme a biological catalyst, i.e. a substance present in small amounts that brings about a chemical reaction; e.g. milk sugar (lactose) is broken down by the enzyme lactase in the small intestine to form GLUCOSE and GALACTOSE.

eosin a red stain used in identifying cells and bacteria.

eosinophil a white blood cell in which the granules can be stained red with eosin.

Epanutin a proprietary preparation of phenytoin sodium, used for the control of epilepsy. *See* Appendix 19.

ephedrine an adrenergic alkaloid; used as a bronchodilator, antiallergic, central nervous system stimulant in narcolepsy, mydriatic and pressor agent.

epicanthus a vertical fold of skin on either side of the nose, sometimes covering the inner canthus (junction of eyelids). Prominent in certain races and in infants with Down's syndrome.

epidemic a situation in which any disease has attacked a large number of people at one time.

epidemiology the study of the distribution of factors determining health and disease in human populations, and the application of this study to the prevention and control of disease.

epidermis the non-vascular outer layer or cuticle of the skin.

epidermolysis bullosa this is a severe, usually fatal, skin disorder characterized by a profusion of fluid-filled blisters resembling PEMPHIGUS NEONATORUM. It is inherited as an autosomal RECESSIVE trait.

epididymis an elongated, cordlike structure along the posterior border of the testis, whose coiled duct provides for the storage, transport and maturation of spermatozoa.

epidural analgesia also known as extradural or peridural anaesthesia. A form of pain relief for both first and second stages of labour, obtained by the injection of a local analgesic, e.g. BUPIVACAINE, into the epidural space (see Figure) in order to block the spinal nerves. It may be approached by two routes: (a) caudal, through the sacrococcygeal membrane covering the sacral hiatus, or (b) lumbar, through the intervertebral space and ligamentum flavum. This is the more satisfactory route. *See* Appendix 8.

epigastrium the upper and middle region of the abdomen, located within the sternal angle. adj. *epigastric*. In patients with severe pre-eclampsia, pain in the epigastric region may herald the onset of eclampsia.

epiglottis the lid-like cartilaginous structure overhanging the entrance to the larynx.

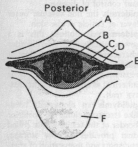

Posterior

A
B
C
D
E

Anterior

Highly diagrammatic cross-section of the spinal cord and vertebra to show the epidural space. A. Epidural space; B. spinal cord; C. cerebrospinal fluid; D. dura; E. spinal nerve; F. vertebral body.

EPIDURAL SPACE

epilepsy paroxysmal transient disturbances of nervous system function resulting from abnormal electrical activity of the brain. Anticonvulsive drugs are required to prevent convulsive seizures. These drugs may have a teratogenic effect on the fetus, most commonly affecting the lip, palate and heart. Maternal fits cause intrauterine hypoxia so must be controlled.

epiphysis the end of a long bone from which in childhood the shaft is separated by a piece of cartilage. The appearance of ossification in the fetal epiphyses may give a rough guide to its maturity. pl. *epiphyses*.

episiorrhapy repair of an EPISIOTOMY. *See* Appendix 10.

episiotomy an incision made into the thinned-out perineal body to enlarge the vaginal orifice during delivery. Prior to the incision the perineum should be infiltrated with local anaesthetic, usually lignocaine 0.5% 10 ml or 1% 5 ml. The incision may be mediolateral or median. There is evidence that the only justifiable indications for episiotomy are: 1. to expedite delivery in cases of fetal distress; 2. prior to an operative delivery such as forceps or ventouse extraction; 3. to minimize the risk of intracranial damage during preterm and breech delivery. The UKCC sanctions midwives to infiltrate the perineum, perform an episiotomy and repair perineal trauma, provided

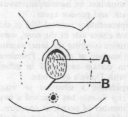

A
B

A. Fetal head; B. mediolateral incision.

EPISIOTOMY

they have been instructed and have attained competence in these procedures.

pispadias a condition in which there is an abnormal urethral opening on the dorsal surface of the penis.

pistaxis nose bleeding.

pithelium a layer of cells covering all outer and lining all inner surfaces, including cavities, glands and vessels.

psilon-aminocaproic acid an anti-fibrinolytic drug used to prevent the breakdown of FIBRIN by PLASMIN. It may be used in cases of severe abruptio placentae.

Epstein's pearls small white epithelial spots seen at the junction of the hard and soft palate.

Equal Opportunities Commission an *ad hoc* body set up in 1975 to help enforce the Sex Discrimination Act and the EQUAL PAY ACT, 1970.

Equal Pay Act, 1970 an Act which came into force in 1975 to eliminate discrimination between men and women with regard to their pay and conditions of employment.

Erb's paralysis paralysis of the upper arm due to injury, during birth, of the upper trunk of the brachial plexus nerves as they leave the spinal cord in the cervical region. A number of muscles are paralysed, so that the arm hangs medially rotated with the elbow extended and the wrist and fingers flexed. It results from traction on the child's neck, as in a breech delivery during the birth of the head or where there

has been SHOULDER PRESENTATION prior to vertex delivery.

erectile having the power of becoming erect. *E. tissue* vascular tissue which, under stimulus, becomes congested and swollen, causing erection of the part, e.g. the nipple of the female breast.

ergometrine an alkaloid which is the active principle of ergot. A valuable oxytocic drug which is effective in preventing or controlling postpartum haemorrhage. It is very commonly used in conjunction with oxytocin as Syntometrine. *See* Appendices 11 *and* 19.

ergot a drug obtained from a fungus which grows on rye. It causes strong sustained contraction of muscle, especially of the uterus.

erosion of the cervix during pregnancy hormonal changes cause softening and an increase in HYGROSCOPIC qualities of the collagen connective tissue. This results in the columnar epithelium near the external os being drawn out to form a red zone around it known as an erosion. Many cervical erosions disappear after delivery.

erythema redness of the skin.

erythroblast an immature, nucleated red blood cell.

erythroblastosis fetalis a condition in which ERYTHROBLASTS are found in the neonatal circulation. More commonly called haemolytic disease of the newborn (HDN). *See* Appendix 17.

erythrocyte a red blood cell. A minute biconcave disc containing haemoglobin which acts as a carrier of oxygen. *E. sedimentation rate* the rate at which red blood cells settle at the bottom of a tube of blood. The normal rate is no more than 10 mm/hour; this is increased in infection and normal pregnancy to an average of 78 mm/hour.

erythromycin an antibiotic with an action similar to that of penicillin.

erythropoiesis the formation of red blood cells.

Esbach's albuminometer a graduated glass tube for estimating the approximate amount of albumin in urine.

Escherichia coli A GRAM-NEGATIVE bacillus normally inhabiting the intestine. Pathogenic strains are the cause of many cases of urinary tract infections and of epidemic diarrhoeal diseases, especially in infants and children. If it enters the blood stream it may cause endotoxic shock.

essential hypertension persistently high blood pressure; cause unknown, but heredity a major predisposing factor.

estimated date of delivery *see* EDD.

ethambutol a tuberculostatic agent.

ether a clear, colourless liquid, extremely volatile and inflammable, used as an inhalation anaesthetic.

ethics rules or principles which govern correct conduct, and personal and social values. Each practitioner, upon entering a profession, is also invested with the responsibility to adhere to the standards of ethical practice and conduct set by that profession. The Code of Professional Conduct for the Nurse, Midwife and Health Visitor, adopted by the UKCC in 1984, provides guidance and advice for standards of practice and conduct that are essential for the ethical discharge of the practitioner's responsibility. Similarly, the Midwives Code of Practice, 1991, provides guidance specifically related to the role of the midwife.

ethnic pertaining to a social group who share cultural bonds or physical (racial) characteristics. *E. minority* a social grouping of people who share cultural or racial factors but who constitute a minority within the greater culture or society.

ethnomethodology a sociological theory which concentrates on the case study using participant or non-participant observation.

ethyl chloride a local anaesthetic applied topically to intact skin.

etiology *see* AETIOLOGY.

eugenics the study of measures which may be taken to improve future generations.

Eugynon 30, Eugynon 50 contraceptive tablets containing oestrogen and progesterone.

euphoria a feeling of well-being, not always justified by the circumstances.

eusol the commonly used name for chlorinated lime and boric acid solution.

eustachian tube the narrow tube which connects the tympanum (middle ear) with the naso-pharynx.

eutocia normal labour, or child-birth.

evacuation an emptying, e.g. of retained products of conception from the uterus.

evaluation a critical appraisal or assessment; a judgement of the value, worth, character or effectiveness of that which is being assessed. In midwifery care, the term is used to try to measure the effectiveness of midwifery care.

eversion a turning inside out; to turn outward.

evisceration a destructive operation, rarely necessary nowadays, involving removal of the organs of the abdomen and thorax of a dead fetus where a tumour or gross ascites has delayed vaginal delivery.

evolution natural development; the process of unfolding or opening out. *Spontaneous e.* a rare delivery without obstetrical aid of a fetus in the transverse lie by shoulder presentation. The shoulder escapes first, the thorax, pelvis and limbs next, and finally the head. cf. Spontaneous expulsion.

ex- prefix meaning 'out of', 'outside', 'away from'.

exacerbation increase in the gravity or seriousness of disease symptoms.

exchange transfusion a method of TRANSFUSION in which a sample of blood is withdrawn from the patient and replaced by the same volume of donor blood. It is used in the newborn to treat severe hyperbilirubinaemia and anaemia, usually resulting from Rhesus incompatibility. It is sometimes called a replacement transfusion. *See* Appendix 17.

excreta any waste matter excreted from the body. Used chiefly of faeces, but applies also to urine, sweat, sputum, etc.

exercises systematic movements to strengthen and to relax the muscles of the body. *Antenatal e.* include toning up the muscles and relaxation, in this way preparing the woman for labour contractions and for rest and relaxation, and so obtain the maximum benefit from the contraction and relaxation of the uterine muscles. *Postnatal e.* are carried out to tone up and strengthen the muscles of the body, particularly those of the abdominal wall and pelvic floor.

exfoliation a falling off in scales or layers. adj. *exfoliative. Lamellar e. of newborn* a congenital hereditary disorder in which the infant is born completely covered with a parchment-like membrane that peels off within 24 hours, after which there may be complete healing, or the scales may re-form and the process repeated. In the more severe form, the baby (harlequin fetus) is completely covered with thick, horny, armour-like scales, and is usually stillborn or dies shortly after birth. Called also ichthyosis congenita, ichthyosis fetalis, and lamellar ichthyosis of newborn.

existentialism an important 20th

century philosophical movement which has influenced psychology and psychiatry. The emphasis is on personal decisions to be made in a world without reason and without purpose. Since there are no objective standards and guides to personal behaviour, the individual may, and must, actively choose his own path. The constant difficult choices of existence are made against the background of the awareness of the inevitability of death. Existentialism emphasizes subjectivity, free will and individuality and has produced a form of psychotherapy that emphasizes 'authentic' experience.

exocrine 1. secreting externally via a duct. 2. denoting such a gland or its secretion.

exogenous of external origin.

exomphalos a herniation of the umbilicus of abdominal contents covered with peritoneum. A midwife must endeavour to avoid damage leading to sepsis by covering it with a sterile non-adhesive dressing and then a pad of cotton wool if medical aid is not immediately available.

exotoxin a potent toxin formed and excreted by the bacterial cell, and found free in the surrounding medium. Bacteria of the genus *Clostridium* are the most frequent producers of exotoxins; diphtheria, botulism, and tetanus are all caused by bacterial toxins.

expression pressing out. 1. pressure on the uterus to facilitate the expulsion of the placenta. *See* CREDÉ'S EXPRESSION. 2. mechan-

ical or digital pressure on the areola to compress the lacteal sinuses so that milk is removed from the breast.

expulsion forcible driving out, e.g. of the fetus from the uterus. *Spontaneous e.* the manner in which a very small macerated fetus can be forced through the pelvis with the shoulder presenting so that the head and trunk are born together.

exsanguinate to deprive of blood, as after a severe haemorrhage.

extension drawing out, lengthening. The opposite of flexion. Used to describe certain movements in the mechanism of labour, e.g. that by which the head is normally born. The occiput of the head escapes under the pubic arch, and, forced downwards by the uterine contractions and forwards by the pelvic floor muscles, the head extends, pivoting under the symphysis pubis.

external os the opening from the cervical canal into the vagina.

external version a manoeuvre designed to convert a breech presentation or a transverse lie to a vertex presentation. The manipulation is carried out through the abdominal wall. *See* VERSION.

extrauterine pregnancy embedding of the fertilized ovum outside the uterine cavity. Theoretically this could be in the abdominal cavity, ovary or fallopian tube. In fact, almost all cases of extrauterine pregnancy are of the tubal variety. *See* Appendix 6.

extravasation the discharge or leaking of fluid from its normal channel into surrounding tissue, e.g. the escape of blood or lymph from a vessel.

extrinsic of external origin. *e. factor* a haematopoietic vitamin that combines with intrinsic factor for absorption and is needed for erythrocyte maturation; called also VITAMIN B$_{12}$ and CYANOBALAMIN.

extubation removal of a tube used in intubation.

exudation the outward flow of a liquid or semi-liquid substance, e.g. of sebum from the sebaceous glands.

F

F abbreviation for FAHRENHEIT.

face in the fetus, that area extending from the mentum or chin to the supraorbital ridges.

face presentation a cephalic presentation in which the spine and head of the child are extended and the face lies lowest in the pelvis. In a mentoanterior position labour may be uncomplicated and delivery spontaneous, especially in a multigravida with a small baby. In a mentoposterior position there is little possibility of spontaneous delivery, unless the chin rotates anteriorly, but a considerable risk of persistent mentoposterior position and obstructed labour. The incidence is 1 in about 500–600 deliveries. *See* Appendix 9.

face-to-pubes persistent occipitoposterior position. An occipitoposterior position of the vertex in which the attitude of the head is military, neither flexed nor extended, and the sinciput, meeting the pelvic floor first, has rotated forwards bringing the

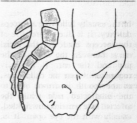

FACE PRESENTATION

occiput to the hollow of the sacrum. Note that face to pubes is a *position* of the vertex presentation, totally different from face PRESENTATION. *See* PERSISTENT OCCIPITOPOSTERIOR *and* Appendix 9.

facial paralysis paralysis of the muscles of the face, usually one side only, resulting from injury to the seventh cranial (facial) nerve. It is not uncommon in newborn infants, and is seen at

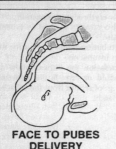

**FACE TO PUBES
DELIVERY**

birth, usually following a forceps delivery. It is due to pressure of the forceps blade on the facial nerve between the angle of the jaw and the ear. It is easily recognized when the child cries, as the mouth is drawn over to the unaffected side while the affected side remains unwrinkled, usually with the eye open. It is, as a rule, a transient condition which clears up within a few hours. It may persist for some days, when spoon feeding may be necessary temporarily.

factor an agent or element that contributes to the production of a result. *Anti-haemophilic f. (AHF)* factor VIII, one of the CLOTTING factors. *Anti-haemorrhagic f.* vitamin K. *Clotting f's, coagulation f's* factors essential to normal blood clotting, whose absence, diminution or excess may lead to abnormality of the clotting mechanism; at least 12 factors have been described. *Extrinsic f.*

see EXTRINSIC. *Intrinsic f.* glycoprotein secreted by the parietal cells of the gastric glands, necessary for the absorption of VITAMIN B_{12}. Its absence results in pernicious anaemia. *Releasing f's* factors elaborated in one structure that effect the release of hormones from another structure. *Rhesus f.* genetically determined antigens present on the surface of erythrocytes. *See* RHESUS.

faeces food residue and other waste products excreted from the bowels.

Fahrenheit a scale of temperature measurement. It registers the freezing point of water at 32°, the normal temperature of the human body at 98.4°, and the boiling point of water at 212°. For comparison with Celsius, *see* Appendix 20.

faint temporary loss of consciousness due to generalized cerebral ischaemia; syncope.

falciform sickle-shaped.

fallopian tubes the uterine tubes or oviducts. Two narrow canals, each 10 cm (4 in) long, leading from the uterine cornua to the ovaries. The tube has four parts: 1. the interstitial part, within the wall of the uterus; 2. the isthmus, a narrow region; 3. the ampulla, where the tube widens; 4. the infundibulum, or fimbriated end, the open extremity. The largest fimbria, the ovarian fimbria, is attached to the ovary and may help to guide the discharged ovum into the tube after ovulation. The tube has an outer incomplete covering of peritoneum, the upper part of the broad ligament; a thin muscle coat consisting of outer longitudinal and inner circular fibres; and a mucous membrane lining which is thrown into deep folds. The epithelium is of the ciliated columnar type, the ciliary current directing the ovum towards the uterus.

Fallot's tetralogy a combination of congenital cardiac defects, namely, pulmonary stenosis, ventricular septal defects, dextroposition of the aorta, so that it overrides the interventricular septum and receives venous as well as arterial blood, and right ventricular hypertrophy.

false labour uterine contractions giving rise to discomfort and simulating labour, but not causing dilatation of the cervix. They are thought to be due to increasing muscle contractility but without the normal FUNDAL DOMINANCE of the uterus.

false pelvis the region between the brim of the true pelvis and the crests of the ilia.

falx a sickle, or a sickle-shaped structure.

falx cerebri the sickle-shaped fold of dura mater which separates the two cerebral hemispheres.

familial occurring in families. The term is applied to such inherited conditions as haemophilia and acholuric jaundice.

family a group of people related by blood or marriage, especially a husband, wife and their children. *Extended f.* a nuclear family and their close relatives such as the children's grandparents, aunts and uncles. *Nuclear f.* a married couple and their children by birth or adoption who are living together and are more or less isolated from their extended family. *Single-parent f.* a lone parent and offspring living together as a family unit. *F. credit* a financial benefit for families whose income falls below a specified level. To be eligible to claim, the parent(s) have to be in full-time work (24 hours per week) and have at least one dependent child. There is an adult credit for each family plus an age-related credit for each child. This is paid on a sliding scale according to income.

family planning the arrangement, spacing and limitation of the children in a family, depending upon the wishes and social circumstances of the parents. *See* Appendix 12.

Family Health Services Authority This replaced the Family Practitioners Committee when the National Health Service and Community Care Act came into force in April 1991. It arranges general practitioner contracts and is the authority to whom patients apply for inclusion on a doctor's list. Dental practitioners, ophthalmic medical practitioners, opticians and pharmacists also contract their services to the authority.

fascia a sheet or band of fibrous connective tissue. The fibres may be arranged loosely as around organs and blood vessels, or in dense strong sheets often between muscles forming their attachments. *Pelvic f.* the fascia of the pelvic cavity is in two layers: a parietal layer, lining the walls and covering the pelvic floor; and a visceral layer, surrounding and supporting the pelvic organs, the part around the uterus being termed the parametrium.

fat 1. adipose or fatty tissue of the body. 2. neutral fat; a triglyceride (or triacyl-glycerol) which is a compound of fatty acids and glycerol.

favism an acute haemolytic anaemia caused by ingestion of fava beans. *See* GLUCOSE-6-PHOSPHATE DEHYDROGENASE.

febrile feverish; pyrexial.

fecundation fertilization.

fecundity the ability to produce offspring.

femoral pertaining to the femur. *F. artery* the principal artery of the thigh, a continuation of the external iliac artery. *F. vein* the main vein of the thigh, a continuation of the popliteal vein. It passes up the leg through the groin, whence it continues as the external iliac vein.

femur the thigh bone, which extends from the hip to the knee, articulating with the innominate bone at the acetabulum.

fenestrated possessing a window-like opening or *fenestra*. The blade of the midwifery forceps is fenestrated. *F. placenta* or *placenta fenestrata. See* PLACENTA.

Fentazin trademark for preparations of perphenazine, a tranquillizer and anti-emetic.

ferment an enzyme, having a specific action.

Fern test cervical cytology undertaken to determine the amount of oestrogen in cervical mucus. When oestrogen is adequate the dried cervical mucus has a fernlike appearance on low power microscopy.

ferritin the iron–apoferritin complex; one of the forms in which iron is stored in the body.

ferrous containing iron in its plus-two oxidation state. *F. fumarate* the anhydrous salt of a combination of ferrous iron and fumaric acid; used as a haematinic. *F. gluconate* a haematinic that is less irritating to the gastrointestinal tract than other haematinics, and generally used as a substitute when ferrous sulphate cannot be tolerated. *F. sulphate* the most widely used haematinic for the treatment of iron deficiency anaemia. It is believed to be less irritating than equivalent amounts of ferric salts and is more effective.

fertile capable of producing offspring. *F. period* 1. the 9 days surrounding ovulation when fertilization of the ovum is theoretically possible. It is usually taken to be the 5 days before, the day of, and the 3 days following ovulation, which is assessed over a period of months by recording the basal temperature. 2. that period of a woman's life during which she has potential for childbearing. Usually taken to be between the ages of 15 and 45.

fertility the ability to produce

young. *See also* SUBFERTILITY *and* INFERTILITY.

ertilization impregnation. The union of the spermatozoon and the ovum. By this event, also called conception, a new life is created and the sex and other biological traits of the new individual are determined. These traits are determined by the combined genes and chromosomes that exist. In vitro *f.* artificial fertilization of the ovum in laboratory conditions. In vivo *f.* that which takes place by artificial means in the living situation, i.e. within the mother's reproductive tract.

etal pertaining to the fetus. *F. abnormalities see* MALFORMATION. *F. alcohol syndrome* a syndrome, described in the USA, resulting from heavy consumption of alcohol in pregnancy (the relevant amount is as yet unknown). Clinical signs seen are abnormalities of facial features, some degree of mental retardation, and these babies are often small for dates. *F. blood sampling* a technique for obtaining a minute quantity of fetal scalp blood to estimate its PH and sometimes the blood gases, to exclude fetal hypoxia, which is indicated by acidosis. *See* Appendix 16. *F. death see* INTRAUTERINE DEATH. *F. distress* fetal hypoxia. *See* Appendix 16. *F. haemoglobin* haemoglobin F. It differs from adult haemoglobin in having a greater affinity for and higher capacity for oxygen. It forms 85 per cent of the haemoglobin of a baby born at full term. *F. heart*

sounds, the heart beat of the fetus, auscultated and counted through the abdominal wall, uterus and liquor amnii. It may be continuously recorded by a fetal heart monitor. *F. maturity* the most satisfactory method of estimating this is by ultrasound CEPHALOMETRY.

fetal skull the bony structure of the head of the fetus. It is divided into three parts. 1. the *vault*, which contains the brain, is composed of 5 bones: 2 frontal, 2 parietal and 1 occipital. These are united by membranes known as sutures and fontanelles, the names of which can be seen in the Figure. The sutures and fontanelles may be felt on vaginal examination during labour, and indicate the position of the occiput and the degree of flexion of the head. 2. the *base of the skull* is composed of 5 bones: 2 temporal, 1 ethmoid, 1 sphenoid and part of the occipital bone. These are firmly fused together. At the base of the skull is an opening known as the foramen magnum, through which passes the spinal cord. Two projections of the occipital bone, the condyles of the occiput, lie alongside this opening. 3. The *face* is composed of 14 bones, all fused together. *Diameters of the f's* 1. *Longitudinal* diameters are taken through the long axis of the skull. They are the diameters which engage in the various vertex presentations, face presentations and the aftercoming head in breech labour. 2. *transverse* diameters are taken

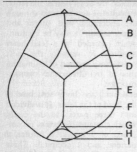

A. Frontal suture; B. frontal bone; C. coronal suture; D. anterior fontanelle or bregma; E. parietal bone; F. sagittal suture; G. posterior fontanelle; H. lambdoid suture; I. occipital bone.

VAULT OF THE FETAL SKULL

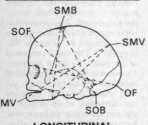

LONGITUDINAL DIAMETERS

through the skull in a transverse direction, the most important being the BIPARIETAL which is about 9.5 cm (3.71 in), taken between the parietal eminences. When this diameter has passed through the pelvic brim the head is said to be engaged. *See also* CEPHALOMETRY. *In utero*, the average measurement at full term is 9.8 cm. *Circumferences* of the fetal skull are measurements taken round the skull at various points. The principal diameters and the presentations in which they engage are given below. The points between which the measurements are taken are shown in the diagrams. Within the skull are the BRAIN and the intracranial membranes: *(a)* the *falx cerebri*, a crescent-shaped fold of dura mater attached to the bone above and running down between the cerebral hemispheres; *(b)* the *tentorium cerebelli*, an almost horizontal fold of dura mater separating the cerebral hemispheres above from the cerebellum below and attached to the posterior part of the falx. These membranes carry the venous sinuses by which blood is drained from the head, namely the superior and inferior longitudinal sinuses between the layers of the falx, the straight sinus at the junction of falx and tentorium, and the transverse sinuses in the tentorium. The vein of Galen or great cerebral vein passes from the midbrain and enters the junction of the inferior longitudinal sinus and straight sinus. In any

Conventional fetal skull measurements

Measurement	Diameter cm	in	Circumference cm	in	Presentation
Longitudinal					
Suboccipitobregmatic (SOB)	9.5	3.75	33.0	13.00	Vertex, head fully flexed
Suboccipitofrontal (SOF)	10.5	4.00	35.0	14.00	Vertex, head almost fully flexed
Occipitofrontal (OF)	11.5	4.50	37.5	15.00	Vertex, deficient flexion
Mentovertical (MV)	13.5	5.25			Brow
Submentobregmatic (SMB)	9.5	3.75			Face, fully extended
Transverse					
Biparietal	9.5	3.75			
Bitemporal	8.0	3.25			
Bimastoid	7.0	3.00			
Bisacromial	10.0	4.00			Measured across shoulders
Bisiliac	10.0	4.00			Breech, between iliac crests
Bitrochanteric	10.0	4.00			Breech, between greater trochanters

form of extreme, rapid or abnormal moulding these membranes with their contained blood vessels may be torn, causing intracranial haemorrhage.

fetoscopy the inspection of a fetus through the uterine wall by means of a fetoscope. *See* Appendix 4.

fetus the unborn offspring of a mammal. The human embryo from the 8th week of pregnancy to the time of birth. *F. papyraceous* one of twins which, dying *in utero* at an early stage of pregnancy, becomes flattened against the uterine wall. It is usually expelled with the placenta and resembles a piece of parchment.

fever pyrexia. A high body temperature. An illness characterized by pyrexia.

fibre a thread-like structure. A muscle cell. *Dietary f.* that portion of ingested foodstuffs that cannot be broken down by intestinal enzymes and juices and, therefore, passes through the small intestine and colon undigested. Vegetables, cereals and fruits are the main sources of dietary fibre. Helps to prevent constipation.

fibrin an insoluble protein formed by the action of thrombin upon fibrinogen. Necessary in the process of blood clotting, where it forms a network of minute long strands in which blood cells get caught.

fibrinogen a protein formed in the liver and circulating in the blood plasma. In tissue injury it is activated by THROMBIN, to form FIBRIN and thus to arrest haemorrhage by clotting. Preparations containing human fibrinogen used to restore blood fibrinogen levels after extensive surgery, or to treat diseases or haemorrhagic conditions that are complicated by AFIBRINOGENAEMIA include fresh frozen plasma and cryoprecipitate. Pure fibrinogen is rarely used because of the risk of transmitting hepatitis.

fibrinolysin 1. PLASMIN. 2. A preparation of proteolytic enzyme formed from profibrinolysin (plasminogen) by action of physical agents or by specific bacterial kinases; used to promote dissolution of thrombi.

fibrinolysis the dissolution of

fibrin by enzymatic action. adj. *fibrinolytic.*

fibrocystic disease see CYSTIC FIBROSIS.

fibroid 1. composed of fibrous tissue. 2. a benign tumour. Uterine fibroids may be submucous, interstitial or subserous. Occasionally a cervical fibroid occurs. In midwifery they are most commonly seen in primigravid women over 30 years of age. In pregnancy they rarely create trouble, but may occasionally be the cause of abortion or undergo red degeneration. In labour, fibroids, unless of the cervix, are usually drawn out of the pelvis as the cervix dilates, and do not cause obstruction. Fibroids in the region of the placental site could interfere with the contraction of the uterus and cause postpartum haemorrhage. In the puerperium and subsequently fibroids may decrease in size so much that operative removal is unlikely to be necessary.

fibromyoma a fibroid.

fibroplasia the formation of fibrous tissue, as in the healing of a wound. *Retrolental f.* a condition characterized by retinal vascular proliferation and tortuosity and by the presence of fibrous tissue behind the lens, leading to detachment of the retina and arrest of growth of the eye, generally attributed to use of excessively high concentrations of oxygen in the care of preterm infants.

fibrosis formation of fibrous tissue; fibroid degeneration. adj.

fibrotic. Cystic f. a generalized hereditary disorder with widespread dysfunction of exocrine glands, chronic pulmonary disease, pancreatic deficiency, high levels of electrolytes in sweat, and sometimes biliary cirrhosis. *See also* CYSTIC FIBROSIS.

ibula the lateral and smaller of the two bones of the leg.

ilter a porous substance which permits fluids and materials in solution to pass through, but which holds back solids in solution, e.g. Millipore. A filter of cellulose acetate which removes bacteria and therefore sterilizes a solution, as in EPIDURAL ANALGESIA.

iltrate fluid which has passed through a filter.

imbria a fringe. The fringe-like extremity of the fallopian tube is described as fimbriated.

irst degree perineal lacerations *see* PERINEAL LACERATIONS.

irst stage of labour the period from the onset of labour until complete or full dilatation of the cervix. *See* Appendix 7.

ission cleavage or splitting. Reproduction by division of a cell into two equal parts. *Nuclear f.* the splitting of the nucleus of an atom.

issure a cleft. This may be normal, e.g. cerebral fissure, or due to disease, e.g. anal fissure.

istula an abnormal passage between two cavities or between a cavity and the surface of the body. *Rectovaginal f.* an opening between the vagina and the rectum, usually resulting from sev-

ere and/or neglected laceration of the perineal body. *Vesicovaginal f.* an opening between the bladder and the vagina, which might result from prolonged pressure in neglected obstructed labour.

fit a seizure. Convulsion, as in eclampsia or epilepsy. *See* Appendix 6.

flaccid limp; without tone. The condition of the muscles in a baby suffering from severe asphyxia.

flagellum the whip-like protoplasmic filament by which some bacteria move. *Trichomonas vaginalis*, a protozoon, is also flagellated. pl. *flagella.*

Flagyl *see* METRONIDAZOLE.

flank the side of the abdomen, between the ribs and the iliac crest.

flat pelvis a pelvis in which the anteroposterior diameter of the brim is much shorter than the transverse diameter. There are two described: the platypelloid and the rachitic. *See* PELVIS.

flatulence the presence of gas or air in the stomach or intestine; sometimes causing severe pain, but as a rule merely discomfort.

flatus gas in the bowel.

fleshy mole CARNEOUS MOLE, a mass of clotted blood surrounding a dead embryo and retained in the uterus.

flexion bending. A movement of a limb or organ out of alignment. *See* ANTEFLEXION *and* RETROFLEXION. Flexion is the normal attitude of the fetus *in utero*.

'flooding' severe bleeding from the uterus. A lay term used to describe menorrhagia, metrorrhagia and severe bleeding in miscarriage.

flora *Intestinal f.* the bacteria normally residing within the lumen of the intestine.

fluid a liquid or gas; any liquid of the body. *Amniotic f.* the fluid within the amnion which bathes the developing fetus and protects it from mechanical injury. *Body f's* the fluids within the body, composed of water, electrolytes and non-electrolytes which are continuously in motion. Fluid within the cell membranes is called intracellular fluid and comprises about two thirds of the total body fluids. The remaining one third is outside the cell and is called extracellular fluid. The extracellular fluid can be further divided into tissue fluid (interstitial fluid) which is found in the spaces between the blood vessels and surrounding cells, and intravascular fluid, which is the fluid component of blood. Intracellular fluid serves as a medium for the basic materials needed by cells for growth, repair and performance of their various functions. Extracellular fluid circulates in the spaces outside the cells and brings to them their nutrients and other substances needed for cell function. A proper balance between intracellular and extracellular fluid volumes is essential to health. In patients with renal failure and heart failure the balance becomes upset, producing either localized or generalized oedema. *Cerebrospinal f.* fluid contained within the ven-

tricles of the brain, the subarachnoid space, and the central canal of the spinal cord. *F. balance* a state in which the volume of body water and its solutes (electrolytes and nonelectrolytes) is within normal limits and there is normal distribution of fluids within the intracellular and extracellular compartments. The total volume of body fluids should be 60 per cent of the body weight. A fluid balance record is kept on each patient who is susceptible or already suffering from a disturbance in the balance of body fluids, e.g. severe pre-eclampsia. All intake and output is accurately recorded on a fluid balance chart.

fluorescent treponemal antibody test a serological test for syphilis; the first to become positive after infection.

'flying squad' an emergency obstetric unit, maintained by a hospital which gives immediate assistance to a woman at home who requires hospital treatment but who, for any special reason, cannot be moved from her home. The services of the unit are obtained very quickly by telephoning the organizing hospital. The commonest reason for a 'flying squad' call is severe postpartum haemorrhage. When the emergency has been dealt with the patient is usually transferred to hospital for further observation. Some hospitals have set up 'flying squads' to transfer an immature or sick baby to a special care unit.

folate a general term used to

describe a large group of compounds, i.e. the folates which are derived from the parent compound, FOLIC ACID. Folates are necessary for a variety of biochemical reactions in the body, the most important of which is required for DNA synthesis. Folate levels in the serum and red blood cells are measurable and are used to assess the body stores; low levels of both are found in megaloblastic anaemia secondary to folate deficiency.

folic acid a constituent of the vitamin B complex, necessary for the development of normal red blood cells. Deficiency in pregnancy causes megaloblastic anaemia as the rapidly dividing fetal cells compete for folic acid to form cell nuclei. Green vegetables, liver and yeast are major sources of folic acid in the diet. It is also produced synthetically. Folic acid deficiency may result from the inability of the body to utilize the vitamin.

follicle a very small sac or gland. *Graafian f.* small vesicles formed in the ovary, each containing an ovum. One follicle matures during each menstrual cycle, which is controlled by pituitary hormones. *See* GONADOTROPHIC.

follicle-stimulating hormone (FSH) a hormone released from the anterior pituitary gland, stimulating one or more GRAAFIAN FOLLICLES to mature, during each menstrual cycle.

fontanelle a membranous space where two or more sutures meet between the cranial bones of the fetus or newborn child. *See* FETAL SKULL.

footling presentation a type of breech presentation in which one or both feet lie in advance of the buttocks. *See* Appendix 9.

foramen an opening or hole, especially in a bone. *F. magnum* the opening in the occipital bone through which the medulla oblongata becomes continuous with the spinal cord. *Obturator f.* the large hole in the os innominatum. *F. ovale* the opening between the two atria of the fetal heart.

forceps surgical instruments with two blades used for lifting or compressing an object: e.g. *dressing f., dissecting f. Artery f.* compress bleeding points during an operation. *Midwifery f.* are used in the second stage of labour to extract the child's head, in cases where this mode of delivery is safer for the mother or child. *Vulsellum f.* have claw-like ends. *See* Appendix 10.

foreskin the prepuce. The skin covering the glans penis.

forewaters the liquor amnii contained in the membranes lying below the presenting part of the fetus.

formaldehyde a powerful disinfectant gas whose solution is formalin.

formalin *see* FORMALDEHYDE.

formula a prescription or recipe, especially for an infant's feed. A group of symbols making a certain statement.

fornix an arch. The vaginal fornices are the recesses at the vault of the vagina in front of (*anterior f.*), behind (*posterior f.*) and at the sides (*lateral f.*) of the cervix. pl. *fornices*.

fossa a pit or hollow, e.g. the iliac fossa, which is a depression on the inner surface of the iliac bone.

foster children children under the care of FOSTER PARENTS.

foster parents persons who undertake for reward the care of children who are not related to them within the meaning of the Children Act. *See* Appendix 5.

Fothergill's operation the Manchester operation for uterovaginal prolapse.

Foundation for the Study of Infant Deaths (SID) a registered charity, founded in 1971, giving support to parents whose child's demise apparently has been a 'cot death'. It also sponsors research into this mysterious syndrome.

fourchette a fold of skin between the posterior extremities of the labia minora.

fracture a break, usually of bone; a possible, though uncommon birth injury. Occasionally in a breech delivery the clavicle, humerus or femur may be fractured, and sometimes after any difficult delivery a depressed fracture of the skull can be found. This normally heals well.

fraenum, frenum, frenulum a small ligament that checks the movement of an organ, e.g. the *f. linguae*, the membranous connection between the floor of the mouth and the lower surface of the tongue. *See* TONGUE TIE.

fragilitas ossium OSTEOGENESIS IMPERFECTA. Fragile brittle bones.

Frankenhauser's plexus a ganglion near the uterine cervix from which sympathetic and parasympathetic nerves supply the vagina, uterus and other pelvic viscera.

friable easily torn, broken or crumbled. The chorion attached to the placenta is friable, and is often torn, portions being retained in the uterus.

Friars' balsam compound tincture of benzoin. This acts as a decongestant when inhaled as a vapour.

Friedman test one of the biological pregnancy tests. The urine of a pregnant woman contains an excess of GONADOTROPHIC HORMONE. If the urine is injected intravenously into female rabbits, on post mortem examination 48 hours later the ovaries will show evidence of ruptured follicles. This test is about 98 per cent accurate, but has largely been superseded by immunological tests.

Fortral trademark for preparations of pentazocine; an analgesic.

frigidity coldness; especially sexual unresponsiveness of the female to physical stimulation, due to psychological causes.

frontal pertaining to the forehead. In the fetus the two frontal bones form the forehead. The frontal suture is the membranous channel between these two bones.

frusemide a diuretic that acts by blocking reabsorption of sodium and chloride in the ascending loop of Henle; used for treatment of oedema and acute renal failure.

FSH see FOLLICLE-STIMULATING HORMONE.

fulminating bursting forth, violently explosive. The term is applied to conditions and diseases that appear with great suddenness and severity. In obstetrics, such conditions include severe pre-eclampsia and eclampsia, when they arise very suddenly.

fundal pertaining to the fundus, usually in obstetrics of the uterus. *F. dominance* normal uterine action is such that the contractions originate from a pacemaker in the fundus, the wave of contraction gradually weakening as it passes over the upper and lower segments of the uterus. *F. pressure* a rarely used method of using the contracted FUNDUS UTERI, following descent of the placenta and membranes into the vagina, as a piston to expel the placenta and complete the third stage of labour.

fundus the base of an organ, or the part farthest removed from the opening. *F. uteri* the top of the uterus—the part farthest from the cervix.

fungus a general term for a group of eukaryotic organisms (mushrooms, yeasts, moulds, etc.). Thrush is a fungal condition.

funic pertaining to the funis, i.e. the umbilical cord. *F. souffle* a soft whispering sound synchronizing with the fetal heart sounds and coming from the umbilical cord.

funis the umbilical cord.

funnel pelvis a pelvis the shape of a funnel, i.e. narrowing from above downwards. This is a characteristic of the ANDROID (or male type of) PELVIS, in which the outlet is considerably smaller than the brim.

Furadantin trademark for preparations of nitrofurantoin, an anti-bacterial agent used in urinary tract infections.

G

g gram (formerly gramme); gravity; the unit of force exerted upon a body during acceleration and deceleration.

G6PD see GLUCOSE-6-PHOSPHATE DEHYDROGENASE.

gag 1. an instrument for holding open the jaws. 2. to retch, or strive to vomit. *G. reflex* elevation of the soft palate and retching elicited by touching the back of the tongue or the wall of the pharynx; called also pharyngeal reflex.

Gairdner headbox a perspex box which is placed over the baby's head into which additional oxygen is provided in order to increase the oxygen concentration of inspired air.

gait walk or carriage. This should be observed in the pregnant woman. It may give rise to the suspicion of a pelvic deformity.

galact-, galacto- word element meaning 'milk'.

galactischia suppression of milk secretion.

galactogogue an agent which is said to increase the secretion of milk.

galactorrhoea an excessive flow of breast milk.

galactosaemia a genetically determined biochemical disorder in which there is a lack of an enzyme necessary for proper metabolism of galactose. Normally the sugar derived from lactose in milk is changed by enzymatic action into glucose. When the conversion of galactose to glucose does not take place, the galactose accumulates in the tissues and blood. At birth the baby appears normal although cataracts may be present. Once milk feeds are given the baby fails to thrive and has an enlarged liver and persistent jaundice. Mental retardation and, in severe cases, death will ensue unless the condition is treated. The condition is diagnosed by finding a high concentration of galactose in blood and urine, which can be found by testing the latter for reducing substances. Treatment consists of exclusion from the diet of milk and all foods containing galactose or lactose. If the disease is detected early, before there is damage to the central nervous system, the symptoms of the disorder can be prevented. The diet has to be continued throughout life.

galactose a MONOSACCHARIDE resulting from the digestion of LACTOSE. The liver converts it to glucose.

galactose-1-phosphate uridyl transferase an enzyme which converts galactose to glucose. Deficiency of the enzyme results in classic galactosaemia.

galea aponeurotica the tendon of the occipitofrontalis muscle, which forms a layer of the scalp.

Galen, vein of the great cerebral vein. A large vein, draining blood from the mid-brain. *See* FETAL SKULL.

gallbladder a sac situated on the under part of the liver, holding and concentrating the bile secreted by that organ.

gamete a male or female reproductive cell.

gamgee tissue absorbent wool covered with gauze and used for dressing wounds, etc.

gamma globulin γ globulin, a class of plasma proteins composed almost entirely of IgG, an IMMUNOGLOBULIN protein that contains most antibody activity. Commercial preparations of gamma globulin are derived from blood serum and are used for prevention, modification, and treatment of various infectious diseases. This type of gamma globulin contains almost all the known antibodies circulating in the blood. It can provide passive immunity, usually for about 6 weeks against infections to which most of the population has antibodies. Certain specific types of gamma globulin may be used to raise the body's resistance to measles, mumps and poliomyelitis. Gamma globulin containing a high concentration of anti-Rhesus antibody can be given to a Rhesus-negative mother within 72 hours of delivery to prevent her forming her own antibody.

ganglion a nerve centre from which nerve fibres proceed.

gangrene death of tissue, usually applied to a large area or definite organ. *Dry g.* is due to failure of arterial blood supply, e.g. the process by which the umbilical cord dries and separates from the umbilicus about 5–7 days after birth. *Moist g.* is caused by putrefactive changes, e.g. infection of the umbilical cord, when it remains moist, becomes offensive and separation is delayed. *See also* GAS GANGRENE.

Gardnerella a genus of Gram-negative rod-shaped bacteria having one species, *G. vaginalis* (formerly called *Haemophilus vaginalis*). It is found in the normal female genital tract and is the causative organism for non-specific vaginitis. *Gardnerella* infection is one of the most common and most infectious of the sexually transmitted diseases. The major symptom is increased vaginal discharge that is thin and grey and has a fishy odour, especially after sexual intercourse. Treatment is with metronidazole for both the woman and her sexual partner.

gargoylism a type of MUCOPOLY-SACCHARIDOSIS.

gas matter in its least dense form,

neither solid nor liquid, where the molecules are in constant movement. A vapour. Air is a mixture of several gases: oxygen, nitrogen, traces of carbon dioxide, argon and helium.

gas gangrene infection of damaged tissues by the anaerobic organism *Clostridium welchii*. The uterus may be thus infected following criminal abortion, and, very rarely, following labour.

'gas and oxygen' analgesia this consists of 50 per cent oxygen and 50 per cent nitrous oxide premixed in the Entonox apparatus which is approved for use to relieve pain in labour, by the UKCC. *See also* Appendix 8.

gastric pertaining to the stomach.

gastritis inflammation of the lining of the stomach.

gastro- a prefix meaning 'relating to the stomach'.

gastroenteritis inflammation of the lining of stomach and intestine. An acute condition of diarrhoea and vomiting particularly dangerous in infants, producing rapid and severe dehydration. Any infant in whom this condition is suspected should be immediately isolated from other babies. The treatment is to administer fluids orally or intravenously, to combat the dehydration, correct the electrolyte balance and treat the infection.

gastrojejunostomy surgical anastomosis of the stomach to the jejunum. It may be performed to bypass the obstruction in cases of duodenal atresia in the newborn.

gastroschisis a congenital fissure of the abdominal wall.

gastrostomy the creation of an opening into the stomach. The procedure is done to provide for the administration of food and liquids when stricture of the oesophagus or other conditions making swallowing impossible.

gate control theory of pain this theory proposes that a neural mechanism in the dorsal horns of the spinal cord acts like a gate which can increase or decrease the flow of nerve impulses from peripheral fibres to the central nervous system. It is the position of the gate which determines how much information is transmitted to the brain and therefore on the amount of pain generated. Influences such as anxiety and anticipation cause the gate to open and therefore increase the level of pain experienced, whereas other factors may cause the gate to close, thereby reducing the pain.

gauze a large-mesh, thin cotton material, used for dressings.

Geiger counter an instrument used to detect radioactive substances.

gemellology the scientific study of twins and twinning.

gender sex; the category to which an individual is assigned on the basis of sex.

gene a single unit of the hereditary factors located in a definite position on a CHROMOSOME. Genes are composed of DEOXYRIBONU-CLEIC ACID (DNA), consisting of a complex double chain of mol-ecules which carry the genetic code of an individual, so governing each characteristic. Through the genetic code of DNA they also control the day-to-day functions and reproduction of all cells in the body. For example, the genes control the synthesis of structural proteins and also the enzymes that regulate various chemical reactions that take place in a cell. The gene is capable of replication. When a cell multiplies by mitosis each daughter cell carries a set of genes that is an exact replica of that of the parent cell. This characteristic of replication explains how genes can carry hereditary traits through successive generations without change. Rarely there may be an abnormal or mutant gene. An example of a condition resulting from two abnormal RECESSIVE genes is PHENYLKETONURIA.

general practitioner obstetrician (GPO) a general practitioner qualified or having experience in obstetrics, who has agreed to provide maternity services on application. This is indicated by the prefix 'M' before the appropriate entry in the Family Practitioner List.

generic 1. pertaining to a genus. 2. non-proprietary; denoting a drug name not protected by a trademark, usually descriptive of the drug's chemical structure.

genetic counselling this is carried out in certain clinics, where the geneticist explains the chances of recurrence of hereditary diseases, and can advise a couple whether there is a risk to future children.

genetics the study of heredity.

genital relating to the organs of reproduction.

genitalia the organs of reproduction.

genitourinary pertaining to the genital and urinary organs.

genotype classification of the genetic makeup of an individual. *See* GENE.

gentamicin an antibiotic complex, effective against many Gram-negative bacteria, especially *Pseudomonas* species, as well as certain Gram-positive bacteria, especially *Staphylococcus aureus*.

gentian violet an anti-bacterial, anti-fungal, and anti-helmintic dye, applied topically in the treatment of infections of the skin and mucous membranes associated with Gram-positive bacteria and moulds and administered orally in pin worm and liver fluke infections.

genu the knee.

genupectoral position knee–chest position, i.e. face downwards and resting on the knees and the chest. *See* POSITION.

genus a classificatory group of animals or plants comprising one or more species.

germ a lay term for a micro-organism. Living substance capable of developing into an organ or a whole organism.

German measles *see* RUBELLA.

germicide an agent capable of destroying micro-organisms.

gestagen any hormone with pro-gestational activity.

gestalt a whole perceptual configuration. *G. therapy* a psychotherapeutic approach which encourages the individual to cease intellectualizing his or her difficulties and instead to focus on feelings and emotions, and thereby to gain emotional insight and balance.

gestation pregnancy. *G. period* in the human species approximately 40 weeks from the first day of the last normal menstrual period or 38 weeks from the date of conception. *Ectopic g.* pregnancy outside the uterus. *See* Appendix 6. *G. sac* the placenta and membranes containing the liquor amnii and the fetus during pregnancy.

gigantism abnormal overgrowth of the whole or part of the body, due to overactivity of the anterior pituitary growth hormone.

Gigli's operation pubiotomy.

Gigli's saw a fine wire instrument for sawing through bone.

Gingerbread a voluntary organization which aims to help one-parent families.

gingivitis inflammation and bleeding of the gums.

girdle a belt. *Pelvic g.* the bony ring of the pelvis formed by the two innominate bones and the sacrum.

glabella the area on the frontal bone above the nose and between eyebrows.

gland a collection of cells specialized to secrete or excrete materials not related to their own metabolic needs. Endocrine glands secrete hormones into the blood stream, e.g. the thyroid gland secretes thyroxine. Exocrine glands discharge their secretion through one or more ducts, e.g. breast or liver.

glans an acorn-shaped body, such as the rounded end of the penis and the clitoris.

globin the protein constituent of haemoglobin; also, any member of a group of proteins similar to the typical globin.

globulin a subdivision of plasma proteins. Globulin is further subdivided into alpha (α), beta (β) and gamma (γ) globulins. *See also* GAMMA GLOBULIN *and* IMMUNO-GLOBULIN.

glomerulus the tuft of capillaries which is invaginated in the kidney tubule at its commencement in the renal cortex.

glossal pertaining to the tongue.

glottis the vocal apparatus of the larynx, consisting of the true vocal cords and the opening between them.

glucagon a polypeptide hormone secreted by the alpha cells of the islets of Langerhans in response to hypoglycaemia or to stimulation by growth hormone. It increases blood glucose concentration by stimulating glycogenolysis in the liver and is administered to relieve hypoglycaemic coma from any cause, especially hyperinsulinism.

glucocorticoid any corticoid substance that increases gluconeogenesis, raising the concentration of liver glycogen and blood sugar, i.e. cortisol

(hydrocortisone), cortisone and corticosterone.

glucose dextrose, a monosaccharide found in many fruits and honey. It is the monosaccharide to which carbohydrates are reduced by digestion, and therefore found in the blood. The metabolism of glucose produces energy for the body cells; the rate of metabolism is controlled by insulin. Glucose that is not needed for energy is stored in the form of glycogen as a source of potential energy, readily available when needed. Most of the glycogen is stored in the liver and muscle cells. The normal fasting level for glucose in the blood is between 70 and 90 mg per 100 ml (5.6–3.9 mmol/l). Unusually high levels of glucose in the blood (hyperglycaemia) may indicate such diseases as DIABETES MEL-LITUS, HYPERTHYROIDISM and HYPERPITUITARISM. A GLUCOSE TOLERANCE TEST is done to assess the ability of the body to metabolize glucose. Glucose is present in the urine of patients with untreated diabetes mellitus. In medicine glucose is used extensively, as it is an excellent source of energy and can be given by mouth or intravenously.

glucose-6-phosphate dehydrogenase (G6PD) an important enzyme, especially in red cells. The absence of this enzyme leads to attacks of HAEMOLYSIS and severe or fatal anaemia. The eating of fava beans can cause such an attack (favism), and the disease is common in coloured races, and in Mediterranean countries. It is inherited as an X-linked RECESSIVE trait.

glucose tolerance test (GTT) a test of the body's ability to utilize carbohydrates. It is used to detect abnormalities of carbohydrate metabolism such as occurs in diabetes mellitus. The client must be in a fasting state when the test is started and a blood sample is taken for measurement of the fasting blood glucose. A dose of 75 g of glucose is given orally. Blood samples are then obtained at intervals for glucose estimation. Abnormal findings would be as follows:

fasting blood glucose over 7.0 mmol/litre

two-hour blood glucose over 10.0 mmol/litre

glucuronyl transferase the liver enzyme which converts fat-soluble or toxic bilirubin to the water-soluble type which is not toxic. See Appendix 17.

gluteal pertaining to the buttocks.

glycogen a polysaccharide. The form in which carbohydrate is stored in the liver and in the muscles.

glycosuria sugar (more strictly, glucose) in the urine. Glycosuria in pregnancy may be: (a) *alimentary*, related to the ingestion of a large quantity of carbohydrate and inability to store it; (b) renal, resulting from a lowering of the renal threshold for sugar—neither is of serious import; (c) due to *diabetes mellitus*, which causes numerous hazards to both mother and child. In order that a differential diagnosis may be made, a midwife should always report the occurrence of glycosuria. See Appendices 6 and 18.

gnathic pertaining to the jaw or cheeks.

goblet cell a goblet-shaped cell, found in the cubical epithelium of the fallopian tubes. These cells produce a secretion containing glycogen to nourish the ovum.

goitre enlargement of the thyroid gland, causing a marked swelling in front of the neck, which sometimes results in pressure on the trachea.

gonad the organ which produces ova or spermatozoa; in the female the ovary and in the male the testis.

gonadotrophic stimulating the gonads. G. *hormones* those of the anterior pituitary lobe or placenta.

gonadotrophin any hormone having a stimulating effect on the gonads. Two such hormones are secreted by the anterior pituitary: follicular-stimulating hormone and luteinizing hormone. *Chorionic g.* a gonad-stimulating hormone produced by the cells of the cytotrophoblast of the chorionic tissue which later forms the placenta. Biological and immunological pregnancy tests depend on the detection of human chorionic gonadotrophin (HGC) in the urine.

gonococcal pertaining to or caused by the gonococcus. G. *ophthalmia* acute conjunctivitis resulting from gonococcal infection. This, occurring in newborn babies, can lead to ulceration of the cornea, and was at one time the commonest cause of blindness in babies and young children. *See* OPHTHALMIA NEONATORUM.

gonococcus *Neisseria gonorrhoeae*. The Gram-negative intracellular diplococcus which causes gonorrhoea.

gonorrhoea a venereal disease due to infection by the gonococcus, usually acquired by sexual intercourse, which infects the mucous membrane of the cervix, urethra and Bartholin's glands. Occasionally, the infection may spread causing salpingitis or septicaemia. The incubation period is 1–16 days. It may cause a purulent discharge from the vagina or urethra and burning pain on micturition, but is more often symptomless. Penicillin will effect a rapid cure. Any vaginal discharge during pregnancy which causes soreness or irritation or is associated with pain, should be investigated without delay. Both smears and cultures may be used in diagnosis.

Goodell's sign softening of the cervix uteri and vagina; a sign of pregnancy.

graafian follicle a cystic structure developing in the ovarian cortex during the menstrual cycle. It has an outer covering or theca folliculi, and a lining of granulosa cells which also surround the ovum, which lies within the follicle. When it is ripe, the follicle ruptures, discharging the ovum (ovulation) and develops into a CORPUS LUTEUM. The graafian

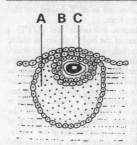

A. *Follicular fluid*; B. *granulosa cells*; C. *ovum*.
GRAAFIAN FOLLICLE

follicle secretes several oestrogenic hormones.

gram the unit of weight of the metric system. Abbreviated 'g'. *See* Appendix 20.

Gram stain a special stain used in bacteriology. Micro-organisms which retain it are said to be Gram-positive (+), and those which lose it Gram-negative (−).

grand mal a major epileptic seizure attended by loss of consciousness and convulsive movements, as distinguished from PETIT MAL, a minor seizure.

grande multipara a woman of high parity. Usually one who has borne 4 or more children.

granulation a process by which healing of a wound may take place. Granulations appear as small red projections on the surface of the wound, bringing a rich blood supply to the healing surface.

granulosa cells the lining cells in the graafian follicle, which secrete oestradiol.

granulosa lutein cells granulosa cells after ovulation. They secrete oestradiol and progesterone.

gravid pregnant.

gravida a pregnant woman. *See* PRIMIGRAVIDA and MULTIGRAVIDA.

Gravigard an intrauterine contraceptive device.

Gravindex an immunological pregnancy test.

gravity weight. The specific gravity of a substance is its weight compared with that of an equal volume of water. The specific gravity of water is 1000, and that of normal urine about 1010–1020. This is increased if more solids are dissolved in the urine, e.g. sugar, and decreased when the normal amount of urea is not being excreted, e.g. chronic nephritis.

grief sorrow, loss, usually caused by death. The normal grieving process may take 2 or 3 years and usually follows a pattern of numbness and denial, followed often by anger, guilt, bargaining and depression, and finally acceptance and readjustment.

grey-scale display a method to show the texture of tissue on ULTRASOUND display. The amplitude of each echo is represented by varying shades of grey. A bright white outline is seen from SPECULAR REFLECTIVE surfaces, a mottled grey from various tissue

areas, and black from collections of fluid such as the bladder and amniotic sac.

grey syndrome a potentially fatal condition seen in neonates, particularly preterm babies, due to a reaction to chloramphenicol, characterized by an ashen grey cyanosis, vomiting, abdominal distension, hypothermia and shock.

Griffiths Report Sir Roy Griffiths was asked by the government to examine the efficiency of the National Health Service and in his Report 'Patients First', published in 1983, recommended the introduction of general management throughout the service. This major reorganization replaced consensus management by placing the overall responsibility on one person, the General Manager at Regional and at District level. Each Health District was divided into Units of Management and each Unit headed by a Unit General Manager. Within the then Department of Health and Social Security a Supervisory Board and a Management Board were set up, the Supervisory Board being a policy-making body and the Management Board's main function being to implement the policies effectively.

groin the junction of the front of the thigh with the trunk.

group practice medical practice carried out by several general practitioners working together.

growth hormone a substance that stimulates growth, especially a secretion of the anterior PITU-ITARY GLAND that directly influences protein, carbohydrate and lipid metabolism, and controls the rate of skeletal and visceral growth. Increased production of growth hormone occurs in the baby of the poorly controlled diabetic mother.

guardian *ad litem* this is a person, usually from the local authority social service department, who is appointed by a court to look after the interests of a child before its full Adoption Order is granted. Meanwhile the prospective adoptive parents have continuous possession of the child, and are visited and interviewed by the guardian *ad litem* to ensure that the home will be satisfactory, and who makes a detailed report to the court.

gum gingiva in pregnancy oestrogen causes the gums to retain fluid and they become enlarged and spongy.

gumma a syphilitic lesion found in the third or tertiary stage of syphilis in any part of the body.

Guthrie test a blood test carried out on a neonate between the 6th and 14th days of life to diagnose PHENYLKETONURIA. The baby must be well established on milk feeds before the test is carried out. If the baby is receiving antibiotics the test is deferred.

gynae- prefix meaning 'woman'.

gynaecoid woman-like. Having feminine characteristics. *G. pelvis* a pelvis of typical female conformation.

gynaecology the branch of medicine which treats diseases of the female genital tract.

gynandroid a hermaphrodite or a female pseudohermaphrodite.

gynandromorphism the presence of chromosomes of both sexes in different tissues of the body, which produces a mosaic of male and female sexual characteristics. adj. *gynandromorphous*.

Gynovlar a contraceptive tablet containing OESTROGEN and PROGESTERONE.

H

H symbol for the element hydrogen.

haem the non-protein, insoluble, iron protoporphyrin constituent of haemoglobin, other respiratory pigments and of many cells. It is an iron compound of protoporphrin and is responsible for

the oxygen-carrying properties of the haemoglobin molecule.

haema-, haemo-, haemato- prefixes denoting or relating to blood.

haemagglutination agglutination of erythrocytes.

haemagglutinin an antibody that

causes agglutination of erythrocytes.

haemangioma a tumour made up of blood vessels, clustered together. Haemangiomas may be present at birth in various parts of the body. They often appear as a network of small, blood-filled capillaries near the surface of the skin, forming a flat red or purple birthmark (a 'strawberry' or 'raspberry' mark), which tends to disappear in childhood. The type of haemangioma known as a 'port-wine' stain tends to persist.

haematemesis the vomiting of blood. In newborn infants it may be a sign of HAEMORRHAGIC DISEASE or a result of swallowed maternal blood. Fetal and maternal blood may be distinguished by SINGER'S TEST.

haematinic 1. improving the quality of blood. 2. an agent that improves the quality of the blood, increasing the haemoglobin level and the number of erythrocytes; examples are iron preparations, liver extract and the B complex vitamins.

haematocele a collection of blood in a cavity. *Pelvic h.* a collection of blood in the pouch of Douglas, generally resulting from tubal abortion or rupture. *See* Appendix 6.

haematocrit *see* PACKED CELL VOLUME.

haematology the science dealing with the nature, functions and diseases of blood.

haematoma a localized collection of extravasated blood in an organ, space or tissue. Haematoma of the vagina, vulva or perineum may occur as a result of trauma during childbirth. Trauma to the fetus in labour may result in a cephal haematoma, which is due to the rupture of small blood vessels between the skull and pericranium. It develops a few hours after birth and does not cross suture lines.

haematometra an accumulation of blood in the uterus.

haematopoiesis the formation and development of blood cells, usually taking place in bone marrow. Also may take place in the spleen, liver and lymph nodes; then called extramedullary haematopoiesis.

haematoporphyrin an iron-free derivative of haem, a product of the decomposition of haemoglobin.

haematosalpinx an accumulation of blood in the fallopian tube.

haematuria blood in the urine, due to injury, infection or disease of any of the urinary organs. *See* Appendix 18.

haemoconcentration loss of fluid from the blood into the tissues, as may occur in shock or dehydration.

haemodialysis a procedure used to remove toxic wastes from the blood of a patient with acute or chronic renal failure.

haemodilution an increase of plasma in the blood in proportion to the cells. This occurs normally in pregnancy, as the blood volume increases (*see* HYDRAEMIA), or in haemorrhage, when fluid is drawn from the tissues into the blood to maintain the volume of circulating blood.

haemoglobin a pigment contained in the red blood cells which enables them to transport oxygen round the circulation. It is a compound of the ferrous-iron containing pigment haem combined with the protein globin. Each haemoglobin molecule contains 4 atoms of ferrous iron, 1 in each haem group, and can unite with 4 molecules of oxygen. Oxygenated haemoglobin (oxyhaemoglobin) is bright red in colour; haemoglobin inbound to oxygen (deoxyhaemoglobin) is darker. *In utero* fetal haemoglobin HbF, which is formed in the liver and spleen, has an increased affinity for oxygen. When erythropoiesis shifts to the bone marrow in the first year of life, the adult haemoglobins HbA and HbA$_2$ begin to be produced.

haemoglobinopathy any haematological disorder due to alteration in the genetically determined molecular structure of haemoglobin, with characteristic clinical and laboratory abnormalities and often overt anaemia. The main haemoglobinopathies which complicate pregnancy are SICKLE CELL DISEASE and THALASSAEMIA.

haemolysin ANTIBODY with COMPLEMENT which releases haemoglobin from the red blood cells.

haemolysis the liberation of haemoglobin from the confines of the red blood cell. In excess, it can cause ANAEMIA and JAUNDICE. Some microbes such as the beta haemolytic streptococcus form substances called haemolysins that have the specific action of destroying red blood corpuscles. In a transfusion reaction or in HAEMOLYTIC disease of the newborn, incompatibility causes the red blood cells to clump together. The agglutinated cells eventually disintegrate, releasing haemoglobin into the plasma. Kidney damage may result as the haemoglobin crystallizes and obstructs the renal tubules producing renal shutdown and uraemia. Other haemolysins include snake venoms, and certain vegetable and chemical poisons. *See* Appendix 17.

haemolytic pertaining to, characterized by or producing HAEMOLYSIS. *H. disease of the newborn* a blood dyscrasia of the newborn characterized by haemolysis of erythrocytes usually due to incompatibility between the baby's blood and the mother's. The fetus has Rh-positive blood and its mother has Rh-negative blood. In Rh incompatibility the mother builds up antibodies against the cells of the fetus; these antibodies pass through the placenta, entering the fetal circulation. There they destroy the fetal erythrocytes very rapidly. To compensate for this rapid destruction of red blood cells, there is increased bone marrow production and early release of immature red blood cells (erythroblasts). The condition is therefore also known as erythroblastosis fetalis. *See* Appendix 17.

haemophilia an inherited disease of delayed clotting of the blood. It is manifested only in males, but transmitted by the female as a sex-linked recessive gene. Over 80% of all patients with haemophilia have haemophilia A which is characterized by a deficiency of clotting factor VIII. Haemophilia B (Christmas disease) which affects about 15% of all haemophiliac patients is caused by a deficiency of factor IX. Treatment aims to raise the level of the deficient clotting factor and maintain it in order to stop local bleeding.

Haemophilus a genus of pathogenic bacteria including *H. ducreyi*, the organism of soft chancre, and *H. influenzae*, associated with influenza.

haemopoiesis the production of red blood cells.

haemoptysis the coughing up of blood. It is distinguishable from vomited blood by its bright colour and frothy character.

haemorrhage an escape of blood from its vessels either externally or within the body. For haemorrhages associated with pregnancy and childbearing, *see* Appendices 6 and 11. *Cerebral h.*, due to rupture of a cerebral blood vessel, may occur in pregnancy associated with any hypertensive condition, e.g. eclampsia, essential hypertension. In the child, *intracranial h.* occurs in difficult delivery as a result of a tear at the junction of the TENTORIUM CEREBELLI and FALX CEREBRI and the blood vessels they contain.

Intraventricular h. occurs in small and preterm babies. *Petechial h.* subcutaneous haemorrhage occurring in minute spots. Sometimes seen in the newborn when the cord has been tightly around the neck, or following a difficult delivery.

haemorrhagic characterized by haemorrhage. *H. disease of the newborn* a condition occurring in the first week of life. The haemorrhage is usually from the gut, showing as haematemesis or melaena. Bleeding can also occur from the umbilicus, puncture sites or internally, as haematuria. It is associated with an unusually low level of blood prothrombin. It is treated by the administration of vitamin K (phytomesadione 1 ml intramuscularly) and, if necessary, blood transfusion. It should be clearly differentiated from haemolytic disease of the newborn (*see* Appendix 17).

haemorrhoids piles. Varicose veins of the lower rectum and canal (internal), or around the anal orifice (external). They commonly enlarge and become painful during pregnancy, due to the relaxing effect of the high secretion of PROGESTERONE on the smooth muscle of the vein walls. Constipation, general increased vascularity and congestion increase the dilatation of the veins and cause discomfort. Symptomatic relief is obtained by applying local analgesic ointment or suppositories, especially if a mild laxative is also used to soften faeces. Vaginal delivery aggravates the condition by direct pressure from the fetal head, increasing venous congestion and stasis. During the puerperium they usually return to the pre-pregnant state and medical or surgical treatment is not often thought necessary.

haemostasis the arrest of bleeding.

haemostatic any drug or other agent capable of arresting bleeding. Those which work by reason of their astringent qualities are called styptics.

hair analysis used as an adjunct to other tests in preconception care to assess nutritional status and detect the concentration of up to 18 metals. High levels of some metals such as lead may be associated with congenital abnormalities. Deficiencies of substances such as zinc can be treated with dietary advice and/or supplements.

hallucination a false perception in which the patient believes he sees, smells, hears, tastes or feels an object or person when there is no basis in the external environmental for the belief. This condition is a PSYCHOSIS, and may be *organic*, resulting from bacterial toxins, drugs, thyrotoxicosis, *psychogenic* or *functional*, where there are no apparent changes in the central nervous system. Any stress, such as childbirth, can precipitate this condition in one who has an inherited susceptibility. *See also* PUERPERAL PSYCHOSIS.

halothane a colourless, non-flammable, volatile liquid whose vapour is inhaled to produce general ANAESTHESIA.

Halsbury Reports reports of a committee, led by Lord Halsbury, on pay and conditions of service for the nursing and midwifery profession in 1974, and NHS paramedical workers in 1975.

hamamelis witchhazel, employed as an astringent, especially for haemorrhoids or oedema of the vulva.

hand presentation the hand may present in labour in uncorrected oblique lie with shoulder presentation and prolapse of an arm, or in COMPOUND PRESENTATIONS. On vaginal examination a hand may be distinguished from a foot by the ability of the thumb to abduct, the absence of the prominent heel and the digits being longer than toes.

handicap a disadvantage for a given individual, resulting from an impairment or a disability that limits or prevents the fulfilment of a role that is normal for that individual.

haploid having half the number of chromosomes characteristically found in the somatic (diploid) cells of an organism.

hard chancre syphilitic ulcer of the first stage. Contagious; may be seen on the labium.

hare lip *see* CLEFT LIP.

Hartmann's solution a solution containing sodium chloride, sodium lactate, and phosphates of calcium and potassium; used intravenously as a systemic alkalizer and as a fluid and electrolyte replenisher.

Hb haemoglobin.

HCG *see* HUMAN CHORIONIC GONADOTROPHIN.

headache pain in the head. A symptom of a great variety of disorders. Headache occurring during pregnancy should never be ignored as it may be associated with pre-eclampsia, though it is usually a late symptom. It is of particular significance if other prodromal signs of eclampsia are present, i.e. raised diastolic blood pressure, spots or flashes before the eyes, or epigastric pain. *Spinal h.* an occasional complication of epidural anaesthesia when the dura mater is inadvertently punctured resulting in the loss of cerebrospinal fluid. The headache may persist for about a week.

headbox a perspex box placed over the baby's head into which additional oxygen can be administered.

head circumference the head circumference of a well-flexed fetus is the suboccipitobregmatic which measures 33 cm, and of a deflexed head, the occipitofrontal which measures 35 cm.

head fitting an attempt to fit the non-engaged fetal head into the brim of the maternal pelvis, whereby disproportion between the head and the brim may be excluded if the head can be made to engage on pressure; or it must be suspected, if this cannot be done. *Methods:* 1. the mother may lie on the couch while the fetal head is palpated. She is helped to a sitting position, when the examiner, keeping his hand on the head, may feel it enter the pelvis. 2. she may be half sitting up, resting backwards on her elbows, her pelvic brim thus being parallel to the couch. The doctor or the midwife then applies gentle, steady pressure to the head straight down towards the couch, when the head may be felt to descend and become engaged. 3. with the woman standing, leaning forwards with her hands resting on the couch, the fetal head is palpated. It may be found to have engaged spontaneously, or a gentle push backwards may effect engagement. In all doubtful cases, X-ray pelvimetry provides much more accurate and detailed information about the pelvis.

Heaf test a form of tuberculin testing.

healing the restoration of structure and function of injured or diseased tissues. The healing processes include blood clotting, inflammation and repair.

health the World Health Organisation (WHO) states that 'health is a state of complete physical, mental and social well-being and not merely the absence of disease or infirmity'.

health authorities (District Health Authorities; DHA) there are about 200 health authorities in England, each of which serves a population of between 150 000 and 500 000. From April 1991 when the NHS and Community Care Act, 1990 came into effect the role of DHAs changed to that of purchasers for populations and the Self-Governing Trusts and Directly-Managed Units to providers.

health care planning teams groups brought together on either a short or long term to plan regularly for service needs, e.g. the district obstetric and gynaecological health care planning teams.

health centre a centre placed strategically in the community, to provide the full range of primary health care, commonly focused around the general practitioner's services. It may also provide facilities for minor surgery.

health education various methods of education aimed at the prevention of disease. Midwives and health visitors have particular responsibilities and opportunities to promote good health, especially with mothers and young babies.

Health Education Authority a special health authority responsible for giving authoritative advice both nationally and locally on a wide range of health education issues through campaigns and publications (formerly the Health Education Council). Now an integral part of the health service and thus participates with other health authorities in planning health service policies and priorities.

health education officer an officer appointed to make health education resources available to the community.

Health and Safety at Work Act, 1974 this Act came into force in 1975. It is comprehensive legislation dealing with the welfare, health and safety of all employers and employees, except domestic workers in a private house.

Health Services Act, 1980 this Act followed the consultation document 'Patients First' which was published in 1979. It resulted in a major re-organization of the NHS when all 90 Area Health Authorities were removed and health districts were replaced by 200 health authorities led by a team of officers. The 14 Regional Health Authorities remained.

Health Service Supervisory Board a policy-making body set up within the Department of Health and chaired by the Secretary of State for Health.

health visitor (HV) A registered nurse who has also obtained the health visitor's qualification following a year's full-time course in social and preventive medicine. The main area of responsibility for the health visitor is health education and preventative care of mothers and children under 5, although some specialize in preventative care of the elderly, the handicapped and other special groups. The midwife liaises with the health visitor when she discharges the mother and baby into her care between 10 and 28 days after delivery.

hearing test see AUDITORY RESPONSE CRADLE. A hearing test is also performed by the health visitor on all babies at 7 months of age.

eart the organ which pumps the blood into the arteries to be conveyed to every part of the body. The cardiac output is considerably increased in pregnancy, since (a) there is much growth in the size and circulation of the uterus, (b) the blood volume is considerably increased, (c) the metabolism is increased, and (d) the body weight increases. *Heart disease in pregnancy. See* Appendix 6. *h. defects* disorders, some of which may be congenital. Fallot's tetralogy and patent ductus arteriosus are examples of congenital heart defects. *H. failure* the inability of the heart to perform its function of pumping sufficient blood to assure a normal flow through the circulation. *H. murmur* any sound in the heart region other than normal heart sounds.

eartburn a burning sensation in the chest, caused by gastroesophageal regurgitation, i.e. regurgitation of stomach contents into the lower oesophagus. It is a very troublesome disorder in pregnancy, caused by the relaxation of the cardia of the stomach. Magnesium trisilicate and other alkaline mixtures give transient relief. Heartburn which is troublesome at night may be relieved if the woman sleeps propped up with several pillows.

eat shield a perspex shield which may be placed over a low birth weight and/or sick baby in an incubator to prevent radiant and convective heat loss.

Hegar's dilators a series of graduated dilators used to dilate the cervix uteri.

Hegar's sign a test for pregnancy, not often used as it is uncomfortable for the woman, and now unnecessary for accurate diagnosis. It may be elicited between the 6th and 10th weeks of gestation when the embryo only occupies the upper part of the uterus. The lower part above the cervix is greatly softened and on bimanual examination almost allows the fingers to meet.

Hellin's law one in about 89 pregnancies ends in the birth of twins; one in 89^2, or 7921, in the birth of triplets; one in 89^3, or 704 969, in the birth of quadruplets. This is roughly correct as the incidence of twin pregnancies in the UK is between 1 in 80 to 1 in 90.

Heminevrin a proprietary preparation of chlormethiazole, a hypnotic and anticonvulsant drug.

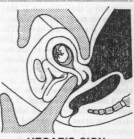

HEGAR'S SIGN

Can be used to control ECLAMP-SIA. *See* Appendix 19.

hemiplegia paralysis of one side of the body.

hemisphere half a sphere. One of the two halves of the cerebrum.

heparin an anticoagulant formed in the liver and circulating in the blood. Injected intravenously it prevents the conversion of pro-thrombin into thrombin, and is used in the prevention and treatment of thrombosis.

hepatic pertaining to the liver.

hepatitis inflammation of the liver. Usually due to a virus infection. There are two forms of viral hepatitis. *Virus A* causes infectious hepatitis which mostly affects children and young adults. It is usually a mild disease which occurs in epidemics and does not cause serious complications in pregnancy. *Virus B* causes serum hepatitis which affects all ages and is a serious complication of pregnancy. The disease is blood-borne and there is a serious risk of midwives and doctors contracting the infection if they have an abrasion which is a portal of entry for infected blood. The incubation period is 50 to 160 days and the disease is charac-terized by a low fever, malaise, marked anorexia, nausea, vomit-ing and jaundice. Bed rest in a single room with separate bath-room facilities is required. If the mother is bleeding or in labour, strict isolation and special pre-cautions to prevent the spread of infection are carried out. Acute hepatic necrosis is a serious com-plication. The baby of a mother with hepatitis B should be given hepatitis B vaccine within 24 hours of delivery and it is repeated at 1 and 6 months of age. Infective jaundice is statutorily notifiable.

hepatomegaly enlargement of the liver.

hepatosplenomegaly enlargement of the liver and spleen.

hereditary transmissible or trans-mitted from parent to offspring; genetically determined.

heredity the inheritance of physi-cal and mental characteristics from the parents and ancestors by the offspring. The science of heredity is termed genetics. The hereditary characteristics are transmitted in the genes, many according to laws first described by Gregor Mendel, a Moravian monk. *See also* INHERITANCE.

hermaphrodite having the charac-teristics of both sexes. In the human subject partial develop-ment of both male and female sex organs may occur. True her-maphrodites are rare, PSEUDO-HERMAPHRODITES relatively more common.

hernia a protrusion of peritoneum and other abdominal structures through a defect in the wall of the cavity. *Diaphragmatic h.* a protrusion into the thorax of any of the abdominal contents, e.g. stomach, gut. It may occur as a serious congenital malformation, in which case an emergency oper-ation will be needed. *Femoral h.* protrusion, usually of a loop of bowel, through the femoral canal.

It is more common in females. *Hiatus h.* protrusion of part of the stomach through the diaphragm into the thorax. This may be responsible for severe heartburn in pregnancy. *Inguinal h.* protrusion of bowel through the inguinal canal into the groin or scrotum. It is much commoner in males, and may be present at birth. *Umbilical h.* protrusion of bowel through the gap in the recti at the umbilicus. It is common in babies of African descent. It almost always heals spontaneously.

heroin a narcotic made from morphine. Used medicinally as an analgesic and abused illicitly for its euphoriant effects. The drug has a great capacity for inducing physical dependence and may be sniffed, smoked or injected subcutaneously or intravenously.

herpes an inflammatory skin eruption characterized by small vesicles. *H. gestationis* a skin eruption of unknown origin occurring occasionally in early or middle pregnancy and causing considerable irritation. *H. simplex* or *labialis*. 'Cold' sore on the face or lip, associated with head colds and fevers. *Genital h.* is usually caused by type 2 virus. Lesions appear on the cervix, vulva and surrounding skin in women and on the penis in men. Caesarean section is recommended for those who have clinical genital tract herpes within 2 weeks of delivery in order to prevent neonatal herpes. Congenital *Herpes simplex* is a very serious condition with a generalized vesicular rash. The baby dies from encephalitis. *H. zoster* shingles. An extremely painful condition, caused by the virus of chicken pox, in which the eruption follows the course of a cutaneous nerve.

heterogeneous dissimilar. Made up of different characteristics.

heterosexual 1. pertaining to, characteristics of, or directed toward the opposite sex. 2. a person with erotic interests directed towards the opposite sex.

heterozygous carrying dissimilar genes. Used commonly to describe a man whose blood is Rhesus positive, but who may transmit to his children either Rhesus-positive or Rhesus-negative genes. cf. homozygous.

heuristic encouraging or promoting investigation; conducive to discovery.

hexachlorophane an antiseptic widely used in midwifery.

Hg symbol for mercury.

hiatus a space or gap. *H. hernia*. See HERNIA.

hibitane a proprietary preparation of CHLORHEXIDINE.

hindwaters in labour the amniotic fluid is divided into the fore and hind-waters. When the well-flexed fetal head descends on to the cervix, it separates the small bag of amniotic fluid in front, the forewaters, from the remainder which surrounds the body, the hindwaters.

Hippocrates Greek physician, 460–370 BC, known as the father of medicine.

Hirschsprung's disease congenital absence of the parasympathetic nerve ganglia in the anorectum or proximal rectum, resulting in the absence of peristalsis in the affected portion of the colon and a consequent massive enlargement of the colon, constipation and obstruction. Severe cases require surgery. Called also aganglionic megacolon and congenital megacolon.

hirsute hairy.

histamine a chemical substance produced when tissue is injured. It is thought to be a factor in the causation of anaphylactic shock, which is characterized by dilatation and increased permeability of capillaries. Antihistamine drugs counteract some of these effects.

histogram a graph in which values found in a statistical study are represented by lines or symbols placed horizontally or vertically, to indicate frequency of distribution.

histology the visualization of the minute structure, composition and function of tissues and organs.

history taking see Appendix 3.

HIV human immunodeficiency virus. *See* AIDS.

Hodge pessary a pessary which is used to maintain the position of the uterus following correction of a retroversion. *See* PESSARY.

Hogben test a pregnancy test, rarely used since the immunological tests were introduced. Injection of pregnancy urine into the dorsal lymph sac of the *Xenopus* toad. If gonadotrophic hormone

is present in the urine, the toad will ovulate in about 8–15 hours after the injection. The test is then said to be positive for pregnancy.

holism a philosophy in which the person is considered as a functioning whole rather than as a composite of several systems.

holistic pertaining to totality, or to the whole. The client's physical, emotional, psychological, social and spiritual needs are recognized as interdependent and he or she is treated as a complete person, rather than focusing only on one problem or condition.

Homan's sign pain felt in the calf when the foot is dorsiflexed with the leg extended. It is a sign of deep vein thrombosis in the calf.

home assessment a visit made by a community midwife to assess the suitability of a home for domiciliary confinement or early transfer home following hospital confinement.

home confinement the delivery of a baby conducted in the home as opposed to a hospital or general practitioner unit.

home confinement box a box containing pre-sterilized pads and dressings, provided in advance for a home confinement.

home help service a branch of the social services department, which provides domestic and housekeeping assistance to those in need. It is on either a short-term or long-term basis, and payment is according to means.

homeopathy a system of therapeutics in which diseases are treated by drugs that are capable of producing in healthy persons symptoms like those of the disease to be treated, the drug being administered in minute doses.

homeostasis a tendency of biological systems to maintain stability while continually adjusting to conditions that are optimal for survival. For instance, it is through homeostatic mechanisms that body temperature is kept within normal range, and nutrients are supplied to cells as needed, to give but two examples. The two basic homeostatic regulators are: 1. negative feedback controls; and 2. on–off switches, in which a response either does or does not occur. Hormonal secretions from the ENDOCRINE glands are typically regulated by the closed-loop feedback control systems, while responses of the nervous system are of the on–off type.

homogeneous having the same nature or being of the same composition throughout.

homologous having the same structure or pattern.

homosexual 1. pertaining to the same sex. 2. an individual who is attracted to a person of the same sex.

homosexuality the attraction for and desire to establish a sexual relationship with a member of the same sex. Female homosexuality is known as lesbianism.

homozygous having a pair of genes which are the same. Used most commonly in midwifery in relation to the genotype of a man who is Rhesus positive. If homozygous, he can transmit only the Rhesus-positive genes to his offspring. All his children will be Rhesus positive even if the mother is Rhesus negative. cf. heterozygous.

hookworm a parasitic roundworm that enters the human body through the skin and migrates to the intestines, where it attaches itself to the intestinal wall and sucks blood from it for nourishment. A large number of worms cause considerable blood loss and anaemia. The infection is found mainly in temperate regions where conditions are very insanitary, and in the tropics and subtropics. Shoes should be worn out of doors as the hookworm usually enters the body through the sole of the foot.

horizon a specific anatomical stage of embryonic development, of which 23 have been defined, beginning with the unicellular fertilized egg and ending 7 to 9 weeks later, with the beginning of the fetal stage.

hormone a chemical substance secreted into the blood stream by an endocrine gland, and exerting an effect on some other part of the body.

hour-glass constriction a constriction ring in the uterus, occurring during the third stage of labour, and imprisoning the placenta. An uncommon cause of retained placenta. It is relieved by the inhalation of amyl nitrite, or by anaesthesia. *See also* CONSTRICTION RING.

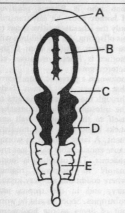

A. *Upper uterine segment*;
B. *placenta*; C. *hour-glass constriction*; D. *lower uterine segment*; E. *vagina*.

HOUR-GLASS CONSTRICTION

Housing Department a department of the local authority, responsible for providing housing.

HPL *see* HUMAN PLACENTAL LACTOGEN.

human chorionic gonadotrophin (HCG) a hormone produced by the TROPHOBLAST. Pregnancy tests can detect its presence in the urine from 30 days after conception.

human placental lactogen (HPL) a hormone secreted by the placenta to aid growth and development of the breast. It is also thought to resemble growth hormone and to affect carbohydrate metabolism.

humerus the bone of the upper arm.

humid moist.

humidity the degree of moisture in the atmosphere.

Huntingdon's disease (chorea) a rare hereditary disease which appears in adulthood between the ages of 30 and 45 years. It is characterized by mental deterioration, speech disturbances and quick involuntary movements caused by degenerative changes in the cerebral cortex and basal ganglia. Total incapacitation and death ensue.

Hutchinson's teeth typical notching of the borders of the upper incisor teeth occurring in congenital syphilis.

hyaline resembling glass. *H. membrane* a protein material found in the alveoli of babies with hyaline membrane disease. This condition is also known as the respiratory distress syndrome (RDS). The baby has increasing difficulty in breathing from birth, with expiratory grunting and rib and sternal recession. Babies who are preterm or born of diabetic mothers are particularly at risk. It is due to a lack of SURFACTANT in the lungs and is demonstrated at post mortem examination. It consists of fibrin with red cells, and necrosed protein and epithelial cells. *See* Appendix 17.

hyaluronidase an enzyme which

can hasten the absorption of drugs into body tissues.

ydatidiform mole vesicular mole. A benign neoplasm of the TRO-PHOBLAST, often the precursor of CHORIOCARCINOMA. It appears like a collection of hydropic vesicles. The incidence is 1 in 2000 pregnancies.

ydraemia a modification of the blood in which there is an excess of plasma in relation to the cells. A degree of this is physiological in pregnancy.

ydrallazine (Apresoline) an anti-hypertensive drug. *See* Appendix 19.

ydramnion, hydramnios excessive accumulation of amniotic fluid. *See* POLYHYDRAMNIOS *and* OLIGOHYDRAMNIOS.

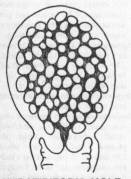

HYDATIDIFORM MOLE

hydro- prefix signifying water or hydrogen.

hydrocele a swelling caused by accumulation of fluid, especially in the tunica vaginalis surrounding the testicles. It is very common in the newborn and usually disappears spontaneously.

hydrocephalus 'water on the brain'. An increased amount of cerebrospinal fluid distending the ventricles of the brain. A congenital malformation, severe degrees of which are incompatible with life, though in milder cases the child may survive and in many cases it can be treated by an operation in which cerebrospinal fluid is diverted from the ventricles into the blood stream. It may be recognized antenatally through an investigation of failure of the head to engage or persistent breech presentation or through observation of an unusually large fetal head. The most accurate method of diagnosis is serial cephalometry by ULTRASOUND.

hydrochloric acid chemical symbol, HCl. A strong acid. It is secreted into the gastric juice. Very acid gastric juice (pH less than 2.0), aspirated into the lungs, is the main cause of bronchospasm in MENDELSON'S SYNDROME.

hydrocortisone one of the hormones secreted by the adrenal cortex.

hydrogen a gas which combines with oxygen to form water (H_2O). Symbol H.

hydrogen ion concentration the proportion of hydrogen ions in the blood, whereby the pH of the blood is determined.

hydrogen ions hydrogen atoms carrying a positive electrical charge. Cations.

hydromeningocele protrusion of the meninges, containing fluid, through a defect in the skull or vertebral column.

hydromyelomeningocele a defect of the spine marked by a protrusion of the membranes and tissue of the spinal cord, forming a fluid-filled sac.

hydronephrosis a collection of urine in the pelves of the kidney, resulting in atrophy of the kidney structure, due to the constant pressure of the fluid, until finally, the whole organ becomes one large cyst. The condition may be (*a*) congenital, due to malformation of the kidney or ureter, or (*b*) acquired, due to any obstruction of the ureter by tumour or stone, or to back pressure from stricture of the urethra.

hydrops fetalis severe oedema of the fetus due to blood incompatibility, usually resulting in either STILLBIRTH or neonatal death. *See* Appendix 17.

hydrosalpinx distension of the fallopian tube by an aqueous fluid.

hygiene the science of health. *Communal h.* the maintenance of the health of the community by provision of a pure water supply, efficient sanitation, good housing, etc. *Personal h.* the cleanliness and care of the body and clothing.

hygroscopic readily absorbing moisture.

hymen a fold of skin, partly occluding the vaginal introitus in a virgin.

hyoscine (scopolamine) a drug with anti-salivary and amnesic properties.

hyper- prefix meaning 'excessive' or 'above normal'.

hyperbilirubinaemia an excess of bilirubin in the circulating blood. *See* Appendix 17.

hypercalcaemia abnormally high concentration of calcium in the blood. *Idiopathic h.* a condition of infants associated with vitamin D intoxication, characterized by elevated serum calcium levels, increased skeletal density, mental deterioration and nephrocalcinosis.

hyperdactyly the presence of supernumerary digits on the hand or foot.

hyperemesis excessive vomiting. *H. gravidarum* an uncommon serious complication of pregnancy, characterized by severe and persistent vomiting, the aetiology of which is not fully understood.

hyperglycaemia excess of glucose in the blood (adult normal 3.3–5.3 mmol/l; 60–95 mg/100 ml). Persistent hyperglycaemia is a sign of DIABETES MELLITUS.

hyperkalaemia an excess of potassium in the blood.

hypernatraemia an excessive concentration of sodium in the blood, usually diagnosed when the plasma sodium is above 150 mmol/l. It can occur if a baby has excessive salt in its feeds or if it becomes dehydrated. Convulsions can occur and can lead to brain damage. The condition can be prevented by giving low-sodium feeds, half or quarter normal strength, to a baby suffering from diarrhoea.

hyperplasia growth by multiplication of cells. Both hyperplasia and HYPERTROPHY occur in the uterus during pregnancy.

hyperprolactinaemia increased levels of prolactin in the blood; in women it is associated with infertility and may lead to galactorrhoea (excessive or spontaneous milk flow), and it has been reported to cause impotence in men.

hyperptyalism abnormally increased secretion of saliva.

hyperpyrexia excessively high body temperature, i.e. over 40°C (104°F).

hypertension abnormally high blood pressure. This may be a sign of any one of a number of diseases, e.g. acute or chronic nephritis, coarctation of the aorta; or it may be raised in an individual who is otherwise healthy, in which case it is termed *essential hypertension*. The cause of essential hypertension is not known, but it is a very common disease in the adult population and, unless treated and controlled, may lead to damage to the blood vessels in such vital organs as the heart, brain and kidneys. In pregnancy, a reading of 140/90 mmHg is regarded as the upper limit of normal, or a rise of 15–20 mmHg or more above the level recorded in the first trimester. Hyperten-sive diseases in pregnancy include pre-eclampsia and eclampsia which are induced by pregnancy, and pre-existing medical conditions such as essential hypertension and renal disease. The cause of pregnancy-induced hypertension is still unknown. In severe cases it is complicated by proteinuria and may develop into eclampsia which is characterized by epileptiform fits. The risk of mortality to both mother and fetus is then greatly increased. *See* Appendix 6.

hyperthyroidism thyrotoxicosis. Excessive activity of the thyroid gland resulting in a raised basal metabolic rate and, often, exophthalmos.

hypertonic 1. relating to hypertonia or to excessive tone or tension as in a blood vessel or muscle. 2. hypertonic action of the uterus is a type of abnormal uterine action in which the muscle tone is excessive. The contractions are extremely painful, the intermissions brief, with inadequate relaxation, labour is prolonged and exhausting to the mother and the fetus often becomes hypoxic. The mother should be under the care of a doctor. She will benefit from EPIDURAL ANALGESIA and intravenous oxytocin but if progress is not made she may need a caesarean section. cf. hypotonic. 3. applied to solutions which are stronger than physiological saline, e.g. hypertonic saline.

hypertrophy growth resulting

from increase in the size of cells. *See also* HYPERPLASIA.

hyperventilation overbreathing, in which an excessive amount of carbon dioxide is removed from the blood. A transient respiratory alkalosis commonly results. Symptoms include 'faintness', palpitations or pounding of the heart, fullness of the throat and tetany, with muscular spasms of the hands and feet. This condition occasionally occurs when a woman is overbreathing in labour. Reassurance and a return to normal breathing is usually sufficient to rectify the situation.

hyperviscosity excessive viscosity of the blood. Occurs in conditions such as polycythaemia when the number of red blood cells is increased. Venesection to remove excess red cells may be necessary.

hypervolaemia abnormal increase in the volume of circulating fluid (plasma) in the body.

hypnosis a state of apparent deep sleep in which a person acts only under the influence of some external suggestion.

hypnotic an agent which produces sleep.

hypo- prefix meaning 'lacking in' or 'below normal'.

hypocalcaemia a low level of calcium in the blood. *Neonatal h.* can occur within 48 hours of delivery or between the 5th and 8th days of life. Convulsions may occur in the latter, especially in babies fed on unmodified cows' milk formula. The high phosphorus content in the formula contributes to this condition.

Since the Report on Infant Feeding (HMSO, 1974), the majority of artificially produced milk is modified to make it as near to breast milk as possible. The condition is also a rare complication of EXCHANGE TRANSFUSION.

hypocapnia diminished carbon dioxide in the blood.

hypochondrium a region of the ABDOMEN.

hypochromic deficient in pigmentation of colouring, as with red blood cells if they are deficient in iron.

hypodactyly less than the usual number of digits on the hand or foot.

hypodermic beneath the skin. Applied to injections into the subcutaneous tissues. *H. syringe* a plastic or glass syringe, used for hypodermic injections.

hypofibrinogenaemia deficiency of fibrinogen in the blood. A rare but serious cause of postpartum haemorrhage, often associated with severe abruptio placentae, amniotic fluid embolism and intrauterine death.

hypogastric arteries branches from the internal iliac arteries, which in the fetus pass out into the umbilical cord to carry deoxygenated blood to the placenta.

hypogastrium *see* ABDOMEN.

hypoglycaemia an abnormally low blood sugar. It may develop in a diabetic patient who is receiving insulin if insufficient carbohydrate is taken. *Neonatal h.* occurs when the blood glucose is less than 1.7 mmol/l in the baby at term and less than 1.2 mmol/l in low birth-weight babies. It may occur very soon after delivery in a baby of a diabetic (or gestational diabetic) mother, where it produces too much insulin (hyperinsulinaemia) for its extrauterine needs. It also may occur within 24–48 hours of delivery in a SMALL FOR GESTATIONAL AGE baby or any baby after severe ASPHYXIA, due to lack of GLYCOGEN in the liver. Fits or APNOEA may occur, when brain damage can ensue. Symptomatic hypoglycaemia may be prevented by early feeding and frequent screening with Dextrostix hourly during the first few days of life in babies at risk.

hypomagnesaemia abnormally low magnesium content of the blood, manifested chiefly by neuromuscular hyperirritability.

hypomenorrhoea menstruation at intervals longer than 1 month.

hyponatraemia deficiency of sodium in the blood; salt depletion. Hyponatraemia is present when the sodium concentration is less than 135 mmol/l. Symptoms include muscular weakness and twitching, progressing to convulsions if unrelieved.

hypopituitarism deficiency of secretion from the anterior lobe of the pituitary gland. It may follow severe postpartum haemorrhage, with failure of lactation and subsequent amenorrhoea and sterility. SHEEHAN'S SYNDROME.

hypoplasia underdevelopment of a part or organ. adj. *hypoplastic*.

hypoprothrombinaemia a lack of prothrombin in the blood. By lessening the clotting power of the blood, it tends to encourage bleeding. *See* HAEMORRHAGIC DISEASE.

hypospadias a malformation in which the urinary meatus opens upon the undersurface of the penis.

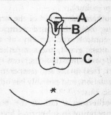

MILD HYPOSPADIAS

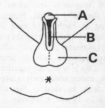

SEVERE HYPOSPADIAS
A. *Glans penis*; B. *urethral orifice*; C. *scrotum*.

hypostatic pertaining to decreased movement. *H. pneumonia* may develop if an ill or elderly patient, or one with eclampsia, lies supine for long periods.

hypotension blood pressure below the normal range.

hypotensive pertaining to low blood pressure. *H. drugs* are drugs which lower the blood pressure, e.g. hydrallazine (Apresoline).

hypothalamus a part of the brain lying near the third ventricle. It controls the activity of the pituitary gland, the sympathetic and parasympathetic nervous system, food intake and temperature regulation, and possibly has other functions.

hypothermia a fall in the body temperature to subnormal levels. Produced artificially as an alternative or an adjunct to local or general anaesthesia. Hypothermia is a particular problem with babies at birth when the temperature will fall markedly unless special measures are taken to keep the baby warm. Extreme chilling at birth or during the subsequent weeks or months may lead to neonatal cold injury when the temperature falls to below 35°C. This is a serious condition which, unless adequately treated, may lead to death. *See also* Appendix 17 *and* SCLEREMA.

hypothesis any theory presented as a basis for argument or discussion.

hypothyroidism the condition produced by deficiency of thyroid

secretion. In the child, cretinism; in the adult, myxoedema.

hypotonia deficient muscle tone, often applied to the abdominal and uterine muscles.

hypotonic describes solutions which are more dilute than physiological saline. *H. uterine action* weak, ineffective contractions with prolongation of labour unless intravenous oxytocin is used when the contractions usually become normal. cf. hypertonic.

hypovolaemia an abnormally low circulating blood volume.

hypoxaemia low oxygen tension in arterial blood; low $P\text{CO}_2$.

hypoxia a diminished oxygen tension in the body tissues. *see also* ANOXIA.

hysterectomy removal of the uterus. *Abdominal h.* removal via an abdominal incision. *Pan-h.* an old term for removal of the uterus and adnexa. *Subtotal h.* removal of the body of the uterus only. *Total h.* removal of the body and cervix. *Vaginal h.* removal *per vaginam. Wertheim's h.* in addition to the uterus, fallopian tubes and ovaries, the parametrium, upper vagina, and all the local lymphatic glands are excised: a successful method of treatment of carcinoma of the cervix.

hysteria a psychoneurosis, with widely varied symptoms, but no organic disease.

hystero-oophorectomy excision of the uterus and one or both ovaries.

hystero-salpingectomy excision of

the uterus and one or both of the uterine tubes.

hystero-salpingography radiography of the uterus and the uterine tubes after instillation of a contrast medium.

hysterotomy an incision into the uterus. An operation which consists of incision of the abdominal wall and the uterus in order to remove the ovum or evacuate the contents of the uterus before the 24th week of pregnancy and after 12 weeks.

I

iatrogenic induced by treatment.

ichthammol an ammoniated coal tar product, used in ointment form for certain skin diseases.

ichthyosis a rare congenital skin abnormality characterized by scaliness and desquamation of the skin of the whole body.

ICM International Confederation of Midwives.

icterus jaundice. Yellow staining of the skin and mucous membranes resulting from an excess of bile pigments in the blood and in the tissues. *I. neonatorum* jaundice of the newborn. *I. gravis neonatorum* severe jaundice of the newborn, usually caused by Rhesus ISOIMMUNIZATION. *See* Appendix 17.

id a Freudian term used to describe that part of the personality which harbours the unconscious, instinctive impulses that lead to immediate gratification of primitive needs such as hunger, the need for air, the need to move about and relieve body tension, and the need to eliminate. Id impulses produce drives aimed at the satisfaction of physiological and bodily needs, as opposed to the EGO and SUPEREGO, which are psychological and social processes.

ideology 1. the science of the development of ideas. 2. the body of ideas characteristic of an individual or of a social unit.

idiopathic of unknown cause.

idiosyncrasy 1. unusual sensitivity to a particular circumstance. 2. a peculiarity of constitution or temperament.

idoxuridine an analogue that prevents replication of DNA viruses; used topically in *Herpes simplex* keratitis.

Ig immunoglobulin of any of the 5 classes: IgA, IgD, IgE, IgG, IgM.

ileocaecal valve the valve at the junction of the ileum with the caecum.

ileum the last part of the small intestine, terminating at the caecum.

ileus paralysis of the wall of the gut, so that it is unable to propel food onward. A functional obstruction. An uncommon complication following caesarean section and other abdominal operations. *Meconium i. see* CYSTIC FIBROSIS.

iliac pertaining to the ilium. *I. crest* the crest of the hip bone. *I. fossa* a large shallow depression forming much of the inner surface of the ilium above the pelvic brim.

iliopectineal pertaining to the ilium and pubes. *I. line* the ridge which crosses the innominate bone from the sacroiliac joint to the *iliopectineal eminence,* a small protrusion marking the fusion of ilium and os pubis.

ilium the upper broad part of the innominate bone.

image 1. the mental recall of a former percept. 2. the optical picture transferred to the brain cell by the optic nerve.

imaging the production of diagnostic images, e.g. radiography, ultrasonography or scintigraphy.

Imferon trademark for a preparation of iron dextran solution, an iron replacement used parenterally.

immature not mature. Not sufficiently developed.

immune protected against infectious diseases, foreign tissue, foreign non-toxic substances and other ANTIGENS. *I.-reactive trypsin (IRT) test* a blood test carried out for the diagnosis of cystic fibrosis.

immunity the resistance possessed by the body to infectious diseases, foreign tissues, foreign non-toxic substances and other ANTIGENS. Immunological responses in humans can be divided into two broad categories: humoral immunity, which takes place in the body fluids and is concerned with antibody and complement activities; and cell-mediated or cellular immunity, which involves a variety of activities designed to destroy or at least contain cells that are recognized by the body as alien and harmful. Both types of response are instigated by lymphocytes that originate in the bone marrow as stem cells and later are converted into mature cells having specific properties and functions. The two kinds of lymphocytes that are important to the establishment of immunity are T-lymphocytes (T-cells) and B-lymphocytes (B-cells). B-lymphocytes mature into plasma cells that are primarily responsible for forming antibodies, thereby providing humoral immunity. Cellular immunity is dependent upon T-lymphocytes which is primarily concerned with a delayed type of immune response as occurs in the rejection of transplanted organs, defence against some slowly developing bacterial diseases, allergic reactions and certain autoimmune diseases. *Acquired i.* is produced specifically in response to an ANTIGEN. It involves a change in the behaviour of cells and in the production of antibody. Antibody is produced as a primary response, and after a short while the body becomes sensitized. The secondary response is produced more quickly and is more marked. *Active i.* this may be (*a*) natural, i.e. from infectious diseases, or (b) artificial, i.e. from injection of living or dead organisms or their products in the form of toxins and toxoids. *Passive i.* this may be: (a) natural, e.g. maternal immunoglobulin G (IgG) via the placenta protects the infant from various infectious diseases for a few months, but undesirable antibodies such as anti-D immunoglobulin may also be transmitted to the fetus; or (b) acquired, e.g. the temporary immunity which follows the injection of antibodies of human (GAMMA GLOBULIN) or, more rarely, animal origin. *Natural or innate i.* is mainly non-specific. It is provided by intact cellular barriers of epithelium and by humoral substances such as COMPLEMENT and LYSOZYME. It is affected by genetic factors, age, race and hormone levels.

immunization rendering immune. *Isoimmunization* immunization from an individual of the same species, e.g. a Rhesus-negative woman may immunize herself against her fetus, if it is Rhesus-positive, by forming specific ANTIBODY.

immunization programme a standard programme for the immunization of children against certain diseases. *See* Appendix 15.

immunoglobulin antibody. A variety of chemical compound found mainly in GAMMA GLOBULIN. Immunoglobulins are major components of the humoral immune response system. They are synthesized by lymphocytes and plasma cells and found in the serum and in other body fluids and tissues. The 5 classes of immunoglobulin (Ig) are: IgA, IgD, IgE, IgG and IgM. There are two types of IgA and both are known to have anti-viral properties. Secretory IgA is present in non-vascular fluids such as colostrum and breast milk. IgD is found in trace quantities in serum. It serves as a B-lymphocyte surface receptor. IgE is called the reaginic antibody and may be increased in persons with allergy. IgG is the most abundant of the five classes of immunoglobulins and is the major antibody in the secondary humoral response of immunity. It is the only immunoglobulin to cross the placenta. IgM is principally concerned with the primary antibody response.

immunological pregnancy test urinary tests using red cells or latex particles covered with human chorionic gonadotrophin (HCG) rather than biological tests using animals such as mice, rabbits or toads. HCG antiserum is added to urine which, if the woman is pregnant, contains HCG. The HCG antibodies are therefore neutralized and when red cells or latex particles covered with HCG are added to the urine there is no agglutination. If the woman is not pregnant there will be agglutination because the HCG antibodies are not neutralized.

impacted driven into, as a wedge; lodged in a narrow strait, e.g. impacted shoulder presentation.

imperforate having no opening. *I. anus* a congenital malformation requiring surgical treatment.

impetigo blisters or raw patches over the skin, especially trunk and buttocks, usually caused by STAPHYLOCOCCI, more rarely by streptococci. In its severe form it is known as PEMPHIGUS NEONATORUM and is highly contagious.

implant the introduction into the body tissues of drugs or tissue.

implantation the act of planting or setting in, e.g. of the fertilized ovum in the endometrium. *I. bleeding* sometimes called nidation or decidual bleeding. Vaginal bleeding at the time and from the site of embedding of the blastocyst. Because this coincides closely with the first missed menstrual period it may lead to an error in the calculation of the expected date of delivery.

implementation a term used in the nursing process meaning that planned care is carried out.

impotence absence of sexual power. The man is unable to achieve or maintain a penile erection of sufficient rigidity to perform sexual intercourse successfully. adj. *impotent*.

impregnate 1. to saturate or instil. 2. to render pregnant.

imprinting a species-specific, rapid kind of learning during a critical period of early life in which social attachment and identification are established.

IMV *see* INTERMITTENT MANDATORY VENTILATION.

in vitro within a glass, observable in a test tube, in an artificial environment.

in vivo within the living body.

incarcerated imprisoned. Held fast.

incarceration of the retroverted gravid uterus the term is applied to a retroverted pregnant uterus which has failed to correct its position spontaneously, and which has, by the 14th week of pregnancy, grown so large that it is now imprisoned under the sacral promontory, and cannot rise out of the pelvis. It may lead to acute retention of urine, abortion or, very rarely, SACCULATION.

incest sexual activity between persons so closely related that marriage between them is legally or culturally prohibited.

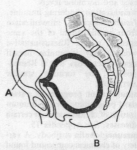

A. *Bladder*, B. *gravid uterus*.
INCARCERATION OF A RETROVERTED GRAVID UTERUS

income support a non-contributory benefit which can be claimed by those over the age of 16 years who are not in full-time work whose income (if any) is insufficient to meet their needs. The main groups who qualify are people over pension age, single parents, the unemployed and those unable to work due to sickness, disability or dependants at home. Those receiving income support are also eligible for other benefits such as free prescriptions, dental treatment and glasses under the NHS.

incompatibility the state of being incompatible, applied to blood or chemicals, etc.

incompatible mutually repellent. Unsuitable for combination.

incomplete abortion an abortion in which some part of the products of conception—usually the placenta—has been retained in the uterus. A cause of serious haemorrhage. *See* Appendix 6.

incontinence inability to control excretory functions. *I. of urine* enuresis. *Stress* i. involuntary escape of urine due to strain on the orifice of the bladder, as in coughing, sneezing or laughing. *Faecal* i. may occur following childbirth if the woman sustains a third degree tear which involves the anal sphincter.

incoordinate lacking in harmony. *Hypertonic* i. *uterine action see* HYPERTONIC.

incubate to place in an optimal situation for the development of living matter, by providing a suitable temperature, humidity and oxygen concentration.

incubation, incubation period the time which elapses between invasion of the body by pathogenic bacteria and the clinical manifestation of the disease. Some common incubation periods are:

Chickenpox	14–15 days
Diphtheria	2–4 days
German measles	17–18 days
Measles	10–14 days
Mumps	14–28 days
Scarlet fever	2–4 days
Smallpox	10–14 days
Whooping cough	7–14 days

incubator 1. an apparatus for providing a suitable environment for low-birth-weight or sick babies. 2. a heated apparatus used to culture micro-organisms in a laboratory.

indigenous occurring naturally in a certain locality.

indomethacin an anti-inflammatory, analgesic and anti-pyretic agent, used in arthritic disorders and degenerative bone disease. Also a prostaglandin inhibitor, thus reduces uterine activity.

induction causing to occur. Used in reference to abortion, anaesthesia or labour. *I. of labour* this may be carried out when the health of the mother or fetus would be impaired by allowing the pregnancy to continue. The method may be (*a*) surgical, i.e. artificial rupture of the membranes (ARM), usually the forewaters (low amniotomy) with forceps, e.g. KOCHER'S, or AMNIOTOMY; or (*b*) medical or hormonal, e.g. oxytocin given intravenously or vaginally as prostaglandins. *See also* Appendix 9.

inertia sluggishness. *Uterine i.* better termed 'hypotonic uterine action'. Inability of the uterine muscle to contract efficiently. A common cause of prolongation of labour. *See* Appendix 9.

inevitable that which cannot be avoided. *I. abortion* the process of abortion at a stage when it is irreversible. *I. (unavoidable) haemorrhage see* PLACENTA PREVIA.

infant a young child from birth to one year of age. *I. feeding* breast and artificial feeding, *see* Appendix 14. *Preterm i.* one born before 37 weeks completed gestation.

infant mortality rate the number of registered deaths of infants under the age of 1 year for every 1000 live births registered in any given year. *See* Appendix 20.

infanticide the murder of an infant.

infantile paralysis POLIOMYELITIS.

infarct an area of necrosis in an organ caused by local ischaemia. In the placenta it is due to an obstruction to the local circulation caused by fibrin deposits in the INTERVILLOUS spaces, so that any VILLI in the area dies from ischaemia. Infarcts occur in ABRUPTIO PLACENTAE and in hypertensive conditions such as pre-eclampsia. Initially in the acute phase they are seen as deep red infarcts, subsequently changing colour, through brown and yellow, to white infarcts, after about a week. If large areas occur, the fetus may die or be

SMALL FOR GESTATIONAL AGE, with all its complications.

infarction the formation of an infarct. *Pulmonary i.* necrosis of the lung tissue, resulting from an embolus.

infection the invasion of tissues by pathogenic micro-organisms. There are several stages in the infectious process: 1. the causative agent, which must be of sufficient number and virulence or capable of destroying normal tissue; 2. reservoirs in which the organism can thrive and reproduce; 3. a portal through which the pathogen can leave the host; e.g. via the intestinal or respiratory tract; 4. a mode of transfer, e.g. the hands, air currents and fomites; 5. a portal of entry through which the pathogens can enter the body, e.g. through open wounds, the respiratory, intestinal and reproductive tracts; 6. susceptible host; not having any immunity to it, or lacking adequate resistance to overcome the invasion by the pathogens. The body responds to the invading organisms by the formation of ANTIBODIES and by a series of physiological changes known as inflammation. *Cross i.* infection transmitted between patients. *Droplet i.* infection due to inhalation of respiratory pathogens suspended on liquid particles exhaled by someone already infected. *Endogenous i.* 1. that due to reactivation of organisms present in a dormant focus, as occurs in tuberculosis; 2. that caused by organisms present in or on the body. *Exogenous i.* that caused by organisms not normally present in the body but which have gained entrance from the body surface of others or from the environment. *Nosocomial i.* hospital-acquired infection.

infertility inability to conceive.

infestation animal parasites on or within the body.

infiltration the entrance and diffusion of some liquid. *I. analgesia* injection of lignocaine into the tissues. *See* Appendix 8.

inflammation a series of changes in tissues indicating their reaction to injury, whether mechanical, chemical or bacterial, so long as the injury does not cause death of the affected part. The cardinal signs are: heat, swelling, pain, redness and loss of function. *Acute i.* the onset is sudden, the signs are marked and progressive. *Chronic i.* a form with slow progress and formation of new connective tissue.

influenza an acute epidemic virus infection of the respiratory tract. It is usually in the form of an acute general illness with fever, generalized aching, pain in the limbs and relatively minor respiratory symptoms. In severe cases pneumonia may follow, usually as a result of secondary bacterial infection.

infra- prefix meaning 'below'.

infundibulum a funnel-shaped structure. The fimbriated end of the fallopian tube.

infusion 1. the process of extracting the soluble principles of substances (especially drugs) by soaking in water. 2. treatment by the introduction of fluid into the body, e.g. dextrose or saline.

ingestion the introduction of food and drugs by the mouth.

inguinal relating to the groin. *I. canal* the channel through the abdominal wall, above Poupart's ligament, through which the spermatic cord and vessels pass to the testicle in the male, and which contains the round ligament of the uterus in the female. *I. hernia, see* HERNIA.

inhalation the breathing of air, vapour or volatile drugs into the lungs. *I. anaesthesia* anaesthesia induced by the inhalation of drugs. *I. analgesia* nitrous oxide and oxygen, or trichlorethylene vapour, inhaled from specially designed machines, and used for the relief of pain in labour. *See* Appendix 8.

inheritance transmission of characteristic or qualities from parent to offspring.

inhibition arresting or restraining.

inhibitor an agent which interferes with or inhibits a reaction.

iniencephaly a congenital malformation with herniation of the brain in the occipital region.

injection the act of introducing a liquid into the body by means of a syringe or other instrument. *Epidural i.* into the EPIDURAL SPACE. *Intradermal i.* into the skin. *Intramuscular i.* into the muscles. *Intrathecal i.* into the theca of the spinal cord. *Intravenous i.* into a vein. *Subcutaneous i.* below the skin.

inlet (pelvic) the brim, the

entrance to the true pelvis. *See* PELVIS.

inner cell mass the group of cells in the cavity of the blastocyst, from which the amniotic membrane and the fetus will develop.

innervation nerve distribution to an organ or part of the body.

innominate without a name. *I. artery* a branch of the arch of the aorta. *I. bone* the hip bone made up of the fused ilium, ischium and os pubis. *See* PELVIS.

inoculation introduction into the body of a protective substance, e.g. antitoxin or vaccine.

inquest a legal or judicial inquiry into some matter of fact. A *coroner's i.* is held in all cases of sudden or unexplained death in order to determine the cause.

insemination introduction of semen into the vagina or cervix. *Artificial i.* insemination by other means than sexual intercourse.

insertion a point of attachment, e.g. of a muscle to a bone or of the cord to the placenta.

insidious a term applied to a disease or condition which develops almost imperceptibly.

insomnia inability to sleep.

inspiration drawing in the breath.

instillation pouring a liquid into a cavity drop by drop, e.g. into the eye.

instruments *see* Appendix 10.

insufficiency a state of inadequate function. *Placental i.* failure of the placenta to fulfil its function adequately. It is often associated with pre-eclampsia, essential hypertension, chronic nephritis, post-maturity and heavy smok-

ing. The effect is to cause the fetus to be SMALL FOR GESTATIONAL AGE or even, in extreme cases, to die *in utero*.

insufflation the blowing of gas, fluid or powder into a cavity. *I. of the fallopian tubes* the blowing of carbon dioxide via the uterus into the fallopian tubes to test their patency. A dye, methylene blue, is now more often used for this purpose.

insulin the HORMONE produced in the islets of Langerhans in the pancreas, which regulates carbohydrate metabolism. Deficiency causes DIABETES MELLITUS. Various preparations of insulin are used in the treatment of diabetes. Overdosage of insulin leads to HYPOGLYCAEMIA.

intelligence quotient (IQ) the assessment of an individual's intelligence, expressed as a ratio of the expected normal for his age.

inter- a prefix signifying 'between'.

interaction the quality, state or process of (two or more things) acting on each other. *Drug i.* the action of one drug upon the effectiveness or toxicity of another (or others).

intercellular between the cells, i.e. the tissue spaces.

intercostal between the ribs. *I. muscles* those of the chest wall.

intermittent having intervals or pauses. Not continuous, e.g. uterine contractions to allow fetal oxygenation.

intermittent mandatory ventilation (IMV) a method used to wean a baby from a ventilator by gradually reducing the ventilator pressure and then the respiratory rate settings.

intermittent positive pressure ventilation (IPPV) a form of respiratory therapy utilizing a VENTILATOR for the treatment of patients with inadequate breathing. Very small babies, or those with severe respiratory distress syndrome, may require virtually all the work of breathing to be done for them. The indications for mechanical ventilation of babies include severe apnoea, a Po_2 of less than 5 kPa despite a high concentration of oxygen in inspired air and a Pco_2 greater than 12 kPa associated with acidosis which fails to respond to treatment. Some paediatricians now ventilate all very-low-birth-weight babies for 24 hours or so in the absence of frank respiratory distress because it is thought to prevent the development of the condition and to avoid such complications as intraventricular haemorrhage. The complications of mechanical ventilation of small babies include pneumothorax, infection, broncho-pulmonary dysplasia and retinopathy of the lens due to high oxygen and possibly carbon dioxide levels. See Appendix 17.

internal os the opening through which the cavity of the cervix communicates with the cavity of the body of the uterus.

internal version usually internal podalic version. Turning the child by intrauterine manipulation to make the breech present.

A manoeuvre once frequently and now occasionally practised during labour to convert the fetus from an oblique to a longitudinal lie or to correct a brow presentation. It consists of inserting a hand into the uterus, grasping one of the child's feet and, with the help of abdominal manipulation, bringing the foot through the cervix to stabilize the presentation.

intersex a person having an abnormality in the sex chromosomes, the gonads, the sex hormones or the genitalia. See KLINEFELTER'S SYNDROME and TURNER'S SYNDROME.

interspinous between the spines. See PELVIS.

interstitial pertaining to a space in the body.

intertrigo an erythematous skin eruption occurring on apposed surfaces of the skin, as the folds of the groin and armpit. It is caused by moisture, warmth, friction, sweat retention and infectious agents. Good hygiene and the application of a talcum containing zinc oxide is the usual treatment.

intervillous between villi. The intervillous spaces allow maternal arterial blood to flow and cascade round the terminal villi of the placenta when gaseous exchange and transport of amino acids, glucose, minerals and vitamins take place.

intestine that part of the alimentary canal which extends from the stomach to the anus. *Small i.* the first 7 m (20 ft) from the pylorus to the caecum, consisting of the duodenum, jejunum and ileum. *Large i.* this is 2 m (6 ft) in length and consists of the caecum, vermiform appendix, ascending, transverse, descending and pelvic colon and rectum. The canal completes the process of digestion and eliminates waste matter.

intra- prefix signifying 'within'.

intracellular within a cell. *I. organisms* those which invade cells, e.g. the gonococcus. *I. fluid* the fluid within the cells of the body.

intracranial within the cranium. *I. membranes* the MENINGES covering the brain. A vertical fold in the midline between the cerebral hemispheres forms the falx cerebri. This joins posteriorly a horizontal fold, the tentorium cerebelli, which separates the cerebellum and cerebrum. *I. pressure* the pressure exerted by the cerebrospinal fluid within the subarachnoid space and ventricles of the brain. It can be measured by monitoring pressure within the cerebral ventricles.

intragastric within the stomach. *I. tube feeding* artificial feeding, usually by naso-gastric tube.

intramuscular within or into muscle.

intrapartum the time between onset of the first stage of labour and completion of the third stage.

intraperitoneal in the peritoneal cavity. By *i. transfusion* it is possible to introduce sufficient Rhesus-negative red cells to replace some of the haemolysed Rhesus-positive cells to prolong the intrauterine life of the affected fetus. *See* Appendix 17.

intrauterine within the uterus. *I. contraceptive device (IUCD)* a mechanical device inserted into the uterine cavity for the purpose of contraception. These devices are made of metallic, plastic or other substances, and are manufactured in various sizes and shapes. Examples include Lippe's loop, Gravigard, Brinberg bow and Hall–Stone ring. Their mode of action is not fully understood but they increase tubal motility, render the endometrium less favourable for implantation and may also increase prostaglandin production, thereby increasing the likelihood of expulsion of the conceptus. *I. death* death of the fetus *in utero*. Generally used to refer to a death during pregnancy rather than one during labour. *I. fetal death (IUFD), see* Appendix 4.

intravascular within a vessel, usually a blood vessel. *I. coagulation* clotting of blood within the circulation.

intravenous within a vein.

intraventricular haemorrhage (IVH) a serious cerebral haemorrhage which occurs in preterm infants below 34 weeks of gestation. It begins on the lateral wall of the ventricle of the brain and causes periods of APNOEA and death. It is now the most common lethal condition in very-low-birth-weight infants (VLBW). It can be diagnosed by COMPUTERIZED AXIAL TOMOGRAPHY (CAT) scan but more con-

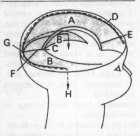

A. *Falx cerebri*; B. *tentorium cerebelli*; C. *great cerebral vein*; D. *superior longitudinal sinus*; E. *inferior longitudinal sinus*; F. *straight sinus*; G. *confluens sinuum*; H. *lateral sinuses leaving skull as internal jugular veins*.

INTRACRANIAL MEMBRANES AND SINUSES

veniently with a portable REAL-TIME ultrasound scanner.

intrinsic relating to a quality of a structure or substance, which is inherent within itself.

introitus the entrance to any cavity of the body. *I. vaginae* the entrance to the vagina.

intubation the introduction of a tube. *Endotracheal i.* introduction of a tube or catheter into the trachea. A doctor or midwife may intubate the trachea of an asphyxiated infant, with the aid of a direct-vision laryngoscope, and insufflate with oxygen or air at a controlled pressure. *See* Appendix 16.

intussusception prolapse of one part of the intestine into the lumen of an immediately adjacent part, causing intestinal obstruction. May occur during the first year of life.

invasion the onset of a disease.

inverse reverse of the normal.

inversion of the uterus a rare condition in which the uterus is partly or completely turned inside out. *Acute i.* occurs in the third stage of labour (*a*) as a result of attempting a CREDÉ EXPRESSION, when the uterus is relaxed; (*b*) by traction on the umbilical cord when the uterus is relaxed and the placenta not completely separated; and (*c*) spontaneously. It causes extreme shock. Replacement should be undertaken as quickly as possible.

involuntary independent of the will.

involution returning to normal size after enlargement, e.g. the uterus after labour. Immediately after labour the uterus weighs about 0.9 kg (2 lb), 1 week later it weighs 0.45 kg (1 lb) and at the end of the puerperium (6–8 weeks) it weighs only about 60 g (2 oz). The length is reduced from about 17.5 cm to about 7.5 cm (from 7 to 3 in). This process is due to ischaemia and AUTOLYSIS of muscle fibre following withdrawal of oestrogen and stimulation of protein synthesis. The soluble end-products are removed by the blood stream. The thrombosed uterine blood vessels also disappear by autolysis and new vessels form. The placental site contracts rapidly at first, then more slowly, and disappears by the 6th or 7th week. *See also* SUBINVOLUTION.

iodide a compound of iodine.

iodine a non-metallic element with a distinctive odour, obtained from seaweed. *Tincture of i.* is the preparation most commonly used. Radioactive iodine is used to evaluate thyroid activity. *See also* ISOTOPE.

ion an electrically charged atom or group of atoms formed when an electrolyte dissolves in water. Hydrogen ions carry a positive charge; hydroxyl ions a negative charge. The hydrogen ion concentration of a fluid determines its reaction, expressed as its pH.

IPPV *see* INTERMITTENT POSITIVE PRESSURE VENTILATION.

iris the coloured part of the eye made of two layers of muscle, the contraction of which alters the size of the pupil.

iritis inflammation of the iris, causing pain, photophobia, contraction of the pupil and discoloration of the iris.

iron a metallic element, which is an important constituent of haemoglobin. Iron compounds ingested in food are converted for use in the body by the action of the hydrochloric acid produced in the stomach. This acid separates the iron from the food and combines with it in a form that is readily assimilable by the body. Vitamin C enhances absorption of iron. The administration of

alkalis hampers iron absorption. The amount of new iron needed every day by an adult is 15 mg. Iron deficiency anaemia is a common problem, especially in pregnancy as a result of increased demands on the mother's blood. Iron-rich foods are advised and, if necessary, iron supplements prescribed.

ischaemia local insufficiency of blood supply.

ischial pertaining to the ischium.

ischium the lower posterior part of the innominate bone of the pelvic girdle.

isoimmunization immunization within the species. This occurs in a Rhesus-negative woman if Rhesus-positive cells from her fetus pass into her circulation via the placenta, causing sensitization and then antibody production (anti-D), to these red cells. When the antibody enters the fetal circulation, HAEMOLYSIS occurs.

isolation the separation of an infected person from those not infected.

isometric maintaining, or pertaining to, the same length; of equal dimensions.

isoniazid an anti-bacterial compound used in treatment of tuberculosis.

isotonic of the same strength or tension. *I. solution* is of the same osmotic pressure as the fluid with which it is compared. Normal, or physiological, saline is isotonic with blood plasma.

isotope an element having the same atomic number, that is the number of protons in the nucleus, but a different number of NEU-TRONS. This leads to instability, often with emission of radioactivity, making even minute quantities identifiable with a Geiger counter.

J

J symbol for joule.

Jacquemier's sign blueness of the lining of the vagina seen from the early weeks of pregnancy due to increased blood supply.

jaundice yellow discoloration of the skin, sclerotics and mucous membranes, due to an excess of bile pigments in the blood and tissues. It may be (*a*) *haemolytic*, when the bile pigment is derived from the haemoglobin of haemolysed red blood cells, or (*b*) *obstructive*, when the bile pigment is present as a constituent of bile. Jaundice may occur in pregnancy from severe HYPEREMESIS GRAVIDARUM, severe pre-eclampsia or eclampsia and acute liver atrophy. It can also be due to coincidental causes such as infective hepatitis, serum hepatitis or drugs. Though rare, these are dangerous conditions, and a midwife observing jaundice during pregnancy in any circumstances should consult a doctor. *Breast milk j.* elevated unconjugated bilirubin in some breast-fed infants due to the presence of a steroid in the breast milk which inhibits glucuronyl transferase conjugating activity.

isoxsuprine a beta-adrenergic stimulant used as a vasodilator in peripheral vascular disease and cerebrovascular insufficiency.

isthmus *see* UTERUS.

Infectious j. 1. infectious hepatitis. 2. leptospiral jaundice. *Physiological j.* mild icterus neonatorum during the first few days of life. For jaundice in the newborn child, *see* Appendix 17.

Jectofer trademark for a preparation of iron sorbitol.

jejunum the portion of the small intestine from the duodenum to the ileum.

jelly a soft, coherent, resilient substance; generally a colloidal semi-solid mass. *Contraceptive j.* a non-greasy jelly used in the vagina for prevention of conception. *Petroleum j.* a purified mixture of semi-solid hydrocarbons obtained from petroleum. *Wharton's j.* the soft, jelly-like intracellular substance of the umbilical cord, which insulates the vein and arteries, preventing occlusion and fetal hypoxia.

joint an articulation. The point of junction of two or more bones. The primary function of a joint is to provide motion and flexibility to the human frame.

joule (J) the international (SI) unit which measures the energy of food, and is replacing CALORIES. One joule = 4.2 calories.

jugular concerning the neck. *J. veins* these are three in number, the *anterior, external* and *internal* jugular veins, and are responsible for carrying blood away from the head.

Jung, Carl Gustav *(1875–1961)* Swiss-born psychologist and psychiatrist; the founder of analytical psychology. Jung's view of the dynamics of personality represents an attempt to interpret human behaviour from a philosophical, religious, and mystical, as well as scientific, viewpoint.

justominor pelvis a small gynaecoid pelvis; all the diameters are reduced but are in proportion.

juxta- word element meaning situated near, adjoining.

juxtaposition apposition; a placing side by side or close together.

K

K chemical symbol, potassium.

k symbol, kilo.

Kabikinase trademark for a preparation of streptokinase used in the treatment of life-threatening venous thrombosis and pulmonary embolism.

Kahn test a blood test to detect syphilis.

kalaemia the presence of potassium in the blood.

kalium potassium (symbol K).

kanamycin a broad-spectrum antibiotic effective against many Gram-negative bacteria, and some Gram-positive and acid-fast bacterial.

kaolin China clay used as a dusting powder and for poultices.

Kaposi's sarcoma a multi-focal metastasizing, malignant reticulosis with angiosarcoma features, involving chiefly the skin. Kaposi's sarcoma is a major feature of AIDS, particularly in homosexuals.

karyo- word element meaning nucleus.

karyotype the chromosomal constitution of the cell nucleus; by extension, photomicrograph of chromosomes arranged in numerical order.

Kegel exercises specific exercises named after Dr Arnold H. Kegel, a gynaecologist who first developed the exercises to strengthen the pelvic–vaginal muscles as a means of controlling stress incontinence in women. The woman is taught the exercises by encouraging her to shut off urine flow while sitting with the legs widely separated. Once the sensation of control is recognized the woman can do the exercises at times other than when she is micturating, and the number of muscle contractions is gradually increased to 300 daily. Strengthening these muscles also aids natural childbirth and contributes to the attainment of orgasm during sexual intercourse.

keloid overgrowth of a fibrous tissue in a scar.

keratin a tough protein which forms the base of all horny tissues.

keratitis inflammation of the cornea.

kernicterus nuclear jaundice. Yellow staining of the basal ganglia of the brain, occurring in infants with severe jaundice, particularly that caused by Rhesus ISOIMMUNIZATION. It is manifested by signs of irritability, fits and athetoid movements of the arms. It may be fatal, or the child may survive but be left with some mental or neurological defect. It may develop in any newborn child in whom the unconjugated serum bile pigment rises above 350 μmol/l (20 mg/100 ml). Infants in whom kernicterus is a danger are treated by one or more replacement transfusions or by phototherapy to prevent development of kernicterus. *See* Appendix 17.

ketoacidosis state of electrolyte imbalance with ketosis and lowered blood pH.

ketone bodies acetone, acetoacetic acid and β-hydroxybutric acid; except for acetone (which may arise spontaneously from acetoacetic acid), they are normal metabolic products of lipids and pyruvate within the liver, and are oxidized by muscles; excessive production leads to urinary excretion of these bodies, as in diabetes mellitus. Called also acetone bodies.

ketonuria the presence of ketones in urine.

ketosis the condition in which ketones are formed in excess in the body. In starvation or in uncontrolled DIABETES MELLITUS, there is a great increase in fatty acid metabolism, and impaired or absent carbohydrate metabolism, which results in greatly increased production of ketone bodies. The production of ketone bodies is reduced to the normal low level and the ketoacidosis is reversed when adequate carbohydrate metabolism is restored. The client with ketosis often has a sweet or 'fruity' odour to his or her breath which is produced by acetone.

key worker a person (commonly a social worker) designated as coordinator for action where several people are involved in the care of a person or family. The key worker is also responsible for calling a CASE CONFERENCE.

kick chart a chart on which the mother herself records fetal movements in a given period of time. Evidence of 10 movements a day is considered acceptable.

kidneys two bean-shaped organs, situated near the lower thoracic and upper lumbar vertebrae and behind the peritoneum. The kidney consists of a cortex and medulla, and is made up of about one million nephrons. The functions of the kidneys are: 1. to maintain the water balance and solute content of the body, thus maintaining the osmotic pressure; 2. to keep the plasma pH constant between 7.35 and 7.45; and 3. to excrete waste products, especially nitrogen from protein metabolism to regulate the blood pressure via the renin–angiotensin–aldosterone mechanism. The kidneys respond to ischaemia by secreting a proteolytic enzyme called RENIN. This acts on a plasma protein (renal substrate) in the blood to produce ANGIOTENSIN I. A converting enzyme from the lungs converts angiotensin I to II, which causes widespread vasoconstriction, increases peripheral resistance and raises the blood pressure. Angiotensin II also effects an increase in blood pressure through its influence on sodium and water retention, by increasing the secretion of aldosterone from the adrenal cortex.

Kielland's forceps obstetric forceps with a sliding lock and no pelvic curve, designed to apply to the fetal head, whatever its position then in the pelvis. The head may then be rotated to an occipitoanterior position with the forceps before it is extracted. *See* Appendix 10.

kilo- the prefix indicating 'one thousand', e.g. kilogram (kg) 1000 grams, kilometre (km) 1000 metres, kilopascal (kPa) 1000 PASCALS, kilocalorie (kcal) 1000 calories.

kiss of life a method of mouth-to-mouth respiration used to resuscitate a person in a state of asphyxia.

Klebsiella a genus of Gram-negative bacteria.

Kleihauer test a microscopic test to detect fetal cells in the maternal circulation, usually done immediately after delivery so that, if the mother is Rhesus-negative and the fetus Rhesus-positive, anti-D immunoglobulin may be given to prevent ISOIMMUNIZATION.

Klinefelter's syndrome an example of intersex. A male with one or more extra X chromosomes. The genitalia appear normal until puberty, when the testes fail to descend and the man is consequently infertile. Development of the breasts also occurs.

Klumpke's paralysis paralysis of the lower arm and hand, resulting in wrist-drop. It is due to injury to the lower part of the BRACHIAL PLEXUS, the eighth cervical and first dorsal nerves. It may occur when bringing down extended arms in a breech labour, or by applying undue traction when releasing the anterior shoulder in a vertex delivery.

knee presentation a type of breech presentation in which one or both knees lie below the buttocks.

Kocher's forceps artery forceps used at birth to clamp the umbilical cord before separation; may also be used for artificial rupture of the membranes.

Konakion trademark for preparation of phytomenadione, a vitamin K preparation.

Koplik's spots small, irregular, bright red spots on the buccal and lingual mucosa, with a minute bluish white speck in the centre of each; they are pathognomonic of beginning measles.

Körner data sets information items for England recommended in a series of reports published from 1982 by the Steering Group on Health Services Information (chaired by Mrs E. Körner). The data sets cover a wide range of hospital and community activity and are designed for use by local managers in planning and monitoring services, and from these, information to meet central requirements are derived. Implementation data relating to the maternity and community services have been collected from April 1988.

Korotkoff's method a method of finding the systolic and diastolic blood pressure by listening to the sounds produced in an artery while the pressure in a previously inflated cuff is gradually reduced.

Kwashiorkor a condition occurring in babies and young children due to severe protein deficiency. Symptoms include oedema, impaired growth and development, distension of the abdomen (pot belly), pathological liver changes and pigmentation changes of skin and hair.

kyphosis posterior curvature of the spine; humpback.

L

labetalol an alpha and beta adrenergic receptor blocker used in the treatment of hypertension.

labial pertaining to the lips or labia.

labile unstable. Liable to variation. *L. hypertension* a term used in reference to a patient whose blood pressure is variable between normal and an appreciably higher level.

labium a lip. *L. majus pudendi* the large fold of flesh surrounding the vulva. *L. minus pudendi* the lesser fold within. pl. *labia*.

labour parturition or childbirth. Literally, the process by which the products of conception are expelled from the uterus via the birth canal. It normally occurs spontaneously at term, that is, between 38 and 42 weeks of pregnancy. The fetus should present by the vertex and, once started, the contractions should increase in length, strength and frequency without interruption or artificial stimulation until the baby, placenta and membranes have been completely expelled by maternal effort via the vagina. The whole process should be completed without undue trauma to mother or baby within 18 hours. Labour takes place in 3 stages: 1. dilatation of the cervix uteri; 2. expulsion of the fetus, following full dilatation of the cervix, from the birth canal; and 3. expulsion of the placenta and membranes. *Obstructed l.* labour in which there is an insuperable obstruction to delivery. *Precipitate l.* one in which the first, second and third stages of labour are completed in unusually short

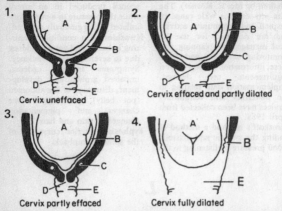

1. Cervix uneffaced
2. Cervix effaced and partly dilated
3. Cervix partly effaced
4. Cervix fully dilated

A. *Fetal head*; B. *membranes*; C. *internal os*; D. *external os*; E. *vagina*.

PHYSIOLOGICAL CHANGES IN THE CERVIX DURING THE FIRST STAGE OF LABOUR

time. A form of abnormal uterine action which may produce extremely powerful but frequently painless uterine contractions. *Premature l.* a loose term for labour occurring after the 24th week of pregnancy and before full term. *Spontaneous l.* that which occurs without being artificially induced or accelerated. *Spurious l.* contractions which occur without any change in the state of the cervix, so that there is no progress towards delivery. Also called false labour. For normal labour, *see* Appendix 7.

laceration tear. *Perineal l. see* PERINEAL.

lacrimal pertaining to tears. *L. ducts* minute openings at the inner end of each eyelid, which convey the fluid into the nose by the nasolacrimal duct to mix with the secretions of the nose. *L. glands* small bodies situated in the orbital cavity at the upper and outer surface of each eyeball, the function of which is to provide the fluid (tears) which keeps the conjunctiva moist and free from infection by LYSOZYME, except in the neonate.

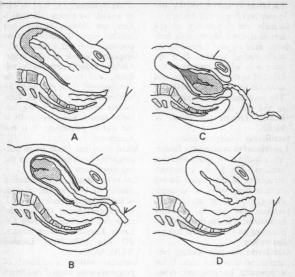

Showing the placenta. A. Before birth of child; B. partially separated immediately after birth; C. completely separated; D. contraction and retraction of uterus after expulsion.

THIRD STAGE OF LABOUR

lactalbumin the main protein in human milk. It is easily digested by the baby.

lactase an enzyme produced by the cells of the small intestine, which splits LACTOSE into the MONOSACCHARIDES GLUCOSE and GALACTOSE.

lactation the secretion of milk by the breasts. *L. period* the period during which a child is suckled. Lactation is brought about by the lactogenic hormone, prolactin, which increases after delivery when the level of oestrogen falls. Milk is produced from about the third day after delivery and is expelled along the ducts of the breast by oxytocin, a hormone released when the baby sucks.

Lactation is maintained by frequent suckling at the breast.

lacteals the lymphatics of the intestine which absorb split fats.

lactic acid an acid formed in the body during hypoxia. It is the main acid which appears in the blood of an asphyxiated baby, and accounts for the high ACIDAEMIA. The acid may also be produced in the gut by fermentation of lactose through the action of bacilli.

lactiferous conveying milk.

Lactobacillus acidophilus Döderlein's bacillus. A GRAM-POSITIVE bacillus, which is a normal inhabitant of the vagina during child-bearing years. It converts glycogen to lactic acid, which inhibits the growth of other organisms; it is also found predominating in the stools of breast-fed babies.

lactoferrin the iron-binding protein found in human milk. It has a powerful bacteriostatic effect on E. COLI.

lactogen any substance that enhances lactation. *Human placental l. (HPL)* a hormone secreted by the placenta, which disappears from the blood immediately after delivery. It has lactogenic, luteotrophic and growth-promoting activity, and inhibits maternal insulin activity during pregnancy.

lactoglobulin a globulin occurring in milk.

lactose milk sugar, a DISACCHAR-IDE. *L. intolerance* this can cause diarrhoea in the neonate, as the lactose may not be split if there is not sufficient LACTASE. It can be treated by giving milk which does not contain lactose, but another sugar. It should not be confused with GALACTOSAEMIA.

lactosuria lactose in the urine. Lactose reduces Benedict's solution, and lactosuria must be distinguished from glycosuria by further tests, e.g. Clinistix. Lactosuria often occurs in the lactation period, and occasionally at the end of pregnancy. It is not significant.

laked describes blood when haemoglobin has separated from the red blood cells.

LaLeche League an organization formed in 1957 for the purpose of helping women to breast feed. Information about the organization can be obtained from La-Leche League of Great Britain, PO Box BM 3424, London WC1V 6XX.

Lamaze method a method of preparation for natural childbirth developed by the French obstetrician Fernand Lamaze, and based on the Russian psychoprophylactic technique of training the mind and body for the purpose of modifying the perception of pain during labour and delivery. Both parents attend classes, and are taught about the process of labour and special exercises that develop neuromuscular control, promote physical conditioning, and eliminate or reduce the need for drugs and instruments during delivery.

lambda the posterior fontanelle of the skull, so called from its resemblance to the Greek letter lambda (λ).

lambdoid suture the suture between the occipital bone and the two parietal bones.

Lancefield classification the classification of haemolytic streptococci into groups on the basis of serological action.

Landsteiner's classification a classification of blood groups in which they are designated O, A, B and AB, depending on the presence or absence of agglutinogens A and B in the erythrocytes; called also international classification.

Langerhans' islets collections of specialized cells in the pancreas, producing insulin which controls carbohydrate metabolism. Disease of the islet cells causes DIABETES MELLITUS.

Langhans' cell layer cytotrophoblast. The inner layer of the TROPHOBLAST.

lanolin wool fat used as a basis for ointments.

lanugo the fine hair covering the fetus *in utero*. Most of it has disappeared by the time the child is born at term.

laparoscope an instrument for examination of the peritoneal cavity.

laparoscopy examination of the interior of the abdomen by means of a LAPAROSCOPE.

laparotomy exploratory opening of the abdominal cavity.

Largactil a proprietary preparation of CHLORPROMAZINE; an anti-emetic and tranquillizer.

laryngoscope an endoscopic instrument for inspecting the larynx and vocal cords and aiding the insertion of an endotracheal tube.

larynx the organ of the voice, situated at the upper end of the trachea. It has a muscular and cartilaginous frame, lined with mucous membrane. Across it are spread the vocal cords of elastic tissue. The space between the cords is termed the glottis.

laser a device that transfers electromagnetic radiation of various frequencies into an extremely intense, small and nearly nondivergent beam of monochromatic radiation in the visible region, with all the waves in phase; from light amplification by simulated emission of radiation. Capable of mobilizing immense heat and power when focused at close range, it is used as a tool in surgery, in diagnosis and in physiological studies.

Lasix trademark for preparations of frusemide, a diuretic.

latent hidden; not manifest. *L. period* a seemingly inactive period.

lateral relating to the side.

'laughing gas' NITROUS OXIDE.

lavage washing out a cavity. *Colonic l.* of the colon. *Gastric l.* of the stomach.

laxative a medicine that loosens the bowel contents and encourages evacuation. A laxative with a mild or gentle effect on the bowels is also known as an aperient; one with a strong effect is referred to as a cathartic or a purgative. It can be dangerous to use purgatives in pregnancy because they may stimulate uterine activity and thereby bleeding.

Leboyer method a method of childbirth advocated by a French doctor, Leboyer. He is especially concerned with the baby being born gently and quietly. The room is darkened for the delivery, and the baby born in quietness and lifted on to its mother's abdomen; the baby is then put into a warm bath. It is claimed that the baby will cry less and become a more contented child and adult because the shock of delivery is minimized.

lecithin a complex molecule of protein and fatty acid which is found in the alveoli of the lung. SURFACTANT is a lecithin and helps to keep the lungs open. The lecithin which is produced in the fetal lung flows out into the amniotic fluid, where it can be measured to give an indication of fetal maturity. *L./sphingomyelin ratio* lecithin, but not sphingomyelin, is produced in greater quantities as pregnancy progresses. Therefore the ratio increases with fetal lung maturity. A ratio of 2 or more indicates that there is little or no risk of respiratory distress in the neonate. Abbreviated L/S ratio.

length an expression of the longest dimension of an object, or of the measurement between its two ends. The internationally accepted (SI) unit of length is the metre (m). *Crown–heel l.* the distance from the crown of the head to the heel in embryos, fetuses and infants; the equivalent standing height in older persons. *Crown–rump l.* the distance from the crown of the head to the breech in embryos, fetuses and infants; the equivalent of sitting height in older persons. Measured by B-mode ultrasound during the first 14 weeks of pregnancy to assess fetal maturity; accurate to within 3 to 4 days.

lesion an injury, wound or morbid structural change in an organ. Used as a general term for a local morbid condition.

Lethidrone a proprietary preparation of NALORPHINE. It was formerly used in the neonate, but was discovered to increase respiratory depression and so has been replaced by NALOXONE (NARCAN). See Appendix 19.

leucocyte a white blood corpuscle.

leucocytosis an increase in the number of leucocytes in the blood, usually as a response to infection.

leucopenia decreased number of leucocytes in the blood.

leucorrhoea a white, mucoid, non-irritating vaginal discharge. The glands of the cervix normally secrete a certain amount of mucus-like fluid that moistens the membranes of the vagina. The discharge is frequently increased at the time of ovulation, before a menstrual period and throughout pregnancy. It is also stimulated by sexual excitement. It should be white, inoffensive and non-irritating. Otherwise infections should be suspected and investigations carried out.

leukaemia an uncommon malignant blood disease. It is characterized by a marked increase in abnormal leucocytes. It is accompanied by a reduced number of erythrocytes and blood platelets, resulting in anaemia and increased susceptibility to infection and haemorrhage. The precise cause of leukaemia is not known. Much research has been directed towards exploring the possibility of a virus or a genetic defect as the cause. Radiation is an established factor in myeloid leukaemia.

levallorphan an analogue of levorphanol, which acts as an antagonist to analgesic narcotics.

levator a muscle which raises a part.

levator ani a broad sheet of muscle, which forms the principal part of the pelvic floor.

libido sexual desire.

Librium trademark for preparation of chlordiazepoxide, a tranquillizer.

lie the relation of the long axis of the fetus to the long axis of the mother's uterus. Normally these are parallel and the lie is said to be longitudinal. Abnormally, the fetus lies across the mother's uterus, the lie is transverse or oblique and, unless this is corrected, labour will become obstructed.

ligament a tough fibrous band of tissue connecting bones or supporting internal organs. The ligaments which support the uterus are (a) transverse cervical or cardinal l., (b) pubocervical l.

and (c) uterosacral l. The round ligaments extend from the cornua of the uterus to the labia majora. The broad ligaments are folds of peritoneum, adjacent to that of the uterus and covering the fallopian tubes so they are not true ligaments.

ligation the process of applying a ligature.

ligature a thread, usually of catgut, nylon or wire, used for tying blood vessels.

light for dates See SMALL FOR GESTATIONAL AGE BABY.

lightening the relief experienced in the late stages of pregnancy when the presenting part sinks into the pelvis and the fundus ceases to press on the diaphragm, usually shortly after 36th week in primigravidae and just before or after the onset of labour in multiparae.

lignocaine (Xylocaine) a drug used for infiltration analgesia and nerve block.

linea a line. L. alba the tendinous area in the centre of the abdominal wall into which the transversalis and part of the oblique muscles are inserted. L. nigra the pigmented line which often appears, during pregnancy, on the abdomen between the umbilicus and pubis, at times extending up to the ensiform cartilage.

lint a loosely woven cotton fabric, one side of which is fluffy, and the other smooth, used for surgical dressings.

lipase an ENZYME, present in pancreatic juice, which splits fat into fatty acids.

Lippe's loop an intrauterine contraceptive device.

liquor amnii the fluid which fills the amniotic sac surrounding the fetus. The composition is similar to that of intracellular fluid: about 99 per cent water, containing proteins, fats and carbohydrates, sodium and potassium in solution, with debris consisting of desquamated fetal epithelial cells, vernix caseosa, lanugo and various enzymes and pigments. Its functions are: (a) it acts as a shock absorber; (b) it allows unhindered growth; (c) it distributes pressure evenly over the whole fetus; (d) it permits the free movement necessary for muscle function; and (e) it prevents diminution of the placental site. The volume is approximately 1 litre at 37–38 weeks' gestation, but this diminishes by nearly half at term. *See also* AMNIOCENTESIS.

Lister, Baron Joseph (1827–1912) Founder of modern antiseptic surgery.

Listeria a genus of Gram-negative bacteria. It produces upper respiratory disease, septicaemia and encephalitic disease.

lithopaedion a dead fetus that has become petrified owing to lime salt deposition. This occurs only in a fetus that has undergone extrauterine development and so is very rare.

lithotomy position the woman lies on her back with thighs and legs flexed and abducted and held in place with lithotomy poles. This position is adopted for forceps or breech delivery and for perineal suturing.

litmus paper blotting paper impregnated with litmus, a pigment which is used to ascertain the reaction of fluids. Blue litmus is turned red by acids and red litmus is turned blue by alkalis.

litre a measure of volume, 1000 ml or about 35 fl. oz.

live birth an infant which is born alive.

liver the large wedge-shaped gland situated in the right hypochondrium and epigastrium. It is essential to life. Its chief functions are: (a) formation of bile; (b) production of plasma proteins except GAMMA GLOBULINS; (c) storage of carbohydrates as glycogen, iron and vitamins A, D, E and K; (d) regulation of metabolism of fat, protein and carbohydrate; (e) detoxication of drugs and other substances; (f) the formation and destruction of ERYTHROCYTES; (g) production of PROTHROMBIN; and FIBRINOGEN; (h) heat production; and (i) phagocytic action on bacteria.

livid cyanotic. The blueness is associated with venous congestion and an inadequate supply of oxygen.

lobe a section of an organ, separated from neighbouring parts by fissures.

lobule a small segment or lobe, especially one of the smaller divisions making up a lobe. adj. *lobular*.

local authority the local government.

local supervising authority the

authority designated to undertake the statutory supervision of midwives, according to the rules of the United Kingdom Central Council (UKCC). Regional Health Authorities in England, District Health Authorities in Wales, Health Boards in Scotland, and Health and Social Services Boards in Northern Ireland are designated as Local Supervising Authorities (LSAs). The LSAs appoint supervisors of midwives, most of whom are the senior midwifery managers within health authorities. A midwife should contact the local supervisor of midwives on all matters as required by the Midwives' Rules and Code of Practice, and for help and advice on any other professional matter.

lochia the discharge from the uterus following childbirth or abortion, consisting of blood from the placental site, shreds of decidua, shed vaginal epithelial cells and, at first, debris from the uterus, e.g. liquor amnii, vernix caseosa and meconium. *L. alba* (whitish) contains white blood cells and mucus. *L. rubra* (red) is largely fresh and then staler blood. *L. serosa* (pinkish) contains fewer red and more white cells. Lochia may be expected to continue for 2–3 weeks or possibly rather longer. Red, profuse lochia should raise the suspicion of subinvolution or infection. An offensive odour is indicative of infection.

locked twins the condition of twins with their bodies and heads so placed that neither can be born naturally; a rare cause of obstructed labour.

locus place; site; in genetics, the specific site of a gene on a chromosome.

lordosis exaggeration of the normal forward curve of the lumbar spine. A moderate degree is common in pregnancy, as a result of faulty posture. The weight of the uterus pulls the body forwards and, to compensate this, the woman leans backwards, thus throwing extra strain on the relaxed sacroiliac joints and causing backache.

Lövset's manoeuvre a manoeuvre whereby the fetal shoulders are delivered when the arms are extended during breech labour. It consists in rotating the fetus through a half circle, keeping the back uppermost, so as to bring the posterior arm into an anterior position below the symphysis pubis, where it can be delivered. The fetus is then rotated a half circle in the reverse direction and the second arm is similarly delivered. *See* Appendix 9.

low-birth-weight baby any baby weighing 2.5 kg or less at birth. Low-birth-weight babies may be: 1. preterm, if born before 37 completed weeks of pregnancy; or 2. small for gestational age, if the birth weight is below the tenth centile for gestational age. Some babies are both preterm and small for gestational age. *See* Appendix 17.

lower uterine segment the part of the UTERUS lying between the vesicouterine peritoneal fold superiorly and the junction of the uterus and cervix inferiorly.

lubricant a cream, jelly or similar substance applied to the hands, gloves or instruments in order to make them slippery and to facilitate manipulations.

lumbar pertaining to the loins. *L. puncture* introduction of a hollow needle into the subarachnoid space, usually between the 4th and 5th lumbar vertebrae, to withdraw cerebrospinal fluid. This may be carried out for diagnostic purposes, to relieve pressure or to introduce drugs.

lumen the space inside a tube.

lumpectomy the surgical excision of only the local lesion (benign or malignant) of the breast.

lungs a pair of conical organs of the respiratory system. Consisting of an arrangement of air tubes (bronchi and bronchioles), terminating in air spaces (alveoli); they occupy most of the thoracic cavity. The lungs supply the blood with oxygen inhaled from the outside air, and they dispose of waste carbon dioxide in the exhaled air, as a part of the process known as respiration.

luteal pertaining to the CORPUS LUTEUM.

lutein the yellow pigment in the corpus luteum.

luteinizing hormone a hormone secreted by the anterior lobe of the pituitary gland acting, with follicular-stimulating hormone, to cause ovulation of mature follicles and secretion of oestrogen by thecal and granulosa cells of the ovary; it is also concerned with formation of the corpus luteum. In the male, it stimulates development of the interstitial cells of the testes and their secretion of testosterone.

lying-in period *see* POSTNATAL PERIOD.

lymph a body fluid, derived from the fluid in the tissue spaces and carried in lymphatic vessels back to the blood stream. It is similar in composition to tissue fluid. Lymph nodes occur at intervals in the course of the lymphatic vessels. Their function is to act as a filter.

lymphatics vessels carrying lymph.

lymphocytes white blood cells, formed mainly from the lymphoid tissue in the bone marrow and thymus.

lyse to cause disintegration of a cell or substance.

lysin a cell-dissolving substance present in blood serum.

lysis 1. a gradual decline, e.g. of a fever. 2. a breaking down, as in haemolysis; a breaking down or destruction of red blood cells.

Lysol a strong proprietary disinfectant and antiseptic, prepared from cresol.

lysozyme an antibacterial (Grampositive) agent present in all tissues and secretions, particularly in tears and breast milk.

lytic cocktail a combination of chlorpromazine, promethazine and pethidine, which can be used in the treatment of severe preeclampsia and eclampsia. Promethazine and pethidine only may be used. It induces deep sleep, aids muscular relaxation and lowers the blood pressure. Less commonly used now. *See* Appendix 6.

M

M 1. an antigen found in the red blood cells of certain persons; hence, a blood group. *See also* N. 2. mil or mille (thousand). 3. symbol, mega. 4. symbol, molar (solution).

m symbol, metre; symbol, milli-.

m- symbol, meta-.

maceration the process of softening a solid by means of soaking. Maceration occurs when a dead fetus is retained in the uterus for more than 24 hours. It is characterized by discoloration, softening of tissues, peeling of the fetal skin and eventual disintegration of a fetus retained in the uterus after its death. It indicates that a stillbirth has been dead *in utero* before the commencement of labour, and may lead to disseminated intravascular coagulation.

Mackenrodt's ligaments the transverse or cardinal ligaments that support the uterus in the pelvic cavity.

macro- prefix meaning 'large'.

macrocyte an abnormally large red blood corpuscle found in the blood in megaloblastic anaemia of pregnancy due to folic acid deficiency.

macrophage any of the large, mononuclear highly phagocytic cells derived from monocytes that occur in the walls of blood vessels and in loose connective tissue. They are components of the reticuloendothelial system and become actively mobile when stimulated by inflammation; they also interact with lymphocytes to facilitate antibody production.

macroscopic discernible with the naked eye.

macrosociology an approach which looks at whole societies, how they are organized and the effects of the organisation on the population. The works of Karl Marx, Max Weber and Emile Durkheim are examples of this perspective.

magnesium an element. Symbol Mg. A bluish white metal. Minute quantities are essential to life, being required for the activity of many enzymes, especially those concerned with oxidative phosphorylation. It is found in intra- and extracellular fluids and is excreted in urine and faeces. The normal serum level is approximately 1 mmol/l. Magnesium deficiency causes irritability of the nervous system with tetany, vasodilation, convulsions, tremors, depression and psychotic behaviour. *M. sulphate* a saline purgative (Epsom salts). *M. trisilicate* an antacid powder used in the treatment of dyspepsia, peptic ulcer and heartburn, and to reduce the acidity of the gastric contents prior to general anaesthesia, particularly during labour to reduce risk of MENDELSON'S SYNDROME.

magnetic resonance imaging (MRI) an imaging technique based on the NUCLEAR MAGNETIC RESONANCE properties of the hydrogen nucleus. Cross-sectional images in any plane may be obtained and the images may represent one or more of several properties.

maintenance order a court order requiring a person to give a regular payment to someone for whom he/she has a responsibility, e.g. a father of a child.

mal- a prefix meaning 'bad', 'wrong', or 'ill'. *Grand m.* a generalized convulsive seizure attended by loss of consciousness. *See also* EPILEPSY. *Petit m.* momentary loss of consciousness without convulsive movements. *See also* EPILEPSY.

malabsorption impaired intestinal absorption of nutrients. *M. syndrome* a group of disorders marked by subnormal intestinal absorption of dietary constituents, and thus excessive loss of nutrients in the stool.

malacia softening of tissues. *Osteomalacia* softening of bone tissue, one effect being deformity of the pelvic bones. It is uncommon in developed countries.

malaise a feeling of general discomfort and illness.

malar pertaining to the malar bone or the region adjacent to it.

male reproductive system consists of two testes (A). These are contained within the scrotum (B) and have the sperm formed within them. A fine tubular system, the epididymis (C), collects the sperm which are then conveyed by a long tube, the vas deferens (D). This passes along the inguinal canal to run by the bladder, for the sperm to be stored in the seminal vesicles (E). When ejaculation occurs, the prostate gland (F) adds fluid to the sperm, which are then passed into the urethra (G) inside the erect penis (H). At intercourse the sperm are deposited in the posterior fornix of the VAGINA.

malformation an anatomical abnormality. Often a deformity, either congenital or acquired.

malignant tending to become progressively worse and to result in death; having the properties of anaplasia, invasiveness and metastasis; said of tumours.

malnutrition the condition in which nutrition is defective in quantity or quality.

Malpighian body the glomerulus and Bowman's capsule of the kidney.

malposition misplaced situation of any organ or part in relationship to neighbouring structures or parts. The term is applied to a fetus with its occiput directed towards one or other posterior quadrant of the pelvis.

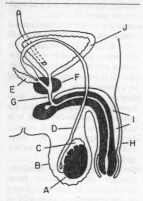

A. *Testes*; B. *scrotum*; C. *epididymis*; D. *vas deferens*; E. *seminal vesicle*; F. *prostate gland*; G. *urethra*; H. *penis*; I. *erectile tissue*; J. *bladder*.

MALE REPRODUCTIVE SYSTEM

malpractice any professional misconduct, unreasonable lack of skill or fidelity in professional duties, or illegal or immoral conduct. Malpractice is one form of negligence, which in legal terms can be defined as the omission to do something that a reasonable person would do, or the doing of something that a reasonable and prudent person would not do. In midwifery malpractice results in injury, unnecessary suffering, or death to the mother or baby.

malpresentation any presentation of the fetus other than the vertex. It may be a breech, face, brow or shoulder presentation.

maltase a sugar-splitting enzyme which converts maltose to glucose. Present in pancreatic and intestinal juice.

maltose a sugar (disaccharide) formed when starch is hydrolysed by amylase.

mamma the breast.

mammal a member of a division of vertebrates, including all that possess hair and suckle their offspring.

mammary pertaining to the breasts.

mammilla the nipple.

mammography radiography of the breast with or without injection of an opaque substance into its ducts. Simple mammography, without the use of contrast medium, is a routine screening procedure for the diagnosis of cancer and other disorders of the breast.

Manchester operation amputation of the cervix, with anterior and posterior colporrhaphy.

mandelic acid a keto acid used as a urinary antiseptic in nephritis, pyelitis, and cystitis.

mandible a horseshoe-shaped bone forming the lower jaw.

mania mental disorder characterized by exaltation and acceleration of all mental processes, often culminating in violence. It may follow childbirth.

manic-depressive psychosis a

mental illness characterized by mania or ENDOGENOUS DEPRESSION. The attacks may alternate between mania and depression or the patient may just have recurrent attacks of mania or depression.

manipulation using the hands in a skilful manner, such as in changing the position of the fetus.

mannitol a sugar alcohol occurring widely in nature, especially in fungi; an osmotic diuretic used for forced diuresis and in cerebral oedema.

manoeuvre similar to manipulation. A procedure carried out with the hands, e.g. to facilitate delivery or to speed the placenta. *See* LÖVSET'S M. *and* MAURICEAU.

manometer an instrument for measuring the pressure or tension of liquids or gases. *See* SPHYGMOMANOMETER.

Mantoux reaction reaction to the *Mantoux test*, which consists of an intradermal injection of old tuberculin to determine susceptibility to tuberculosis. A weal developing in hours indicates a positive reaction. This signifies that a previous infection has conferred some degree of immunity.

manual with the hand. *M. removal of the placenta* introducing a hand into the uterus to remove a retained placenta.

maple syrup urine disease a genetic disorder involving deficiency of an enzyme necessary in the metabolism of branched-chain amino-acids, marked clinically by mental and physical handicap, feeding difficulties and a characteristic odour of urine.

marasmus severe malnutrition and weight loss in babies associated with a form of protein-calorie deficiency, but usually with retention of appetite and mental alertness. It is considered to be related to KWASHIORKOR.

Marcain (Bupivacaine) a local anaesthetic, commonly used for epidural anaesthesia when it is usually effective for 2–3 hours.

Marevan trademark for preparations of WARFARIN, an anticoagulant.

Marfan's syndrome a hereditary disorder of connective tissue characterized by abnormal length of the extremities, especially of the fingers and toes, subluxation of the lens, congenital anomalies of the heart and other deformities.

marijuana, marihuana a preparation of the leaves and flowering tops of *Cannabis sativa*, the hemp plant, which contains a number of pharmacologically active principles. Hashish, also derived from the hemp plant, is obtained from the clear resin secreted by the flowering tops of the plant and is thought to be more potent than marijuana. Both drugs are used for their euphoric properties and are 3 or 4 times more potent when smoked and inhaled than when ingested. Its possession is illegal in many countries, including the UK. There is some evidence that marijuana increases the risk of miscarriage and birth defects.

marrow the soft, organic, sponge-like material in the cavities of bones. Its chief function is to manufacture erythrocytes, leukocytes and platelets. The bone marrow is occasionally subject to disease, as in aplastic anaemia, which may be caused by the destruction of the marrow by chemical agents or excessive X-ray exposure. Other diseases that affect the bone marrow are leukaemia, pernicious anaemia, myeloma and metastatic tumours.

mask a covering for the nose and mouth, worn to prevent the spread of droplet infection.

massage systematic therapeutic stroking or kneading of the body. *Cardiac m.* intermittent compression of the heart by pressure applied over the sternum (closed cardiac massage) or directly to the heart through an opening in the chest wall (open cardiac massage).

mastitis inflammation of the breast. Puerpural mastitis is an infection resulting usually from the presence of staphylococci and occasionally streptococci, which usually enter through cracked nipples. A wedge-shaped area of the breast becomes tender, red and warm and the woman feels generally unwell. The condition responds quickly to antibiotic treatment. Delay in treatment may lead to the development of an abscess which needs to be incised and drained.

materia medica the science of the source and preparation of drugs used in medicine.

maternal pertaining to the mother. *M. mortality* death due to pregnancy or childbearing. *M. mortality rate see* Appendix 20.

maternity pertaining to childbearing. *M. benefits see* Appendix 5.

matrix the intercellular substance of a tissue, as bone matrix, or the tissue from which a structure develops, as hair or nail matrix.

Matthews Duncan expulsion of placenta the placenta is expelled maternal side first at the end of the third stage of labour. There is rather more bleeding and the placenta was probably lying lower in the uterus than in the SCHULTZE EXPULSION.

maturation ripening or developing. In biology, a process of cell division during which the number of chromosomes in the germ cell is reduced to one-half the number characteristic of the species.

Mauriceau a famous French male midwife. *M.–Smellie-Veit manoeuvre* a method of delivering the aftercoming head in a breech delivery. Flexion is increased, and jaw and shoulder traction applied. *See* Appendix 9.

Maxolon trademark for a preparation of metoclopramide, an anti-emetic.

MCH mean corpuscular haemoglobin; an expression of the average haemoglobin content of a single cell in picograms. Normal range 27–33 pg.

MCHC mean corpuscular haemoglobin concentration, an expression of the average haemoglobin concentration in grams per decilitre (g/dl). Normal range 32–35 g/dl.

MCV mean corpuscular volume; an expression of the average volume of individual red cells in femtolites.

mean an average; a numerical value intermediate between two extremes.

measles a highly infectious disease caused by a virus; called also rubeola or morbilli. Routine immunization with live attenuated vaccine (in combination with mumps and rubella vaccines) is given in the UK in the second year of life.

meatus an opening or passage. *Auditory m.* the opening leading into the auditory canal. *Urinary m.* where the urethra opens to the exterior.

mechanism of labour the sequence of movements whereby the fetus adapts itself to pass through the maternal passages during the process of birth.

meconium the material present in the fetal intestinal tract, which is passed per rectum during the first few days of life. It is greenish black in colour and contains bile pigments and salts, mucus, intestinal epithelial cells and, usually, liquor amnii. *M. aspiration* the inhalation of liquor containing meconium, which can occur in babies who have been hypoxic in *utero*, especially those who are growth-retarded. *See* Appendix 16. *M. ileus* gross distention of the bowel with inspissated meconium found in CYSTIC FIBROSIS.

median situation in the median plan or in the midline of a body or structure. *M. nerve* a nerve that originates in the brachial plexus and innervates muscles of the wrist and hand. *M. plane* an imaginary plane passing longitudinally through the body from front to back and dividing it into right and left halves.

mediastinum. 1. a median septum or partition. 2. the mass of tissues and organs separating the sternum in front and the vertebral column behind, containing the heart and its large vessels, trachea, oesophagus, thymus, lymph nodes and other structures and tissues. It is divided into anterior, middle posterior and superior regions.

medical pertaining to medicine. *M. aid* The services of a doctor can be obtained, and should be sought by the midwife, for any complication which may arise during pregnancy, labour or the puerperium. *M. audit* an evaluation process applied to the quality of clinical practice, often by peer review of routine or specially collected records of individual cases. *M. certificate* replaced (since 1976) by medical statement. *M. statement* provided by a doctor to advise how long a patient should refrain from work. When claiming sickness benefit the statement must be sent to the local social security office.

medicine 1. any drug or remedy. 2. the art and science of the diagnosis and treatment of disease and the maintenance of health.

3. the non-surgical treatment of disease.

medium 1. an agent by which something is accomplished or an impulse is transmitted. 2. a substance providing the proper nutritional environment for the growth of micro-organisms; also called culture medium.

MEDLARS acronym for Medical Literature Analysis and Retrieval System, a computerized bibliographic system of the National Library of Medicine (Bethesda, MD, USA), from which the *Index Medicus* is produced. The system is available in major national libraries.

MEDLINE acronym for MEDLARS on-line, a computerized bibliographical retrieval system, an on-line segment of MEDLARS.

medulla the central or inner portion of an organ. *M. oblongata* the lowest part of the brain-stem, lying between the pons varolii and the spinal cord. It is the seat of the vital centres, i.e. the cardiac, respiratory and vasomotor centres.

mega (M) word element meaning 'large'; used in naming units of measurement to designate an amount of 10^6 (one million) times the size of the unit to which it is joined, as in megacuries (10^6 curies).

megalo- a prefix meaning 'great'.

megaloblastic anaemia an anaemia which occurs in pregnancy, in which immature red cells circulate in the blood. It is due to a deficiency of folic acid.

megaloblasts large nucleated

immature red blood cells, normally present in the bone marrow.

meiosis the process by which the germinal epithelium in either ovary or testis gives rise to a gamete containing only one CHROMOSOME from each pair. This number is called the haploid and is 23 in man; the normal number is the diploid, and is 46 in man.

melaena the presence of dark, altered blood in the stools. It occurs in haemorrhagic disease of the newborn and may be accompanied by HAEMATEMESIS.

melanin dark pigment found in hair, choroid coat, etc. It is sometimes deposited in malignant tumours.

melanocyte-stimulating hormone (MSH) a peptide from the anterior pituitary that influences the formation or deposition of melanin in the body.

membrane a thin tissue covering the surface of certain organs and lining the cavities of the body. *Mucous m.* contains secreting cells, and lines all cavities connected directly or indirectly with the skin. *Membranes* the fetal membranes, the CHORION and AMNION.

menarche the first sign of menstruation.

Mendel's laws the pattern, first demonstrated by Gregor Mendel, a Moravian monk, whereby inherited characteristics are transmitted, some being dominant and others recessive.

Mendelson's syndrome this occurs when even a small volume of acid gastric juice is inhaled during general anaesthesia. It causes marked irritation of bronchi and alveoli, giving severe bronchospasm and pulmonary oedema. The signs are extreme dyspnoea, cyanosis and tachycardia. It may lead to hypotension and death.

meninges the membranes covering the brain and spinal cord. There are three: the dura mater, arachnoid and pia mater.

meningitis inflammation of the meninges.

meningocele a congenital deformity of the fetus, characterized by protrusion of the meninges through the skull or spinal column, appearing as a cyst filled with cerebrospinal fluid. *See also* SPINA BIFIDA.

meningoencephalocele hernial protrusion of the meninges and brain substance through a defect in the skull.

meningomyelocele hernial protrusion of the meninges and spinal cord through a defect in the vertebral column.

meniscocyte a sickle cell.

menopause the normal cessation of menstruation. *Artificial m.* a cessation induced by operation or irradiation.

menorrhagia an excessive menstrual discharge.

menses menstruation.

menstrual pertaining to menstruation. *M. cycle* the series of events which occurs in the endometrium between the 1st day of one menstrual period and the 1st day of the next, normally 28 days. It is

governed by the changes in the ovarian cycle which in turn are controlled by the gonadotrophic hormones of the anterior pituitary lobe.

menstruation a discharge of blood from the uterus, at approximately 4-week intervals commencing at puberty and lasting until the menopause.

mental 1. pertaining to the mind. 2. pertaining to the chin. *M. handicap* faulty or inadequate development of the brain which causes some degree of impaired adaptation in learning, social adjustment or maturation, or in all these areas.

mentoanterior with the chin directed anteriorly in the pelvis. Similarly, mentolateral and mentoposterior.

mentum the chin; the denominator in face presentation.

meptazinol a newer narcotic analgesia claimed to cause less respiratory depression. It has a relatively quick onset of action but a short duration of action of 2–4 hours. Nausea and vomiting are quite common side-effects.

Meptid trademark for a preparation of meptazinol.

mercury an element. Symbol Hg. A heavy liquid metal. It is used in thermometers because it expands with heat, and in SPHYGMOMANOMETERS because it is much heavier than water, so a short tube only is needed to record a wide variation in pressure.

mesentery a membranous fold attaching various organs to the body wall, especially the peritoneal fold attaching the small intestine to the dorsal body wall. adj. *mesenteric*.

nesoderm cells lying between ectoderm and entoderm cell layers in the embryo, from which are developed bone, muscle, heart, blood, blood vessels, gonads, kidneys and connective tissues.

mesosalpinx the peritoneum covering the fallopian tubes.

mesovarium a fold of peritoneum connecting the ovary to the broad ligament.

metabolism the process of life, by which tissue cells are broken down by combustion (catabolism) and new protein is built up from the end products of digestion (anabolism). *Basal m. Inborn error of m.* a genetically determined biochemical disorder in which a specific enzyme defect produces a metabolic block that may have pathological consequences at birth, as in phenylketonuria, or in later life. *See* BASAL METABOLIC RATE.

metastasis the transfer of disease from one organ to another not directly connected with it. pl. metastases. A growth of malignant cells or pathogenic microorganisms distant from the primary site.

metatarsum the part of the foot between the ankle and the toes, its skeleton being the 5 bones (metatarsals) extending from the tarsus to the phalanges.

methadone a synthetic compound with pharmacological properties qualitatively similar to those of morphine and heroin.

methotrexate folic acid antagonist used as an anti-neoplastic agent; it is also used in the treatment of psoriasis.

methoxyflurane (Penthrane) a volatile liquid which was used for inhalation analgesia.

methyldopa a hypotensive drug, sometimes used in essential hypertension in pregnancy. *See* Appendix 19.

metopic suture the frontal suture.

metra the uterus.

metra-, metro- word element meaning 'uterus'.

metre (m) the Système International (SI) unit which measures length and distance; the equivalent of 39.371 inches.

metritis inflammation of the uterus.

metronidazole (Flagyl) an antimicrobial drug effective for anaerobic infections, especially *Trichomonas vaginalis*.

metropathia haemorrhagica a disease characterized by painless excessive menstrual and intermenstrual bleeding and failure of ovulation, hence failure of corpus luteum development.

metrorrhagia haemorrhage from the uterus independent of menstruation.

metrostaxis persistent slight haemorrhage from the uterus.

Michel's clips small metal clips for closing skin wounds.

miconazole an anti-fungal agent used topically for dermatophytic infections such as athlete's foot or vulvovaginal candidiasis, orally for candidiasis of the mouth and gastrointestinal tract, and systemically by intravenous infusion for systemic fungal infections.

micro- 1. prefix meaning 'small', of microscopic size. 2. the prefix indicating 'one-millionth', e.g. microgram (μ), one-millionth of a gram.

microbe a micro-organism, especially a pathogenic bacterium. adj. *microbial, microbic*.

microcephaly possessing an abnormally small head. A microcephalic infant has markedly ossified skull bones and is always mentally subnormal.

microcytic having unusually small cells. See ANAEMIA.

micrognathia an unusually small mandible or lower jaw, with a receding chin. See PIERRE–ROBIN SYNDROME.

Micronor a proprietary contraceptive pill composed only of progesterone, used (*a*) during breast-feeding and (*b*) for patients with a risk of thrombosis or who suffer severe side effects from pills containing oestrogen.

micro-organism a minute living organism, animal or vegetable (such as a virus or bacterium), visible under a microscope.

microphage a small phagocyte; an actively mobile neutrophilic leukocyte capable of phagocytosis.

micturition the act of passing urine.

midwife 'a person who, having been regularly admitted to a midwifery education programme, duly recognized in the country in which it is located, has successfully completed the prescribed course of studies in midwifery and has acquired the requisite qualifications to be registered and/or legally licensed to practice midwifery. She [or he] must be able to give the necessary supervision, care and advice to women during pregnancy, labour and the postpartum period, to conduct deliveries on her [or his] own responsibility and to care for the newborn and the infant. The care includes preventative measures, the detection of abnormal conditions in mother and child, the procurement of medical assistance and the execution of emergency measures in the absence of medical help. She [or he] has an important task in health counselling and health education, not only for the patients, but also within the family and the community. The work should involve antenatal education and preparation for parenthood and extends to certain areas of gynaecology, family planning and child care. She [or he] may practise in hospitals, clinics, health units, domiciliary conditions or in any other service.' Definition adopted by the International Confederation of Midwives, and International Federation of Gynaecologists and Obstetricians in 1972 and 1973, respectively, following amendment of the definition formulated by the World Health Organisation.

midwifery dealing with childbirth. OBSTETRICS.

midwifery process a systematic,

cyclical method of organizing midwifery care. It is carried out by the assessment of actual and potential problems, and the planning, implementation and evaluation of care.

Midwives Acts a number of Acts of Parliament, to regulate the practice of midwives, passed in the years 1902, 1918, 1926 and 1936. All this legislation was consolidated by the Midwives Act 1951. The Nurses, Midwives and Health Visitors Act of 1979 replaced the former Midwives Acts, and established a new statutory structure for Nursing, Midwifery and Health Visiting in the UK.

Midwives' Code of Practice a code issued by the UKCC as guidance to the midwife and applicable to all midwives practising in the UK. The Code of Practice was issued in 1991 and can be revised as required because it is not secondary legislation.

Midwives' Rules all practising midwives are responsible for complying with the UKCC rules approved in 1991. Failure to do so is likely to result in an allegation of professional misconduct.

miliaria a cutaneous condition with retention of sweat, which is extravasated at different levels in the skin; called also prickly heat or heat rash.

milk the secretion of the mammary gland. The average composition of cows' and human milk, as a percentage, is:

	Cows' milk	Human milk
Protein	3.5	1.5
Fat	4.5	3.5
Carbohydrate	4.0	7.0
Mineral salts	0.75	0.2
Water	87.3	87.8

These percentages in human milk, particularly of fat, vary according to the time of day and the time during a feed. *Pasteurized m.* may be prepared in two ways: (*a*) high temperature short time (HTST), where the milk is held at 73°C (162°F) for 15 seconds and then cooled quickly; or (*b*) where the milk is kept at 63°–66°C (145°–150°F) for 30 minutes then rapidly cooled and bottled. *Sterilized m.* this has been heated to 100°C (212°F) for 15 minutes to render it free from bacteria. *Tuberculin-tested m.* milk from cows certified free from tuberculosis and subject to strict bacteriological tests.

milk flow mechanism, milk ejection reflex this occurs about 30–40 seconds after the baby takes the AREOLA of the breast between its jaws. Oxytocin is released from the posterior lobe of the pituitary in response to the nervous stimulation, which causes contraction of the MYOEPITHELIAL CELLS so that milk is driven out of the ALVEOLI into the ducts and lacteal sinuses, so becoming available to the baby.

milli- the prefix indicating 'one-thousandth', e.g. milligram (mg) one-thousandth of a gram, millilitre (ml) one-thousandth of a litre, millimetre (mm) one-thousandth of a metre.

Millipore filter trademark for a device used to filter nutrient solutions as they are administered intravenously.

Milton a proprietary antiseptic consisting of a standardized 1 per cent solution of electrolytic sodium hypochlorite. It is used especially for the sterilization of babies' feeding bottles.

mineral any naturally occurring non-organic homogeneous solid substance. There are 19 or more minerals forming the mineral composition of the body, of which at least 13 are essential to health. These minerals are supplied in a mixed and varied diet of animal and vegetable products.

Minilyn a contraceptive pill of oestrogen and progesterone combined.

Ministry of Agriculture, Fisheries and Food (MAFF) a government department which undertakes research and takes advice from scientific bodies into topics relating to agriculture, fisheries and food. The ministry can make recommendations and introduce legislation for changes in policy relating to food and nutrition in the United Kingdom.

Minovlar, Minovlar ED proprietary contraceptive pills containing oestrogen and progesterone.

miscarriage ABORTION. The expulsion of the fetus before the 24th week of pregnancy, i.e. before the fetus is legally viable, the fetus not being born alive. *See* Appendix 6.

Misuse of Drugs Act, 1971 came into effect in 1973, to control the possession and supply of certain drugs. Narcotic drugs such as papaveretum (Omnopon), cocaine, morphine, diamorphine and those which affect the central nervous system (e.g. LSD and amphetamines) are included. *See* Appendix 19.

mitosis the normal process of cell multiplication, where nuclear division occurs, with each chromosome dividing into two, so that two identical cells are formed. cf. meiosis.

mitral shaped like a mitre. *M. incompetence* a term which describes a defective mitral valve, usually the result of scar tissue following endocarditis. *M. regurgitation* the result of mild endocarditis, when the valve is puckered and closes imperfectly. *M. stenosis* a more serious condition in which fibrous tissue causes a narrowed orifice. Both regurgitation and stenosis may be present together. Mitral stenosis is the commonest cardiac lesion occurring in childbearing women. *M. valve* the bicuspid valve between the left atrium and left ventricle of the heart. *M. valvotomy* cutting into, and therefore widening, the narrowed mitral valve, performed to relieve mitral stenosis.

mittelschmerz abdominal or pelvic pain occurring between menstrual periods, and possibly related to ovulation.

Mogadon trademark for a preparation of nitrazepam, a hypnotic.

MOH Medical Officer of Health.

mole a dead and degenerate ovum. *See* Appendix 6.

molecule the smallest particle of an element or compound consisting of a varying number of atoms. Water, as seen from the symbol H_2O has a molecule consisting of two hydrogen atoms and one oxygen atom.

mongolian spot a smooth, brown to greyish blue naevus consisting of an excess of melanocytes, sometimes found at birth in the sacral region. This is found in babies of African and Asian parents and sometimes in those of Mediterranean origin. It usually disappears during childhood.

mongolism *see* DOWN'S SYNDROME.

Monilia a former name for the genus of fungi now known as *Candida*. *Candida albicans* is the common cause of thrush in infants, and of monilial vaginitis. Particularly common in pregnant women.

moniliasis candidiasis.

Monitor an adaptation for the UK of the USA Rush Medicus system of assessing quality of nursing care. It consists of 'checklists' for quality leading to a scoring system. The closer the score to 100% the better the care being given. The master list has over 200 criteria which are divided into 4 categories based on patient dependency levels.

monitor to check constantly on a given condition or phenomenon, e.g. blood pressure, or heart or respiration rate.

monoamine an amine containing only one amino group. *M. oxidase inhibitors (MAO inhibitors)* substances that inhibit the activity of monoamine oxidase, increasing catecholamine and serotonin levels in the brain; they are used as anti-depressants and anti-hypertensives. Pethidine should not be given to patients receiving amino oxidase inhibitors as these drugs potentiate the action of pethidine about 10 times, thus the combination is highly dangerous.

monosaccharide the simplest form of sugar, e.g. dextrose, glucose.

monozygotic pertaining to or derived from a single zygote (fertilized ovum); said of TWINS.

mons veneris the area covered with hair over the pubes in a woman.

monster a malformed fetus.

Montgomery's glands or tubercles sebaceous glands around the nipple, which enlarge during pregnancy.

morbid diseased, or relating to diseased parts.

moribund dying.

morning sickness nausea, sometimes accompanied by vomiting, which occurs in greater or lesser degree in 50 per cent of normal pregnant women between the 4th and 12th weeks of pregnancy. Despite its name, morning sickness is not always limited to the morning. It is thought to be due to a disturbance in the metabolism of glucose, or as a result of the increased metabolism of pregnancy causing a low blood sugar and accompanying feeling of nausea on rising. In rare cases, HYPEREMESIS GRAVIDARUM may develop which results in such symptoms as dehydration and weight loss. This condition may threaten the life of both mother and fetus.

Moro reflex in response to any sudden movement or noise near by, a normal newborn child will quickly extend his arms and bring them together again. Variously called the 'embrace' or 'startle' reflex. Absence of the Moro reflex is noted in sick and preterm babies.

morphine the principal alkaloid obtained from opium, and given hypodermically as an analgesic. Can be given only on medical orders.

mortality death. *M. rate* death rate. *See* Appendix 20.

morula the fertilized ovum, about 4 days after fertilization when it resembles a small mulberry.

mosaicism a condition in which a person has several different types of cell within his body. An example is mosaicism for Down's syndrome. Here the individual may have some cells with 47 chromosomes.

motivation the reason or reasons, conscious or unconscious, behind a particular attitude or behaviour.

motor nerves those which convey an impulse of motion from a nerve centre to a muscle.

mould a species of fungus, e.g. *Penicillium*.

moulding the process of overriding of the cranial bones at the sutures and fontanelles whereby the fetus adapts itself to the pelvis through which it is passing. The head is squeezed to a different shape, with alteration to various diameters. In normal moulding the head is well flexed with suboccipitobregmatic and biparietal diameters presenting and as the bones overlap these diameters are decreased, while the one at right angles (i.e. mentovertical) is slightly lengthened. Conversely, in face presentation the submentobregmatic diameter is squeezed and the occipitofrontal lengthened. In persistent occipitoposterior moulding the occipitofrontal diameter is squeezed and the submentobregmatic increased. This upward moulding puts a greater strain on the intracranial membranes. The head returns to its normal shape within 3 days of birth. Moulding which is abnormal in direction, excessive in amount, or extremely rapid may cause tearing of the falx cerebri and tentorium cerebellum, leading to intracranial haemorrhage and possible death.

movements (fetal) *see* QUICKENING.

MSU mid-stream specimen of urine.

mucoid resembling mucus.

mucopolysaccharoidosis gargoylism. A serious inborn error of metabolism. There are several types, but in all of them mucopolysaccharide builds up within

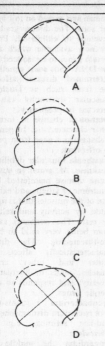

The unmoulded head is indicated by the heavy line: A. *Moulding in the occipitoanterior position*; B. *moulding in the persistent occipitoposterior position*; C. *face moulding*; D. *brow moulding*.
MOULDING

the body. The children look ugly and have large spleens, difficulty in joint movements and mental retardation.

mucopurulent containing mucus and pus.

mucosa mucous membrane.

mucous pertaining to or secreting mucus. *M. membrane see* MEMBRANE.

mucoviscidosis *see* CYSTIC FIBROSIS.

mucus the viscid secretion of mucous membranes.

müllerian duct either of the paired embryonic ducts developing into the vagina, uterus and uterine tubes in the female, and becoming largely obliterated in the male. Called also paramesonephric duct.

multicultural an adjective relating to a society, a community or country consisting of a number of different cultural and/or ethnic groups.

multifactorial 1. of, or pertaining to, or arising through the action of, many factors. 2. in genetics, arising as a result of the interaction of several genes.

multigravida a pregnant woman who has previously had more than one pregnancy. *Grand m.* a pregnant woman who has had 4 or more previous pregnancies. *See also* MULTIPARA.

multipara a woman who has borne more than one VIABLE infant.

multiple pregnancy a pregnancy of more than one fetus. Twin pregnancy is relatively common, occurring in England about once in 80 pregnancies. The incidence of triplet pregnancy is said to be about 1 in 80^2, i.e. 1 in 6400; and that of quadruplet pregnancy 1 in 80^3, i.e. 1 in 512 000.

mumps a communicable paramyxovirus disease that attacks one or both of the parotid glands. Occasionally the submaxillary glands are also affected. Immunization in the first 2 years of life (with measles and rubella—MMR) is recommended.

Munro Kerr's manoeuvre *see* HEAD FITTING.

murmur an auscultatory sound, particularly a periodic sound of short duration of cardiac or vascular origin. May be associated with disease or abnormality.

muscle a bundle of long, slender cells, or fibres, that have the power to relax and contract and hence to produce movement. Uterine muscle, the myometrium, also has the power of retraction, whereby the muscle fibres retain some of the shortening of the fibres that occurs with contractions. This property of retraction assists in the progressive passage of the fetus down the birth canal.

muscular dystrophy a group of genetically determined, painless, degenerative myopathies that are progressively crippling because muscles are gradually weakened and eventually atrophy. *Duchenne m. d.* a sex-linked recessive disease carried by the woman and passed on to 1 in 2 of her sons. The disease gradually develops in childhood. Probes are now available which allow certain genes to be isolated from the DNA, thus some genetically determined diseases affecting the fetus such as Duchenne muscular dystrophy can be detected in pregnancy.

mutation a change in form or other characteristic. In genetics a change in a gene from parent to offspring.

myasthenia muscular debility or weakness. *M. gravis* an autoimmune disease manifested by a syndrome of fatigue and exhaustion of the muscles that is aggravated by activity and relieved by rest. The weakness ranges from being very mild to being life-threatening. The disease characteristically affects the ocular and other cranial muscles, tends to fluctuate in severity, and responds to cholinergic drugs.

Mycobacterium a GRAM-POSITIVE bacterium distinguished by acid-fast staining, e.g. *M. tuberculosis*.

myocardium the middle and thickest layer of the heart wall, composed of cardiac muscle. adj. *myocardial*.

myoepithelial cells branched contractile epithelial cells which curve round each ALVEOLUS in the breast tissue. *See also* MILK EJECTION REFLEX *and* BREAST.

myoma a tumour of muscle tissue.

myomectomy removal of a

myoma—usually referring to a uterine tumour.

myometrium the uterine muscle.

myxoedema hypothyroidism. A disease caused by a lack of thyroid hormones being secreted by the thyroid gland. Marked by oedematous swelling of face, limbs and hands; dry and rough skin; loss of hair; slow pulse; subnormal temperature; slowed metabolism, and mental dullness. It is treated with preparations of thyroid gland. Congenital hypothyroidism causes CRETINISM.

N

N 1. an antigen found in the red blood cells of certain persons; hence, a blood group. *See also* M. 2. symbol, newton. 3. chemical symbol, nitrogen. 4. symbol, normal (solution).

Naboth's cysts (follicles) cyst-like formations due to occlusion of the lumina of glands in the mucosa of the uterine cervix causing them to be distended with retained secretion. Called also nabothian cysts or follicles.

Naegele's pelvis a very rare abnormal pelvis which is asymmetrical due to a congenital failure of one sacral ala to develop fully.

Naegele's rule a rule for calculating the estimated date of labour: subtract 3 months from the first day of the last normal menstrual period and add 7 days.

naevus a birthmark; a circumscribed area of dilated superficial blood vessels.

nalorphine a drug, related to morphine, previously used in asphyxia neonatorum but now replaced by NALOXONE.

naloxone (Narcan) the specific antidote to a narcotic drug. It may be administered to an asphyxiated neonate if the mother has been given a narcotic recently in labour. *See* Appendices 16 and 19.

nano- the prefix indicating 'one-thousand-millionth', e.g. nanogram (ng) one-thousand-millionth of a gram. *See* Appendix 20.

napkin rash any rash which occurs in the area usually covered by the napkin. There are several types, the most common being ammoniacal dermatitis. This is not likely to occur in the neonatal period, but later produces erythema and vesicles. Other causes are thrush, napkin psoriasis and perianal erythema.

Narcan trademark for preparations of naloxone, an opiate antagonist.

narco- a prefix denoting 'stupor'.

narcosis a state of unconsciousness produced by a narcotic drug.

narcotic 1. a drug that produces narcosis. 2. a drug that produces insensibility or stupor. Medically the term narcotic includes any drug that has this effect. By legal definition, however, the term refers to habit-forming drugs, e.g. opiates such as morphine and heroin, and synthetic drugs such as pethidine. Narcotics can be legally obtained only with a doctor's prescription. The sale or possession of narcotics for other than medical purposes is strictly prohibited by the Misuse of Drugs Act, 1971.

nares the nostrils. *Posterior n.* the opening of the nares into the nasopharynx. sing. *naris*.

nasal pertaining to the nose.

Naseptin trademark for a combination preparation containing chlorhexidine and neomycin, a nasal cream for the treatment of staphylococcal infections.

nasogastric tube a tube of soft rubber or plastic that is inserted through the nostril and into the stomach. The tube is inserted for the purpose of instilling liquid food or other substances, or as a means of withdrawing gastric contents. Before insertion the length from the bridge of the nose to the xiphoid process is measured with the tube which is then marked. Once the tube is inserted its position is checked by aspirating stomach contents with a syringe and testing for acidity with litmus paper, or alternatively injecting air into the stomach which can be heard as a 'whooshing' sound through a stethoscope. Having ascertained that the tube is correctly positioned it is firmly anchored to the face.

nasojejunal feeding a method in which a silicone-coated or Silastic catheter is passed through the nose into the jejunum, to provide sufficient nutrition to a sick baby on a ventilator or receiving CONTINUOUS INFLATING PRESSURE (CIP) by mask or nasal tube. It is used to prevent the dangers of aspiration with a nasogastric tube feed. *See* Appendix 17.

nasopharynx the part of the pharynx above the soft palate.

National Boards for Nursing, Midwifery and Health Visiting set up in England, Wales, Scotland and Northern Ireland by the 1979 Nurses, Midwives and Health Visitors' Act. For structure and functions, *see* Appendix 22.

National Childbirth Trust (NCT) a charitable organization concerned with education for pregnancy, birth and parenthood, with over 300 branches and groups in the UK. Primarily through these local groups, it runs antenatal classes, breastfeeding counselling and postnatal support. *See* Appendix 25.

National Health Service (NHS) the provision of health care in hospital or the community on a national basis which is freely available at the point of delivery to all residents in the UK. The health service was established in 1948 when the National Health Service Act of 1946 was implemented. This Act set up a tripartite structure for health care which included hospitals, general practitioners (GPs) and local authorities, and remained in force until 1974. The National Health Service Reorganisation Act of 1973 was then implemented, which integrated the hospital and local authority health services under a single management structure. The health service was then managed by Regional and Area Health Authorities and health districts. The National Health Service Act of 1980 abolished the Area Health Authorities and established 200 District Health Authorities (DHA), each with a team of officers and management was by consensus. In 1983, following the publication of the Griffiths Report, consensus management was abolished with the introduction of general management at Regional, District and Unit level. The National Health Service and Community Care Act of 1990 is being implemented from April 1991 and allows some hospitals and/or other services to become self-governing trusts (SGTs) and the remaining services are known as directly managed units (DMUs). The DHAs are now purchasers of services and the SGTs and DMUs are the providers. Some GP practices have opted to have their own budgets and will purchase services for their patients. Despite these changes, the provision of health care is still free at the point of delivery.

natural childbirth a term used to describe an approach to labour and delivery in which the parents are well prepared in pregnancy for the event by learning about the process of childbirth, exercises that develop neuromuscular control, physical conditioning exercises, specific breathing patterns, relaxation and their expected roles. The parents aim for a pleasurable, fulfilling experience of childbirth in which they have autonomy, and avoid medical intervention and the need for analgesic preparations. Many of the techniques learned in natural childbirth classes can be applied to reduce the effects of stress and relieve discomfort associated with tension in situations not related to childbirth.

nausea a sensation of sickness with inclination to vomit. A common disorder of early pregnancy which normally resolves by about the 14th week. The cause is not fully understood, but could be associated with the hormonal or metabolic changes of early pregnancy.

navel the umbilicus.

Necator a genus of HOOKWORM.

necro- prefix meaning 'dead'.

necrobiosis degeneration and death of tissue. Uterine fibroids may undergo this process in the middle trimester. The treatment is rest in bed and the administration of analgesic drugs.

necropsy a post-mortem examination.

necrosis death of tissue.

necrotizing enterocolitis an inflammatory disease of the bowel of the neonate which is associated with septicaemia. It is thought to be due to bacteria proliferating in the bowel and penetrating the bowel wall at points where it has suffered ischaemic damage. Oedema, ulceration and haemorrhage of the bowel wall are found and may progress to perforation and peritonitis. Babies at risk of this condition include those with a history of asphyxia, respiratory distress, hypoglycaemia, hypothermia or cardiovascular disease. The condition is treated with parenteral nutrition, antibodies and, in cases of perforation, surgery.

need something that is required or necessary. Basic human needs are things that are required for complete physical and mental well-being. Abraham H. Maslow classifies needs according to their relative urgency as follows: physiological, food, fluid and air; safety and security; belonging and love; esteem; self-actualization. Those listed first must be met before attention can be paid to the others.

negligence in law, the failure to do something that a reasonable person of ordinary prudence would or would not do in a certain situation. Negligence may provide the basis for a law suit when there is a legal duty, as the duty of a midwife or doctor to provide reasonable care to clients, and when negligence results in damage to the client.

Neisseria gonorrhoeae the microorganism which causes GONORRHOEA. It is difficult to culture outside the human body.

nem a unit of nutrition equivalent to the nutritive value of 1 g of breast milk.

Nembutal a proprietary preparation of pentobarbitone, a barbiturate.

neo- prefix meaning 'new'.

neomycin a broad-spectrum antibiotic; used as an intestinal antiseptic.

neonatal pertaining to the first 4 weeks after birth. *N. mortality rate* the number of deaths of infants up to 4 weeks old per 1000 live births in a year.

neonate a newborn child up to 4 weeks old.

neoplasm any new growth, e.g. a tumour.

Nepenthe a proprietary preparation of MORPHINE.

nephrectomy excision of a kidney.

nephritis inflammation of the kidneys. *Acute n.* a kidney lesion which may follow a streptococcal infection such as scarlet fever or tonsillitis, characterized by pain in the lumbar region, pyrexia and oedema. Renal function is impaired, the urine contains albumin, blood and casts of the renal tubules, but little urea, while the blood urea rises. Most patients recover completely, while some develop chronic nephritis. *Chronic n.* renal function is permanently impaired and the patient has oedema, proteinuria and often hypertension, with a raised blood urea. *N. in pregnancy* a woman with severe nephritis is often infertile. If pregnant, she is more prone to abort and to develop PRE-ECLAMPSIA and all its complications, so needs frequent and specialized care during the antenatal period.

nephron the glomerulus, Bowman's capsule and the tubule system which is the functioning unit of the kidney. Each kidney contains about one million nephrons.

nephropathy any disease of the kidneys.

nephrosis any renal disease.

nephrotic syndrome any kidney disease, especially disease marked by purely degenerative lesions of the renal tubules. The disease may follow acute nephritis and is marked by excessive accumulation of fluid in the body, due to a great loss of protein in the body and decreased serum albumin. Diuretics, a high protein diet, possibly steroids and, recently, the possible administration of immunosuppressive drugs are the methods of treatment.

nerve a bundle of nerve fibres enclosed in a sheath called the epineurium. Its function is to transmit impulses between any part of the body and a nerve centre. *Motor (efferent) n.* conveys impulses causing movement from a nerve centre to a muscle. *N. fibre* the prolongation of the nerve cell, which conveys the impulse to or from the part which it controls. *Sensory (afferent) n.* conveys sensations from an area to a nerve centre. *Vasomotor n.* either dilator or constrictor to blood vessels.

nerve block a block by local analgesic drugs, to impulses passing along nerves, e.g. EPIDURAL ANALGESIA.

nervous 1. pertaining to, or composed of, nerves. 2. unduly excitable. *N. breakdown* a common term used to describe any type of mental illness that interferes with a person's normal activities. Can be used to describe any of the mental disorders. *N. system* the organ system which, along with the endocrine system, correlates the adjustments and reactions of an organism to internal and environmental conditions. It has 2 main divisions: the central nervous system, composed of the brain and spinal cord; and the peripheral nervous system, which is subdivided into the voluntary and autonomic systems.

nettle rash a vascular reaction characterized by sudden outbreaks of itching and burning swellings on the skin; called also URTICARIA.

neural tube defect a structural anomaly of the brain or spinal cord causing anencephaly or spina bifida. In anencephaly there is absence of the cranium, thus the brain tissue is exposed and the condition is incompatible with life. A defect of the posterior laminae and spinous processes of one or more vertebrae may present clinically as a hairy patch or dimple on the midline of the infant's back and requires no treatment (spina bifida occulta); if the defect allows herniation of the meninges (meningocele) surgery is required; herniation of both meninges and spinal cord (meningomyelocele) is a serious condition which requires expert assessment to decide whether operative treatment is possible and likely to improve the quality of life. Many of these babies have other defects and complications which are incompatible with life.

neuritis inflammation of a nerve.

neuromuscular pertaining to nerves and muscles, and particularly to their coordination.

neuron, neurone nerve cell; any of the conducting cells of the nervous system, consisting of a cell body, containing the nucleus and its surrounding cytoplasm, and the axon and dendrites. *N. thermal environment* environmental temperature in which energy losses and oxygen consumption required to maintain body temperature within normal limits will be minimal.

neurosis a functional disturbance of the nervous system characterized by emotional instability but without any obvious structural change in the nerve substance.

neutral neither acid nor alkaline. A hydrogen ion concentration (pH) of 7 is neutral.

neutron a neutral particle found with protons in the nucleus of an atom.

Neville Barnes forceps obstetric forceps for operative vaginal delivery; these forceps have axis traction handle attachments to allow downward traction of a high head into the pelvis. These attachments are not used now and the forceps are used for low-cavity deliveries.

niacin a water-soluble vitamin of the B complex found in various animal and plant tissues, especially liver, yeast, bran, peanuts, lean meats, fish and poultry. It is required for the synthesis of some enzymes.

nicotine a very poisonous alkaloid. The nicotine in tobacco, though small in amount, can cause indigestion, increase in blood pressure and dull the appetite. It also acts as a vasoconstrictor.

nidation the embedding of the fertilized ovum in the endometrium of the uterus.

nikethamide a cardiac and respiratory stimulant of short duration. Coramine is a proprietary preparation of it.

nipple the small conical projection in the centre of the AREOLA of the breast which gives outlet to the milk from the breast. The areola increases in size and becomes darker in colour in pregnancy, especially in brunettes. Small sebaceous glands called Montgomery's tubercles open on to the areola, and secrete a sebum to lubricate and protect the nipple. The tip of the nipples contains 15–20 small depressions that are the openings of the lactiferous ducts. To breast feed successfully and prevent sore nipples the baby should have both the nipple and the areola in his mouth. *Accessory n.* a rudimentary nipple anywhere in a line from the breast to the groin. *N. shield* a shield fitted with a rubber teat which covers the areola of a nursing mother when her nipple is sore or not sufficiently protractile for the baby to suck. *See also* WOOLWICH SHELL.

nitrazepam a hypnotic and sedative drug used to treat insomnia with early morning wakening.

nitrofurantoin (Furadantin) an antibacterial agent used in the treatment of urinary tract infection.

nitrogen an element. Symbol N. A gas which forms nearly 80 per cent by volume of atmospheric air. A constituent of all protein foods and substances.

nitrous oxide N_2O. Laughing gas. A general anaesthetic inducing a brief spell of unconsciousness, and used largely for dental operations. With oxygen it is used extensively as an anaesthetic. With 50 per cent oxygen it relieves pain without producing loss of consciousness, and this mixture, self-administered by inhalation, is used to relieve pain in labour. The gases are premixed in a single cylinder with a simple valve, tubing and face mask in the Entonox apparatus, which is approved by the United Kingdom Central Council for use by midwives.

node a small mass of tissue in the form of a swelling, knot or protuberance, either normal or pathological. adj. *nodal*.

nodule a small boss or node that is solid and can be detected by touch.

non-accidental injury (NAI) the variety of injury caused to a 'battered baby'. There may be fractures of bones, especially of the skull, with intracranial haemorrhage and other physical injuries. The term also includes the giving of poisons and dangerous drugs, sexual abuse, starvation and any other form of physical assault. The parents, or other persons looking after the child, are usually responsible for inflicting the injuries. These cases need careful investigation and handling.

non-shivering thermogenesis the use of brown adipose tissue by the neonate to produce heat in times of cold stress. Brown fat is stored in the mediastinum, around the nape of the neck, between the scapulae and around the kidneys and suprarenal glands.

noradrenaline a catecholamine which is the neurotransmitter of most sympathetic postganglionic neurons and also of certain tracts in the nervous system. It is released from the adrenal medulla in response to sympathetic stimulation, primarily in response to hypotension. It produces vasoconstriction, an increase in heart rate, and elevation of blood pressure.

Noriday a proprietary contraceptive pill composed of progesterone alone and therefore suitable for use while breast-feeding.

Norinyl a proprietary combined oestrogen and progesterone contraceptive pill.

normoblasts immature nucleated red blood cells normally remaining in the bone marrow until maturity, but released into the circulation in certain anaemias.

normotensive having a normal blood pressure.

notifiable a term applied to certain transmitted diseases, the occurrence of which must be statutorily notified to the Director of Public Health in the health authority. Notification is the doctor's responsibility. A midwife suspecting any notifiable disease should immediately inform a doctor. Notifiable diseases include infective jaundice, leptospirosis, scarlet fever, whooping cough, measles, smallpox, diphtheria and tuberculosis. Ophthalmia neonatorum remains notifiable but puerperal pyrexia, notifiable for many years, is no longer so.

notification a midwife must notify the officer designated by the regional health authority (NHS Reorganisation Act 1974, schedule 4, section 64) of the following: (*a*) intention to practise; (*b*) change of name or address.

notification of birth *see* BIRTH, NOTIFICATION OF.

nucha the nape of the neck.

nuchal displacement a complication of breech labour, when an arm is displaced behind the child's neck.

nuclear family parents and their children living together in a household without members of the extended family such as grandparents, aunts and uncles living with them, or in the same locality.

nuclear magnetic resonance a phenomenon exhibited by atomic nuclei having a magnetic moment, i.e. those nuclei that behave as if they are tiny bar magnets. When disturbed from equilibrium by a radiofrequency pulse their alignment changes but, at the termination of the pulse, the nuclei return to their position of equilibrium. Signals elicited can be analysed and used for chemical analysis (NMR spectroscopy) or for imaging (MAGNETIC RESONANCE IMAGING; MRI).

nucleic acids extremely complex, long-chain compounds of high molecular weight that occur naturally in the cells of all living organisms. They form the genetic material of the cell and direct the synthesis of protein within the cell. There are 2 major classes of nucleic acids: DEOXYRIBONUCLEIC ACID (DNA) AND RIBONUCLEIC ACID (RNA).

nucleus the essential part of a cell containing the chromosomes, its division being essential for the formation of new cells. *Basal n.* group of nerve cells in the brain which, in severe jaundice in the newborn, may become stained with bilirubin, causing KERNICTERUS.

nullipara a woman who has never given birth to a viable child.

nulliparous never having borne a child.

nurse 1. a person who is qualified in the art and science of nursing, and meets certain prescribed standards of education and clinical competence. 2. to provide services that are essential to, or helpful in the promotion, maintenance or restoration of, health and well-being. 3. to nourish at the breast. *Registered n.* in the UK, one whose name is on the Register held by the United Kingdom Central Council for Nurses, Midwives and Health Visitors (UKCC).

nursery, day a nursery for children under school age, for working mothers—especially those who are unsupported or parents who are sick. Provision is made, under the National Health Service Act, 1977, by the local authority social services department. Day nurseries may also be run by private or voluntary bodies, provided they are registered and supervised by the local authority. *N. school* schools for children between the ages of 2½ and 5 years provided by the local education authority. There are a limited number of places available in nursery schools and thus priority is given to children with special needs.

Nurses, Midwives and Health Visitors Act, 1979 this Act brought together nurses, midwives and health visitors in one statutory structure for the whole of the UK. It established the United Kingdom Central Council (UKCC) for Nursing, Midwifery and Health Visiting and the 4 National Boards, 1 for each of the 4 countries, England, Wales, Scotland and Northern Ireland. Under the Nurses, Midwives and Health Visitors Act, Midwifery Committees were established at UKCC and National Board level in order to give midwives control over their practice.

Nurses, Midwives and Health Visitors Act 1992 is being implemented in April 1993. *See* Appendix 22.

nursing process a systematic approach to individualized nursing care involving 4 main steps: 1. assessment—gathering information; 2. planning—identifying problems and setting realistic goals, involving 3. implementation—care giving; and 4. evaluation—measuring the effectiveness of nursing care.

nutrition the process by which food is assimilated into the body in order to nourish it. Nutrition is particularly concerned with those properties of food that build sound bodies and promote health. Good nutrition means a balanced diet containing adequate amounts of the essential nutritional elements that the body must have to function normally. The essential ingredients of a balanced diet are proteins, vitamins, minerals, fats and carbohydrates. The body can manufacture sugars from fats, and fats from sugars and proteins, depending on the need. But it cannot manufacture proteins from sugars and fats.

nylon a synthetic material of exceptional strength, used for sutures.

nystagmus involuntary, rapid, rhythmic movement (horizontal, vertical, rotatory, or mixed, i.e. of 2 types), of the eyeball.

Nystan trademark for a preparation of NYSTATIN, an anti-fungal agent.

nystatin an antibiotic effective in the treatment of superficial fungal infections, e.g. candidiasis.

O

O chemical symbol, oxygen.

obesity excessive development of fat throughout the body; increase in weight beyond that considered desirable with regard to age, height and bone structure. Obesity can affect physical and mental health. In pregnancy, complications such as hypertension are more common in obese women.

objective signs those which are noted by the observer, e.g. the midwife, as distinct from symptoms which the patient reports (subjective).

oblique slanting. *See* PELVIS, diameters of the.

oblongata, medulla oblongata the area of the brain below the midbrain, the continuation upwards of the spinal cord. This portion of the brain contains the centres that activate the heart, blood vessels and respiratory system.

observational study an epidemiological study of events without the intervention of the investigator.

observation register a register of children whose development may be adversely affected by problems occurring during the fetal or neonatal period. They should be carefully followed up by the health visitor, general practitioner and special paediatric department.

obsession an unwanted idea or impulse that repeatedly intrudes into consciousness. Morbid obsession may dominate the mind and lead to irrational actions that are an attempt to escape the obsessional thoughts.

obstetric pertaining to obstetrics, the branch of medicine dealing with pregnancy, labour and the puerperium. *O. conjugate* the pelvic diameter extending from the sacral promontory to the upper inner border or the symphysis pubis. It measures approximately 11 cm and is the first narrow strait through which the fetal head has to pass. *O. flying squad* an emergency team from a consultant maternity unit comprising obstetrician, midwife and, if required, anaesthetist and/or paediatrician, who go out by ambulance to emergencies in the home or small maternity hospitals. They take emergency equipment such as O-negative blood, equipment for blood transfusion, operative delivery, manual removal of the placenta, anaesthesia (if required) and resuscitation of both mother and baby. After treatment the patient is transferred to hospital in the ambulance. *O. history* information about all previous pregnancies, and abortions, including details of labour, the puerperium and the baby, which is taken and recorded when a woman books with her midwife or doctor for a subsequent pregnancy *O. pulser* an appliance used for transcutaneous electrical nerve stimulation (TENS). *O. shock* collapse associated with childbirth owing to circulatory failure which occurs most commonly as a result of haemorrhage, or trauma such as acute inversion of the uterus, or septicaemia caused by Gram-negative organisms.

obstetrician a person skilled in the art and practice of obstetrics.

obstetrics the branch of medicine dealing with pregnancy, labour and the puerperium.

obstructed labour a state in which it is mechanically impossible for the child to be born. There is no advance of the presenting part despite strong uterine contractions. Obstruction most commonly occurs at the brim of the pelvis but may occur at the outlet, e.g. deep transverse arrest in an android pelvis. *See* Appendix 9.

obturator anything that closes an opening. *O. foramen* the opening in the anterolateral aspect of the os innominatum closed by fascia and muscle.

occipital relating to the occiput.

occipitoanterior when the back of the head, the occiput, is to the front of the mother's pelvis as the child's head comes through the birth canal. *Occipitoposterior* is where the occiput is towards the sacrum. Occipitolateral is where the occiput is to the lateral area of the mother's pelvis.

occiput the back of the head. The area extending from the lambdoid suture to the nape of the neck.

occlusive cap a rubber cap which covers the cervix and mechanically obstructs the entrance of spermatozoa. It should be used in conjunction with a spermicidal agent to increase its effectiveness.

occult obscure or hidden from view. *O. blood test* examination, microscopically or by a chemical test, of a specimen of faeces, urine, gastric juice, etc. to determine the presence of blood not otherwise detectable.

ocular pertaining to the eye.

Odent, Michel a French obstetrician who advocates a natural approach to childbirth.

odynometer an instrument for measuring pain.

oedema an excess of fluid, either because an excess is formed or because there is a failure of absorption. It may first be recognized by excessive weight gain only (occult oedema), then by pitting on pressure. It may be physiological, as in pregnancy, where the pregnant uterus presses on the pelvic veins, or in varicose veins. PATHOLOGICAL oedema occurs with chronic renal disease, PRE-ECLAMPSIA, ECLAMPSIA, severe heart disease, severe anaemia and malnutrition.

Oedipus complex a term used originally in psychoanalysis to signify the complicated conflicts and emotions felt by a boy when, during a stage of his normal development as a member of a family circle, he becomes aware of a particularly strong, sexually tinged attachment to his mother; the term **also** applies to a similar attachment felt by a girl to her father (called also *electra complex*).

oesophageal pertaining to the oesophagus. *O. atresia* absence of the opening of the oesophagus. May occur in a pregnancy complicated by POLYHYDRAMNIOS. As the baby will be unable to swallow its saliva, this will come out of the mouth continuously as clear mucus. Any baby showing this sign must have a stiff tube passed to ensure that the oesophagus is patent, as soon after delivery as possible. Any delay increases the mortality from the corrective operation. This condition is almost always accompanied by TRACHEO-OESOPHAGEAL FISTULA.

oesophagus the canal which extends from the pharynx to the stomach. It is about 22.5 cm (9 in) long in the adult.

oestradiol one of the ovarian hormones; the most potent naturally occurring OESTROGEN in humans.

oestriol an ovarian hormone; a relatively weak human oestrogen.

oestrogen a generic term used to describe any hormone with OESTROGENIC activity, including oestradiol, oestriol and oestrone. It can be produced by the ovary, the adrenal gland and, in small amounts, the testis, and fetoplacental unit. Oestrogens are responsible for female secondary sexual characteristic development, and during the menstrual cycle act on the female genitalia to produce an environment suitable for fertilization, implantation and

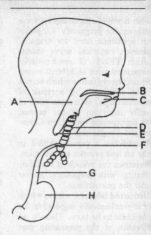

A. *Pharynx*; B. *palate*; C. *tongue*; D. *trachea*; E. *oesophageal atresia*; F. *tracheo-oesophageal fistula*; G. *distal oesophagus*; H. *stomach*.

OESOPHAGEAL ATRESIA WITH TRACHEO-OESOPHAGEAL FISTULA

nutrition of the early embryo. During pregnancy oestrogens stimulate the growth of the uterus and the duct system of the breasts. They are also responsible for water and electrolyte retention, for the suppression of ovulation and inhibition of lactation in pregnancy.

oestrogenic producing secondary

sex characteristics in a female at puberty, and some changes during the menstrual cycle and pregnancy, particularly development of the ducts in the breast and the uterine muscle.

estrone an OESTROGEN isolated from urine in pregnancy, the human placenta, and also prepared synthetically.

lfactory pertaining to the sense of smell.

ligaemia deficiency in volume of the blood.

ligohydramnios deficiency in the amount of amniotic fluid. It is associated with fetal malformations, e.g. renal agenesis, and intrauterine growth retardation of the fetus.

ligomenorrhoea scanty menstruation.

ligospermia deficiency of spermatozoa in the semen.

liguria diminished secretion of urine. It may be associated with impaired renal function following severe abruptio placentae, severe postpartum haemorrhage, severe pre-eclampsia or eclampsia.

mbudsman a person appointed to receive complaints about unfair administration. The officer in the National Health Service, appointed as 'ombudsman' or Health Service Commissioner, investigates complaints about failures in the health services. He is not able to pass judgement on clinical matters.

mentum fold of peritoneum extending from the stomach to adjacent abdominal organs.

omnivorous eating both plant and animal foods.

Omnopon a proprietary preparation of PAPAVERETUM, an opiate analgesic.

omphalocele umbilical hernia.

omphalus the umbilicus.

onco- word element meaning 'tumour', 'swelling', 'mass'.

oncology the sum of knowledge regarding tumours; the study of tumours.

onych(o)- word element meaning 'the nails'.

onychia inflammation of the nail bed.

ooblast a primitive cell from which an ovum ultimately develops.

oocyte the immature ovum.

oophor(o)- word element meaning 'ovary'.

oophorectomy removal of an ovary.

oophoritis inflammation of an ovary.

OPCS Office of Population Censuses and Surveys.

operant conditioning a form of behaviour therapy in which a reward is given when the subject performs the action required of him. The reward serves to encourage repetition of the action.

operculum the plug of mucus which fills the cervical canal during pregnancy and is shed at the beginning of labour. See 'SHOW'.

ophthalmia neonatorum any purulent discharge from the eyes of an infant within 21 days of birth. The causes of severe ophthalmia may be the GONOCOCCUS, *E. coli* or the staphylococci, but now is more commonly due to CHLAMYDIA TRACHOMATIS. Blindness can occur if the infection is gonococcal. It is therefore a condition NOTIFIABLE to the Director of Public Health.

ophthalmic pertaining to the eye.

ophthalmoscope an instrument for inspecting the interior of the eye.

opiate a class of drugs including: 1. the naturally occurring opiates, all of which are derived from the opium poppy. This group includes opium and its alkaloids (morphine and codeine); 2. the semi-synthetic opiates, including heroin and various other preparations; 3. the synthetic opiates, including methadone, meperidine and phenazocine; 4. the narcotic antagonists which, when used in conjunction with an opiate, block its effects but, when used alone, have opiate-like properties. Naloxone is an important exception, being an opiate antagonist but having no narcotic properties. The opiates have powerful analgesic and narcotic effects, and also produce both drug tolerance and drug dependence.

opium a susbtance derived from poppy juice and used to relieve pain. *Alkaloids of o.* morphine and codeine. *Tincture of o.* laudanum. *See also* Appendix 19.

opportunistic 1. denoting a microorganism which does not ordinarily cause disease but becomes pathogenic under certain circumstances. 2. denoting a disease or infection caused by such an organism.

opsonin any substance which coats bacteria and so makes them more easily phagocytosed. Antibody is therefore an opsonin.

optic pertaining to vision.

oral pertaining to the mouth. *O. contraceptive pill* 1. the combined oral contraceptive pill contains both oestrogen and a synthetic form of progesterone and has a very low failure rate, 0.1–1 per hundred women years (HWY), i.e. the number who would become pregnant if 100 women used the method for one year. 2. the progestogen only pill is usually prescribed for breast feeding women, for those over the age of 35 years and in other selected cases when the combined pill is contraindicated. The failure rate is 0.3–5 per HWY.

orbit the bony cavity containing the eyeball.

orbital ridge the bony rim of the orbit.

orchi(d)(o)- word element meaning 'testis'.

orchitis inflammation of a testis.

organ a part of the body which performs a particular function.

organic pertaining to the structure of an organ.

organism an individual animal or plant.

organogenesis the origin or development of organs.

orgasm the apex and culmination of sexual excitement.

orifice any opening in the body.

oropharynx the part of the pharynx between the soft palate and the upper edge of the epiglottis.

-orrhaphy suffix meaning 'repair'

or 'suturing', e.g. perineorrha-phy.

rthostatic standing erect. *O. albuminuria* albuminuria occur-ring when the individual is upright, but not after rest in bed.

rtolani's test one method of diagnosing CONGENITAL DISLO-CATION OF THE HIP. A 'click' or popping sensation is felt on reversing the movements of abduction and rotation of the hip while the child is lying with knees flexed.

s 1. a bone. *O. calcis* the heel bone or calcaneum. *External o.* The opening of the cervix into the vagina. *O. innominatum* nameless bone. The right and left innomi-nate bones articulate with the sacrum to form the pelvic girdle. *O. uteri* the opening of the uterus into the vagina which dilates progressively as labour advances. 2. a mouth or opening. *Internal* ɔ. the junction of the cervical canal and cavity of the uterus.

ɔsiander's sign pulsation of the uterine arteries through the lat-eral fornices which can be detected on examination *per vaginam* in early pregnancy. This is one of the signs which may assist in the diagnosis of preg-nancy.

smolality the concentration of a solution in terms of osmoles of solutes per kilogram of solvent. *Serum o.* a measure of the number of dissolved particles per unit of water in serum. Used in assessing status of hydration. *Urine o.* a measure of the number of dis-solved particles per unit of water in the urine.

osmosis the passage of a solvent through a semi-permeable mem-brane into a more concentrated solution. The process of osmosis and the factors that influence it are important clinically in the maintenance of adequate body fluids and in the proper balance between volumes of extracellular and intracellular fluids.

osmotic pressure the power of a fluid, dependent on its molecular content, to draw another fluid towards it.

ossification the formation of bone. *O. centres* the appearance of these on X-ray at the distal end of the fetal femoral epiphysis between 35 and 40 weeks gestation, and the proximal tibial epiphysis at 37–42 weeks may be helpful in determining fetal maturity if other methods are unsuitable or not available. *See also* ULTRA-SOUND.

osteoblasts cells which mature and form bone.

osteogenesis the formation of bone. *O. imperfecta* an inherited condition of extreme fragility of the bones, in which spontaneous fractures are liable to occur. The gene is dominant.

osteomalacia adult rickets. A dis-ease characterized by painful softening of bones. Due to gross vitamin D deficiency.

osteomyelitis inflammation of bone, localized or generalized, due to a pyogenic infection. It may result in bone destruction, in stiffening of joints if the infection spreads to the joints, and, in extreme cases occurring before the end of the growth period, in the shortening of a limb if the growth centre is destroyed.

otitis inflammation of the ear. *O. externa* of the external ear. *O. media* infection of the middle ear, which occasionally occurs in newborn babies. *O. interna* labyrinthitis.

-otomy suffix meaning 'cutting into', e.g. hysterotomy, incision into the pregnant uterus.

ounce (oz.) a measure of weight in both the avoirdupois and the apothecaries' system. *Fluid o.* a unit of liquid measure of the apothecaries' system, being 8 fluid drams, or the equivalent of 29.57 ml.

outlet a means or route of exit or egress. *Pelvic o.* the inferior opening of the pelvis; literally that bounded by the ischial spines, lower border of the symphysis pubis and the sacrococcygeal joint.

output the yield or total of anything produced by any functional system of the body. *Cardiac o.* the effective volume of blood expelled by either ventricle of the heart per unit of time (usually volume per minute); it is equal to the stroke output multiplied by the number of beats per the time unit used in the computation.

ova plural of ovum.

ovarian pertaining to an ovary *O. cyst* a tumour of the ovary containing fluid. *O. pregnancy* a fertilized ovum developed in the ovary. *O. vein syndrome* obstruction of the ureter due to compression by an enlarged or varicose ovarian vein; typically the vein becomes enlarged during pregnancy, the symptoms being those of obstruction or infection of the upper urinary tract. The right side is usually affected.

ovariotomy usually taken to mean removal of an ovary but, literally, incision of an ovary.

ovary one of a pair of glandular organs in the cavity of the female pelvis, attached to the posterior fold of the broad ligament near the fimbriated end of the fallopian tube. Their function is the production of ova and of the hormones (oestrogens and progesterone) which cause various changes in the body at the time of puberty and during pregnancy.

oviduct a passage through which ova leave the maternal body or pass to an organ communicating with the exterior of the body.

oviferous producing ova.

ovulation the process of liberating an ovum from the ovary by rupture of a graafian follicle. Normally, in an adult woman, ovulation occurs at intervals of about 28 days and alternates between the 2 ovaries. Usually only 1 ovum is produced, but occasionally ovulation produces 2 or more ova which, if fertilized, may result in multiple births, such as twins or triplets.

Ovulen a proprietary contraceptive pill containing both oestrogen and progesterone.

ovum an egg. The reproductive cell of the female. pl. *ova*.

oxidase any of a class of enzymes that catalyse the reduction of molecular oxygen independently of hydrogen peroxide.

oxidation a process of combining with oxygen.

oxprenolol a beta-blocking drug used in the treatment of angina, hypertension and cardiac arrhythmias.

oxygen an element. Symbol O. A colourless, odourless gas, essential to life. It constitutes 21 per cent of the atmosphere. In combination with hydrogen, it forms water; by weight, 90% of water is oxygen. Oxygen is essential in sustaining all kinds of life. Among the higher animals, it is obtained from the air and drawn into the lungs by the process of respiration. For therapeutic purposes it is stored in black and white cylinders. CYANOSIS is a sign of lack of oxygen (hypoxia). ANOXIA is the commonest cause of neonatal death. There are many predisposing causes, most of which are aggravated by labour, when the fetal heart beat may alter because of the acidaemia resulting from the hypoxia (fetal distress). In an asphyxiated baby, oxygen is used during resuscitation by ventilation through an endotracheal tube. When nursing the neonate, very careful monitoring of oxygen concentration is necessary, preferably by serial measurements of the Po_2 or visually by watching skin colour, to ensure that the amount of oxygen given is sufficient to prevent brain damage, but not so much as to cause retinopathy of prematurity leading to blindness in the preterm infant. *See* Appendix 17.

oxyhaemoglobin haemoglobin combined with molecular oxygen, the form in which oxygen is transported in the blood.

oxytetracycline a broad-spectrum antibiotic of the tetracycline group.

oxytocic term applied to any drug which stimulates contractions of the uterus in order to induce or accelerate labour.

oxytocin that part of posterior pituitary lobe extract which stimulates contraction of the uterus muscle, now produced synthetically. Oxytocin also causes milk to be expressed from the alveoli into the lactiferous ducts during suckling. Oxytocin may be administered intravenously to induce or augment labour, or intramuscularly or intravenously to contract uterine muscle after delivery of the placenta, and to control post-partum haemorrhage.

P

P 1. chemical symbol, phosphorus. 2. symbol peta-.

P probability.

Pco₂ carbon dioxide partial pressure or tension.

Po₂ oxygen partial pressure (tension).

Pₐco2 symbol for partial pressure of carbon dioxide in the arterial blood.

Pₐo₂ symbol for partial pressure of oxygen in arterial blood.

Pa 1. chemical symbol, protactinium. 2. symbol, pascal.

pack 1. a large swab used to control abdominal contents during operation, or to control bleeding in any wound. 2. a tampon.

packed cell volume (PCV) the percentage of blood cells to PLASMA. The normal PCV is about 45 per cent.

paediatrician a specialist in the study of infant and child in health and disease.

paediatrics that branch of medicine dealing with the care of babies and children.

paedophilia abnormal fondness for children; sexual activity of adults with children. adj. *paedophiliac*.

Paget, Rosemary (*1855–1948*) a midwife who joined the Midwives Institute in 1886 (now the Royal College of Midwives) and was instrumental in developing the educational activities of the College.

pain suffering and distress, caused by stimulation of specialized nerve endings. All receptors for pain stimuli are free nerve endings of groups of small myelinated or unmyelinated nerve fibres abundantly distributed in the superficial layers of the skin and in certain deeper tissues. Following stimulation, nerve endings in the skin transmit nerve impulses along sensory nerve fibres to the spinal cord. They then travel upward along the sensory pathways to the thalamus, which is the main sensory relay station of the brain. The conscious perception of pain probably takes place in the thalamus and lower centres; interpretation of the quality of pain is probably the role of the cerebral cortex. The perception of pain by an individual is highly complex and individualized. The cerebral cortex is concerned with the appreciation of pain, its quality, location, type and intensity, but the perception of pain is influenced by psychological and cultural responses to pain-related stimuli. The brain also produces morphine-like analgesic susbtances known as ENDORPHINS and ENKEPHALINS. The release of enkephalins inhibits the transmission of pain in small nerve fibres. The discovery of endorphins and the inhibition of pain by tactile signals explains the effectiveness of such techniques as relaxation, massage and acupuncture in the control of pain and discomfort. *P. in childbirth* this is caused by contractions of the upper uterine segment which first dilate the cervix and then expel the fetus through the birth canal. Although these contractions are present during pregnancy (Braxton Hicks contractions) they are then painless, but usually they become painful during labour because they are stronger and therefore render the uterine muscle ischaemic. This pain is felt intermittently in the lower abdomen and back, occurring with increasing frequency and intensity as labour proceeds. At the same time pain may be felt in the sacral region. This originates in the cervix and if it is severe it indicates that the cervix is not relaxing well and labour may be abnormal. The intensity of the pain which the woman feels during labour varies considerably due to some of the factors already considered. Women who are well prepared for childbirth and have learned breathing, relaxation and coping techniques usually experience less pain, and remain in control.

palate the roof of the mouth. *Hard p.*, in front, is of bone. *Soft p.*, continues from it, and is of muscle. *See also* CLEFT PALATE.

palliative an agent which relieves, but does not cure disease.

palpation examination by touch; the application of the fingers with light pressure to the surface of the body for the purpose of determining the condition of the parts beneath in physical diagnosis. *See* ABDOMINAL EXAMINATION *and* VAGINAL EXAMINATION.

palpitation abnormally rapid beating of the heart of which the patient is conscious.

palsy paralysis. *Bell's p.* facial paralysis due to lesion of the facial nerve, resulting in characteristic facial distortion. *Cerebral p.* a persisting qualitative motor disorder appearing before age 3. *Erb's palsy* a limp inwardly rotated arm with half-closed hand turned outwards; caused by damage to the upper roots of the brachial plexus. *Klumpke's p.* paralysis of the hand and wrist drop; caused by damage to the 8th cervical and 1st thoracic nerve roots.

Panadol trademark for preparations of paracetamol, an analgesic and anti-pyretic.

pancreas a racemose gland about 15 cm (6 in) long, lying behind the stomach, with its head in the curve of the duodenum and its tail in contact with the spleen. It secretes digestive juice, which enters the duodenum by the pancreatic duct which joins the common bile duct. The pancreas also secretes the hormone INSULIN from the islets of Langerhans.

pancreatic duct the main excretory duct of the pancreas, which usually unites with the common bile duct before entering the duodenum at the major duodenal papilla.

pancuronium a neuromuscular blocking agent used as a muscle relaxant during surgery, or during mechanical intermittent positive pressure ventilation, when it has been shown to prevent pneumothorax in babies actively expiring against ventilator inflation.

pandemic an epidemic spreading over a wide area.

panhysterectomy total hysterectomy, i.e. removal of the body and cervix of the uterus.

Papanicolaou test (smear) a simple test used most commonly to detect cancer of the uterus and cervix; often called the smear test. Malignant epithelia shed their surface cells more rapidly than normal cells. A blunt wooden spatula (Ayre's spatula) is passed through the cervix and rotated 360° near the internal os to scrape off surface cells. These cells are transferred on to a glass slide and examined microscopically.

papaveretum (Omnopon) an analgesic drug; a mixture of opium alkaloids.

papilla a small nipple-like eminence. pl. *papillae*.

papilloma a benign tumour derived from epithelium. *P. virus* a sexually transmitted infection causing anogenital warts (condylomata acuminata). It is associated with an increased incidence of cervical carcinoma. Rarely neonates may develop laryngeal papillomas due to infection acquired during vaginal delivery.

papule a small solid raised elevation of the skin.

papyraceous like paper. *Fetus p* may occur early in a multiple pregnancy when one fetus die and becomes flattened. It is disco vered at delivery.

para used to describe a woman who has produced one or more viable offspring. adj. *parous* Numerals designate the number of pregnancies that have resulted in the birth of viable infants, a para 0 (none = nullipara), par I, para II, para III, etc. The number is not indicative of the number of infants produced in the event of multiple birth, o synonymous with the number o pregnancies.

para- prefix meaning 'near', e.g. parametrium connective tissue near the uterus.

para-aminosalicylic acid (PAS PASA) a derivative of benzoi acid used in the treatment o tuberculosis. It enhances th potency of streptomycin an delays development of bacill resistant to streptomycin.

paracentesis puncture of the wal of a cavity in order to draw off fluid. *P. uteri* amniocentesis Puncture of the abdominal an uterine wall to gain access to th uterine cavity in pregnancy. *Se* HYDRAMNIOS.

paracervical block infiltration o Lee–Frankenhauser's plexus wit local anaesthetic performe through the lateral fornices t relieve the pain of cervical dila tation in labour. Only effectiv for up to 3 hours. Inadverten injection into the uterine artery which is in close proximity to the plexus may cause fetal bradycardia and possibly intra-uterine fetal death.

paracetamol an analgesic and antipyretic drug commonly used instead of aspirin for relief of moderate pain and reduction in fever. Acute paracetamol overdosage can cause severe and potentially fatal hepatic necrosis.

paraesthesia disorder of sensation, e.g. a feeling as of 'pins and needles'. It may occur with the CARPAL TUNNEL SYNDROME and is occasionally felt in the feet following epidural analgesia.

paraldehyde a powerful hypnotic, sedative and anti-convulsant drug, quick in action and generally safe, but having a strong and unpleasant smell.

paralysis palsy. Failure of function of a nerve, especially of a motor nerve, and therefore failure or impairment of the muscles (voluntary or involuntary) supplied by the affected nerves. *Facial p. see* BIRTH INJURY. *Infantile p.* POLIOMYELITIS. *See also* ERB'S PARALYSIS *and* KLUMPKE'S PARALYSIS.

paralytic pertaining to or affected by paralysis.

paramedical, paramedic having some connection with or relation to the science or practice of medicine; adjunctive to the practice of medicine in the maintenance or restoration of health and normal functioning. The paramedical services include physiotherapy, and occupational and speech therapy, etc., and the services of social workers.

parametric 1. situated near the uterus; parametrial. 2. pertaining to or defined in terms of a parameter.

parametritis inflammation of the PARAMETRIUM; pelvic cellulitis.

parametrium the pelvic connective tissue surrounding the lower part of the uterus and filling in the spaces between it and the related organs.

paranoia a mental disorder characterized by well systematized delusions of persecution, illusions of grandeur, or a combination of both. adj. *paranoic*. It is a chronic disease that develops over months and years and for which usually there is no cure.

paranoid 1. resembling paranoia. 2. paranoiac.

paraplegia paralysis of the legs and, in some cases, the lower part of the body. adj. *paraplegic*. Paraplegia is a form of central nervous system paralysis, in which the paralysis affects all the muscles of the parts involved.

parasite a plant or animal which lives within or upon another living organism, termed the host, upon which it satisfies all its needs without compensation.

parasympathetic nervous system part of the autonomic NERVOUS SYSTEM; post-ganglionic fibres are distributed to the heart, smooth muscles, and glands of the head and neck, and thoracic, abdominal and pelvic viscera. Almost ⅔ of all parasympathetic nerve fibres are in the VAGUS nerves, which serve the entire thoracic and abdominal regions of the body. The predominant secretion of the nerve endings of the parasympathetic nervous system is acetylcholine, which acts on the various organs of the body to either excite or inhibit certain activities.

parathyroid glands four small endocrine glands—two associated with each lobe of the thyroid gland, and sometimes embedded in it. Its hormone plays an important role in maintaining the plasma calcium level.

paratyphoid a notifiable infection caused by *Salmonella*.

parenteral outside the alimentary tract. Used to describe the introduction of a substance into the body by any route but the alimentary tract.

parenthood education a series of classes held in the antenatal period for parents to help them prepare for labour and parenthood. The midwife and other professionals such as the health visitor and physiotherapist are usually involved in facilitating these sessions which aim to meet the needs of those participating.

paresis partial paralysis affecting muscular action but not sensation.

parietal related to or attached to the wall of a cavity. One of two thin flat bones forming the major part of the vault of the skull.

parity 1. para; the condition of a woman with respect to her having borne viable infants. 2. equality;

close correspondence or similarity.

Parlodel trademark for a preparation of bromocriptine mesylate, a dopamine receptor agonist.

paronychia inflammation of the folds of skin surrounding the fingernail. A fairly common infection in newborn babies, almost always staphylococcal in orgin.

parotid near the ear. *P. glands* the largest of the 3 main pairs of salivary glands, located on either side of the face, just below and in front of the ears.

parous having borne one or more viable offspring. *See also* NULLIPAROUS *and* PRIMIPAROUS.

paroxysm 1. a sudden recurrence or intensification of symptoms. 2. a spasm or seizure. adj. *paroxysmal*.

partial pressure *See* PCO_2 *and* PO_2.

partogram a record of the progress of labour, particularly the dilatation of the cervix. *See* Appendix 7.

parturient being in labour; relating to childbirth.

parturition giving birth to a child.

pascal (Pa) the international (SI) unit of pressure, which corresponds to a force of 1 newton per square metre.

passive not active. *P. immunity see* IMMUNITY. *P. movements* manipulation by a physiotherapist without the help of the patient.

Pasteur, Louis (*1822–1895*) French chemist and bacteriologist, founder of microbiology and developer of the method of vaccination by attenuated virus.

pasteurization heating of milk or other liquids to a temperature of 60°C (140°F) for 30 minutes, killing pathogenic bacteria and considerably delaying other bacterial development.

Patau's syndrome trisomy 13 syndrome; a relatively rare chromosomal abnormality characterized by certain clinical features affecting facies, hands and feet and mental retardation.

patella the small, circular, sesamoid bone forming the knee-cap.

patent open. *P. ductus arteriosus* abnormal persistence of an open lumen in the ductus arteriosus, between the aorta and pulmonary artery, after birth. It places special burdens on the left ventricle and causes a diminished blood flow in the aorta. Closure of the patent ductus arteriosus can be produced in preterm infants by administration of an inhibitor of prostaglandin formation, such as indomethacin. Conversely, in neonates suffering from severe congenital heart defects in which an open ductus arteriosus could be beneficial, prostaglandins are given to keep the channel open.

paternity can now be proved by analysis of DNA in blood. The unsupported mother can apply for an affiliation order against the man she alleges to be the father of her child and, providing the court is satisfied about the paternity of the child, the putative father can be required to pay a fixed weekly sum for the maintenance of the child. *See* Appendix 5.

patho- a prefix denoting 'disease'.

pathogen any micro-organism or material which causes disease.

pathogenic causing disease.

pathological pertaining to the study of disease.

pathology the branch of medicine treating the essential nature of disease, especially the structural and functional changes in tissues and organs in the body.

patulous distended or open. Used in reference to the external os in a multiparous woman and during pregnancy when the cervix is incompetent.

Paul–Bunnell test a method of testing for the presence of heterophil antibodies in the blood for the diagnosis of infectious mononucleosis.

Pawlik's grip a method of estimating the mobility and engagement or non-engagement of the presenting part by palpation of the lower pole of the uterus. It can cause discomfort if not performed gently and slowly, ensuring that the patient is well relaxed. It is particularly useful to feel under the apron of fat in a very obese patient.

PCO_2 partial pressure of carbon dioxide. In the blood it is about 40 mmHg. The value is raised in respiratory failure. *See also P*O_2.

PCV packed-cell volume, the volume of packed red cells in litres per litre of blood.

pectineal pertaining to the os pubis.

pectoral 1. of or pertaining to

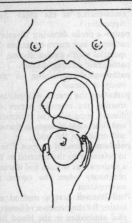

PAWLICK'S GRIP

the chest or breast. 2. relieving disorders of the respiratory tract, as an expectorant.

pedicle the stem of a tumour.

pediculosis infestation with lice of the skin or hair.

pediculus a louse.

pedigree a table, chart, diagram or list of an individual's ancestors, used in genetics in the analysis of mendelian inheritance.

peduncle a large stalk or pedicle.

PEEP positive end-expiratory pressure. A background pressure (the PEEP) which is applied during mechanical ventilation to prevent alveolar collapse.

peer review the basic component of a QUALITY ASSURANCE pro-

gramme in which the results of health and/or midwifery care given to a specific client population are evaluated according to defined criteria established by the peers of the professionals delivering the care.

pellagra a syndrome caused by a diet seriously deficient in niacin (or by failure to convert tryptophan to niacin). Most patients with pellagra also suffer from deficiencies of vitamin B2 (riboflavin) and other essential vitamins and minerals. The disease also occurs in people suffering from alcoholism and drug addiction.

pelvic Pertaining to the pelvis. *P. bone* hip bone, comprising the ilium, the ischium and pubis. *P. cellulitis see* PARAMETRITIS. *P. diameter* any diameter of the pelvis, Table (p. 204) shows the pelvic measurements at the level of the brim, the cavity and the outlet of the pelvis. The diagonal conjugate is measured from the apex of the pubic arch to the sacral promontory and is about 12.25 cm. The obstetric conjugate extends from the upper, inner border of the symphysis pubis and measures about 11 cm. The true or anatomical conjugate measures slightly more than the obstetric conjugate because it extends from the promontory of the sacrum to the centre of the upper surface of the symphysis pubis, but the extra space is not available for the passage of the fetus. *P. floor*, or diaphragm, consists of strong sheets of muscle fibres, the chief of which are the levatores ani, which form the principal support of the pelvic organs. *P. girdle* the ossa innominata and sacrum. *P. inflammatory disease (PID)* infection involving the uterine tubes, ovaries and parametrium. Other organs in the pelvis, especially the gut, may also be involved. The infection may follow delivery or abortion, may be secondary to infection elsewhere in the pelvis or abdomen, e.g. appendicitis, or in the genital tract, e.g. gonorrhoea, or may be due to blood-borne infection, e.g. tuberculosis. Acute PID causes abdominal pain, fever and vaginal discharge and is treated with antibiotics, rest and analgesia. Surgery may be required in cases of severe, chronic PID. Secondary infertility due to blocked uterine tubes is a common complication. *P. peritonitis see* PERITONITIS.

pelvimeter calipers for measuring the diameters of the pelvis.

pelvimetry measurement of the capacity and diameter of the pelvis, either internally or externally or both, with the hands, with a pelvimeter, or by radiography.

pelvis a bony girdle formed anteriorly and laterally by the innominate bones, and posteriorly by the sacrum and coccyx. It has a muscular floor, and contains the uterus, fallopian tubes, ovaries, urinary bladder and rectum. *False p.* the part lying above the brim (*see below*) bounded by the iliac fossae laterally, with the lumbar spine

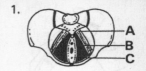

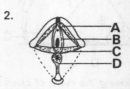

1. *Superior view of deep layer (levator ani):* A. *ischiococcygenus*; B. *iliococcygeus*; C. *pubococcygeus.* 2. *Superficial layer from below:* A. *ischiocavernosus*: B. *bulbocavernosus*; C. *transverse perinei*; D. *anal sphincter.*
PELVIC FLOOR MUSCLES

posteriorly and the abdominal wall anteriorly. Of little importance in obstetrics. *True p.* the part including and below the level of the brim. Of great importance, as it forms the bony canal through which the fetus must pass to be born normally. *Divisions. Brim* or *inlet*, bounded by the sacral promontory and alae, upper part of the sacroiliac joints, iliopectineal lines, and upper inner borders of the upper rami of the

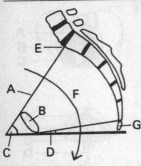

Showing the curve of carus and angles of inclination: A. plane of pelvic brim; B. symphysis pubis; C. angle of inclination of brim 55°; D. angle of outlet 5°; E. sacral promontory; F. curve of carus; G. coccyx.

SECTION OF BONY FEMALE PELVIS

pubes and symphysis pubis. *Cavity*, bounded by the hollow of the sacrum, the sacrospinous ligaments, the ischial and pubic bones and the symphysis pubis. *Outlet*, bounded anatomically by the coccyx, the sacrotuberous ligaments, the ischial tuberosities and the pubic arch. An *obstetrical outlet* is bounded posteriorly by the lower aspect of the sacrum and laterally by the ischial spines, this being the lowest level at which the fetus has bone sur-

rounding it within the birth canal. *See* table of average measurements. *Inclination of p.* the brim slopes at an angle of approximately 55° to the horizontal, and the bony outlet slopes at an angle of about 15°. The *axis of the brim*, an imaginary line drawn at right angles through the centre of the plane, thus in a backwards and downwards direction. Similarly, the axis of the bony outlet is almost horizontal. The axis of the birth canal (sometimes called the curve of Carus) is a curved line passing downwards and backwards at the brim, changing direction deep in the cavity, and (on account of the concavity of the sacrum and the arrangement of the pelvic floor muscles) directed downwards and forwards at the outlet. This is the direction followed by the fetus as it passes through the birth canal, and it is thus a direction to be followed in conducting any obstetric manipulation, e.g. head fitting, vaginal examination, application of forceps. *Android p.* this has masculine characteristics, including a roughly triangular or heart-shaped brim. *Anthropoid p.* this has a brim which is long anteroposteriorly and narrow transversely. *Gynaecoid p.* this is the normal female pelvis. It is as nearly as possible round at the brim, cavity and outlet. It is roomy and shallow, and ideally shaped for the transmission of the fetus. *Platypelloid* or *flat p.* this has an oval brim, small anteroposteriorly and wide transversely. All these types

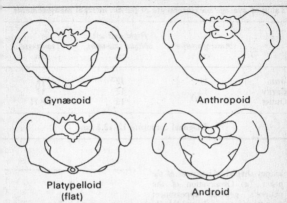

Gynæcoid   Anthropoid

Platypelloid
(flat)   Android

CALDWELL AND MOLOY'S CLASSIFICATION OF THE BRIM OF THE PELVIS

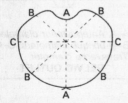

A–A. *anteposterior diameter*;
B–B. *oblique diameters*;
C–C. *transverse diameter*.
PELVIC BRIM

of pelvis are normal, and only cause difficult labour if they are extreme or small. The pelvis may also be deformed as a result of rare inherited characteristics, disease or accident. Examples are: the Naegele pelvis, in which one sacral alae has failed to develop, producing asymmetry; the Robert pelvis (an extremely rare type) in which both sacral alae are undeveloped and the symphysis pubis is sometimes split; the spondylolisthetic pelvis, in which the 5th lumbar vertebra has slipped forwards on the sacrum, creating a false promontory; the rachitic pelvis, the brim of which is markedly flattened and

Table of average measurements of pelvis: internal measurements

	Anteroposterior cm	Right and left oblique diameters cm	Transverse cm
Brim	11	12	13
Cavity	12	12	12
Outlet	13	12	10–11

Diagonal conjugate 12–12.5 cm

kidney-shaped. *Assessment of the pelvis.* (*a*) Observation of the patient's general appearance; sometimes a rough guide. (*b*) Previous obstetric history may be very valuable. (*c*) Measurement of the pelvis.

The pelvis can be assessed accurately by VAGINAL EXAMINATION. The ability of the fetal head to engage is a most valuable guide to the capacity of the pelvis. In cases of doubt, e.g. a head which fails to engage and cannot be made to do so, breech presentation or an obstetric history suggesting mechanical difficulty in labour, radiological pelvimetry is accurate and valuable.

pemphigus an acute or chronic skin disease, characterized by watery blisters. *P. neonatorum* bullous impetigo. It is an extremely infectious disease, and is usually due to infection with *Staphylococcus aureus*. The midwife should immediately report any blister. The child should be

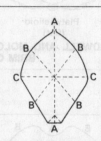

A–A *Antepoterior diameter*;
B–B *oblique diameters*; C–C
Transverse diameter.
PELVIC OUTLET

strictly isolated until the cause of the condition has been found. *Syphilitic p.* may, rarely, occur in the neonate.

Penbritin trademark for preparations of ampicillin; an antibiotic.

pendulous hanging down. *P. abdomen* a condition seen in multigravid women with extreme laxity of the abdominal muscles. The uterus falls forwards so much that the abdomen may hang below the symphysis pubis. Apart from the marked discomfort, this causes malpresentation of the fetus.

penicillin an antibiotic substance obtained from cultures of the mould *Penicillium*.

penis the male organ of copulation.

pentazocine a synthetic narcotic analgesia developed as an attempt to produce a narcotic without abuse potential. It is used orally and by infusion.

Penthrane *see* METHOXYFLURANE.

pepsin a proteolytic enzyme that is the principal digestive component of gastric juice. It acts as a catalyst in the chemical breakdown of protein to form a mixture of polypeptides. It also has a milk-clotting action similar to that of RENNIN and thereby facilitates the digestion of milk protein.

peptide the peptides form the constituent part of proteins; known as di-, tri-, tetra-, etc., peptides, depending on the number of amino acids in the molecule.

per through (Latin), e.g. in *per vaginam*: through the vagina.

percentile a term used in statistics to show how common some characteristic is. The line represents the percentage of the population who have this. The 90th percentile (or centile) for height means that 90 per cent of the population will be no taller than the figure. The 50th percentile is the median or average. The charts are widely used in midwifery to show the birth weight of babies at different gestations.

perception the conscious mental registration of a sensory stimulus. adj. *perceptive*. Extrasensory *p.* (*ESP*) knowledge of, or response to, an external thought or objective event not achieved as the result of stimulation of the sense organs.

percussion tapping a surface with the fingers to determine, by the sound, the condition of the underlying organs.

perforation a hole or break in the containing walls or membranes of an organ or structure of the body. Perforation occurs when erosion, infection, or other factors create a weak spot in the organ and internal pressure causes a rupture.

perforator an instrument for perforating the fetal skull. Formerly used in obstructed labour, to facilitate delivery, but rarely employed nowadays.

performance indicators 'package' of routine statistics derived nationally and presented visually in ways which highlight the relative efficiency of health services in each health authority compared with other authorities.

peri- prefix meaning 'around'.

pericardium the smooth membranous sac enveloping the heart, consisting of an outer fibrous and an inner serous coat. Inflammation of this membrane is called *pericarditis*.

pericranium the external periosteum of the cranial bones.

perimetrium the peritoneum of the uterus.

perinatal around the time of birth. *P. mortality rate* the number of stillbirths plus deaths of babies under 1 week old per 1000 total births in any 1 year. *See* Appendix 20.

perineal pertaining to the perineum. *P. lacerations* are classified as: (*a*) first degree, a tear of skin only, the muscle being intact; (*b*) second degree, a tear of skin and muscle which may be slight or severe, but which does not include the anal sphincter; (*c*) third degree or complete, where the tear extends through the whole of the perineal body, and through the anal sphincter into the rectum. *P. repair see* Appendix 10.

perineorrhaphy repair of the perineal body following injury sustained during childbearing. *See* Appendix 10.

perineum anatomically, the area extending from the pubic arch to the coccyx, with the underlying tissues. Obstetrically, the perineal body is the fibromuscular pyramid between the lower third of the vagina anteriorly and the anal canal posteriorly, and ischial tuberosities laterally. For composition, *see* PELVIS.

periosteum a specialized connective tissue covering all bones of the body, and possessing bone-forming potentialities. It also serves as a point of attachment for certain muscles.

peripheral relating to the periphery.

periphery the outer surface or circumference.

peristalsis a wave-like contraction which travels along the walls of a tubular organ, tending to press its contents onwards. It occurs in the muscle coat of the alimentary canal and in the fallopian tubes. Sometimes visible peristalsis occurs in PYLORIC STENOSIS.

peritoneum the serous membrane lining the abdominal cavity and forming a covering for the abdominal organs. *Parietal p.* that which lines the abdominal cavity. *Pelvic p.* that which covers the pelvic organs, in the female forming a pouch between the rectum and the uterus, the pouch of Douglas, and a shallow pouch between the uterus and the bladder, the uterovesical pouch. The peritoneum which hangs over the fallopian tubes is known as the broad ligament. *Visceral p.* the inner layer which closely covers the organs, and includes the mesenteries. adj. *peritoneal*.

peritonitis inflammation of the peritoneum, due to infection. *General p.* the whole of the abdominal cavity is affected. *Pelvic p.* the infection is restricted to the peritoneum of the pelvic cavity. It is an occasional complication of puerperal sepsis.

periventricular haemorrhage a serious complication occurring in preterm babies, especially those under 34 weeks gestation. The haemorrhage can be graded from 0 to 3, with 3 being the most extensive.

periventricular leukomalacia cystic, ischaemic lesions occurring in the periventricular region. This condition is associated with periventricular haemorrhage and is diagnosed by ultrasound scanning. It is associated with a high incidence of spastic cerebral palsy.

permeable able to be penetrated. Applied to membrane which allows fluid to pass through, e.g. the walls of the capillaries (also semipermeable).

pernicious highly destructive; fatal. *P. anaemia* a megaloblastic anaemia occurring in middle-aged people and caused by failure of the gastric secretion of intrinsic factor, and treated by the administration of vitamin B12. Not to be confused with megaloblastic anaemia of pregnancy, which is due to lack of folic acid in the diet.

peroxide a compound of any element with more than the normal quantity of oxygen required to form an oxide. *P. of hydrogen* a compound of hydrogen and oxygen.

persecution a symptom of schizophrenia and paranoia. A fear of being harmed when there is no just cause.

persistent mentoposterior a face presentation in which the sinciput has rotated forwards and the chin has been rotated backwards to the hollow of the sacrum. A rare cause of obstructed labour, when the thorax must present at the pelvic brim with the head.

persistent occipitoposterior a deflexed vertex presentation in which the sinciput has rotated forwards and the occiput has been rotated backwards to the hollow of the sacrum; this may cause delay in the second stage of labour. Spontaneous FACE-TO-PUBES delivery is possible. *See also* Appendix 9.

persona Jung's term for the personality 'mask' or facade presented by a person to the outside world, as opposed to the anima, the unconscious, or inner being, of a person.

personality that which constitutes, distinguishes, and characterizes a person as an entity over a period of time; the total reaction of a person to his environment. Many factors that determine personality are inherited; they are shaped and modified by the individual's environment. The early years of life influence personality development.

perspiration 1. sweating; the excretion of moisture through the pores of the skin. 2. sweat; the salty fluid, consisting largely of water, excreted by the sweat glands in the skin. In cystic fibrosis the sweat shows a raised level of sodium chloride.

pertussis whooping cough. A potentially serious infection of the respiratory tract, usually caused by the organism *Bordetella pertussis*. The incidence declined until the mid-1970s. It is now higher than 20 years ago, and has risen in parallel with the fall in immunization rate. It is particularly serious in babies under 3 months and in children with asthma. *See also* Appendix 15.

pessary an object inserted into the vagina. It may be a device to maintain anteversion of the uterus in early pregnancy, or a drug in a solvent base, e.g. anti-fungal or contraceptive.

petechiae small spots caused by minute subcutaneous haemorrhages, seen in purpura and sometimes on the face of the normal newborn child, due to venous congestion during delivery. When seen over the whole body it is a feature of congenital RUBELLA, TOXOPLASMOSIS and CYTOMEGALOVIRUS infection.

pethidine an analgesic and antispasmodic drug, very effective in relieving pain in labour. Under the Misuse of Drugs Regulations, 1973, registered midwives who have notified their intention to practise are authorized to be in possession of pethidine as long as it is necessary for the practice of their profession and has been obtained in the recognized manner. This applies only to midwives working in the community or in independent practice. Because of depression of the fetal respiratory system and its adverse effect on neonatal behaviour, including breast feeding, for the first few days of life, pethidine is now less popular for use in labour. *See* Appendix 19.

Pethilorfan a proprietary preparation of pethidine and levallorphan, now rarely used to relieve pain in labour.

petit mal a relatively mild epileptic attack, contrasting with GRAND MAL, a major attack. In petit mal, the affected person loses consciousness only momentarily.

Pfannenstiel's incision a transverse abdominal incision just above the symphysis pubis. *See* Appendix 10.

PG prostaglandin.

pg picogram.

pH the symbol used to express the hydrogen ion concentration or reaction of a fluid. In a scale ranging from 0 to 14, 7 is neutral, below 7 acid and above 7 alkaline. Blood, with a pH of 7.4, is slightly alkaline. It may be measured with an Astrup machine. The pH is used as a measure of whether the body is maintaining a normal ACID–BASE BALANCE. A favourable pH is essential to the functioning of enzymes and other biological systems.

phaeochromocytoma a rare growth of the adrenal medulla, associated with an increased production of adrenaline and consequent hypertension. The test considered most reliable to diagnose phaeochromocytoma is direct assay of adrenaline and noradrenaline in the plasma and urine. Another test involving measurement of vanillylmandelic acid (VMA) and of metanephrine and normetanephrine in urine may be carried out. The level of these substances in the urine in patients with phaeochromocytoma is almost twice the upper limits of normal. Surgical removal of the tumour is necessary.

phage a virus which kills certain micro-organisms. Viruses have differential susceptibility, which enables them to be distinguished into phage types.

phagocytes polymorphonuclear leucocytes and monocytes which engulf and digest bacteria and foreign particles.

phagocytosis the action of PHAGO-CYTES.

phalanx any bone of a finger or toe. adj. *phalangeal*.

phallic pertaining to the penis.

phantom 1. an image or impression not evoked by actual stimuli. 2. a model of the body or of a specific part thereof. 3. a device for simulating the *in vivo* interaction of radiation with tissues.

pharmaceutical relating to drugs.

pharmacology the science of the nature and preparation of drugs.

pharmacopoeia an authoritative publication which gives the standard formulae and preparation of drugs as used in a given country. *British Pharmacopoeia (BP)*; that authorized for use in Great Britain.

pharmacy the art of preparing, compounding and dispensing medicines.

pharynx the back of the mouth leading to the oesophagus and the larynx and communicating with the nose through the posterior nares, and the ears through the Eustachian tubes.

Phenergan a proprietary preparation of promezathine hydrochloride, an anti-histamine drug often given in labour with pethidine. *See* Appendix 19.

phenobarbitone a barbiturate drug which depresses the cerebral cortex. It is used in the treatment of epilepsy. *See* Appendix 19.

phenol a powerful and very poisonous antiseptic.

phenothiazine a group of major tranquillizers, the phenothiazine derivatives.

phenotype 1. the outward, visible expression of the hereditary constitution of an organism. 2. an individual exhibiting a certain phenotype; a trait expressed in a phenotype.

phenylalanine an essential amino acid, normally converted to tyrosine by an enzyme from the liver.

phenylketonuria the presence in the urine of phenylketones resulting from the incomplete breakdown of PHENYLALANINE to tyrosine. A high blood level of phenylalanine leads to mental retardation, fits and poor muscular coordination. Early diagnosis should be achieved by routine screening of infants' blood by the GUTHRIE TEST, for example, as urine tests are less accurate. A diet containing only a little phenylalanine must be given. The incidence is about 1 in 10 000. The inheritance is autosomal RECESSIVE. Persons with phenylketonuria are usually blue-eyed and blond, with defective pigmentation, the skin being excessively sensitive to light and tending to eczema.

phenytoin (Epanutin) an anticonvulsant drug used to control epilepsy. *See* Appendix 19.

phimosis constriction of the orifice of the prepuce so that it cannot be drawn back over the glans.

phlebitis inflammation of a vein. It is usually a vein of the leg, and a deep or superficial vein may be involved. Phlebitis in a deep vein can be a cause of THROMBOSIS and EMBOLISM.

phlebothrombosis clotting of blood in a vein, not associated with infection. The clot is loosely attached to the wall of the vein and there is considerable risk of separation of all or part of it, and, therefore, EMBOLISM. cf. THROMBOPHLEBITIS.

phlebotomy venesection.

phlegmasia inflammation. *P. alba dolens* white leg. A condition, uncommon nowadays, of puerperal femoral THROMBOPHLEBITIS or PHLEBOTHROMBOSIS, associated with venous obstruction and/or reflex arterial spasm. The leg is swollen and very painful. Treatment consists of elevating the leg without immobilization and giving antibiotics only if the condition is caused by thrombophlebitis; in other cases anticoagulants may be given in addition.

phlegmatic of dull and sluggish temperament.

phobia any persistent abnormal dread or fear that appears to result from repressed inner conflicts of which the affected person is unaware. Used as a word ending designating abnormal or morbid fear of, or aversion to the subject indicated by the stem to which it is affixed. A person with a phobia reacts uncontrollably and unreasonably to the situation of which he or she is afraid, e.g. acrophobia, fear of heights; claustrophobia, morbid fear of closed places.

phocomelia congenital absence of the proximal portion of a limb or limbs, the hands or feet being attached to the trunk by a small, irregularly shaped bone.

phospholipid any lipid that contains phosphorus, including those with a glycerol backbone (phosphoglycerides and plasmalogens) or a backbone of sphingosine or a related substance (sphingomyelins). They are the major lipids in cell membranes.

phosphorus a chemical element. Symbol P. It is an essential element in the diet. In the form of phosphates it is a major component of the mineral phase of bone and is involved in almost all metabolic processes. It also plays an important role in cell metabolism. It is obtained by the body from milk products, cereals, meat and fish, and its use by the body is controlled by vitamin D and calcium.

photophobia intolerance of light.

phototherapy treatment using fluorescent light, containing a high output of blue light, to reduce the amount of unconjugated bilirubin in the skin of a neonate. Complex changes occur and the non-toxic photodegradation products are excreted without the help of the enzyme system in the liver. Side effects are skin rashes and loose green stools. The latter requires an extra fluid intake of about 30 mg/kg per 24 hours to compensate, and conventionally the eyes and gonads are covered in case the light may cause problems. Phototherapy also may be used prophylactically in preterm infants with bruising, and in babies affected by Rhesus incompatibility. It is used therapeutically with levels of bilirubin of 340 μmol/l at term, 210 μmol/l at 34 weeks, and about 150 μmol.l at 28 weeks.

phrenic pertaining to the diaphragm or to the mind. *P. nerve* a major branch of the cervical plexus. Nerve impulses from the inspiratory centre in the brain travel down the phrenic nerve, causing contraction of the diaphragm, and inspiration occurs.

phthisis pulmonary tuberculosis.

physiology the science of the function of living organisms.

physique the body organization, development, and structure.

phytomenadione a preparation of vitamin K, effective in treating haemorrhage occurring during anticoagulant therapy, and due to vitamin K deficiency. Prophylactic vitamin K is given orally or intramuscularly to the newborn to prevent haemorrhagic disease.

pia mater the innermost membrane enveloping the brain and spinal cord.

pica a craving to eat unnatural substances, sometimes occurring during pregnancy.

pie chart a circular diagram divided into segments showing the proportional distribution of observations of particular events.

Pierre–Robin syndrome a congenital abnormality where there is MICROGNATHIA and a cleft palate. If it is not recognized at birth, severe respiratory obstruction may occur, as the tongue occludes the pharynx. The baby should be nursed prone, with the tongue pulled forwards if necessary to clear the airway.

pigment any dye or colouring agent. *Bile p.* BILIRUBIN and biliverdin. *Blood p.* haematin.

piles HAEMORRHOIDS.

pilonidal having a nest of hairs. *P. cyst* an implantation dermoid in the natal cleft. The cyst results from penetration of hairs in the natal cleft through the skin of the fold thus causing a sinus (pilonidal sinus) and epithelium cell implantation. Prone to recurrent infection. *P. depression* a depression in the midline near the coccyx, seen in the newborn child. It is of no significance. *P. sinus* a small sinus, opening near the coccyx. It is seen on routine examination of the newborn child soon after birth. It is a remnant of the neural canal and may become infected necessitating excision.

Pinard's stethoscope a trumpet-shaped instrument which can be placed on the maternal abdomen over the fetal chest to hear the fetal heart sounds. Called also fetal or monoaural stethoscope.

pineal 1. shaped like a pine cone. 2. pertaining to the pineal body.

P. body, p. gland a small conical structure attached by a stalk to the posterior wall of the third ventricle of the cerebrum, believed to be an endocrine gland.

pinna the projecting part of the ear lying outside the head.

Piriton trademark for chlorpheniramine maleate; a preparation used for the relief of allergy and the emergency treatment of anaphylactic reactions.

Pitressin a proprietary preparation of vasopressin.

pituitary gland an endocrine gland lying in the pituitary fossa of the sphenoid bone. It has an anterior and a posterior lobe. The anterior lobe produces GONADOTROPHIC hormones, GROWTH HORMONE, lactogenic hormone (prolactin), ADRENOCORTICOTROPHIC HORMONE and thyrotrophic hormone. The posterior lobe secretes OXYTOCIN and antidiuretic hormone.

PKU phenylketonuria.

place of safety order a court order whereby a child was arbitrarily removed from the care of its parents in the interests of his/her safety has now been replaced by the emergency protection order.

placebo a substance given to a patient as medicine or a procedure performed on a patient that has no intrinsic therapeutic value and relieves symptoms or helps the patient in some way only because the patient believes or expects that it will. Placebos are used in controlled clinical trials of new drugs. While some patients selected at random are given the new drug, others are given a placebo. Neither the patients nor those administering the drug, but the effects are closely monitored on all patients.

placenta the afterbirth. A flat organ measuring 17.5–20 cm (7–8 in) in diameter and 2.5 cm (1 in) in thickness tapering to 1.2 cm (0.5 in) at the periphery. It weighs approximately one-sixth of the baby's birth weight at full term. The placenta is developed from the trophoblastic layers with a lining of mesoderm in which the blood vessels develop. It is formed by the 12th week of pregnancy and is composed of large numbers of chorionic villi grouped together in cotyledons, and embedded in the decidua basalis of the uterus. The villi contain the fetal blood vessels (which ultimately join together to form the umbilical vessels), whilst they are separated by intervillous spaces through

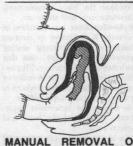

MANUAL REMOVAL OF THE PLACENTA

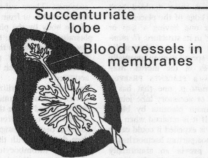

Succenturiate
lobe

Blood vessels in
membranes

PLACENTA WITH SUCCENTURIATE LOBE

which the maternal blood circulates. The branches of the umbilical vessels can be seen on the fetal surface, radiating from the insertion of the cord which is usually placed centrally. This surface is covered by the amnion, which can be stripped from it up to the insertion of the cord. The chorion is continuous with the edge of the placenta. The placenta functions to transmit oxygen and nutrients from the maternal blood to the fetus and to excrete carbon dioxide and other waste products of metabolism from the fetus to the mother. It also acts as a barrier to some infections, e.g. tuberculosis and pneumonia, but the treponema of syphilis and the tubercle bacillus can penetrate the placenta. Viruses can cross the placenta freely and may cause congenital abnormalities. Most drugs cross the placenta and may

have a beneficial effect on the fetus, e.g. antibiotics administered to a woman with syphilis. Some drugs, however, are teratogenic, e.g. thalidomide. Antibodies also cross and some are beneficial, e.g. immunoglobulin G (IgG), which confers immunity on the baby for about 3 months after birth, while others, e.g. anti-D Rhesus antibody, are harmful. It manufactures hormones, namely OESTROGENS, PROGESTERONE and CHORIONIC GONADOTROPHIN. *Abruptio p.* premature separation of a normally situated placenta. *Battledore p.* one in which the cord is attached to its margin and not the centre. *Bipartite p.* one having 2 lobes. *P. accreta* one abnormally adherent to the myometrium, with partial or complete absence of the decidua basalis. *P. circumvallata* one encircled with a dense, raised, white nodular ring, the attached membranes being doubled back over the edge of the placenta. *P. fenestrata* one having a gap or 'window' in its structure. *P. membranacea* one that is abnormally thin and spread over an unusually large area of the uterus. May occur as a PLACENTA PRAEVIA. *Succenturiate p.* one that has a separate or accessory lobe joined to the main placenta by blood vessels. If it is retained when the placenta is expelled it could cause serious postpartum haemorrhage.

placenta previa an abnormally situated placenta in the lower segment of the uterus, either completely or partially covering the internal os. *See* Appendix 6.

placental lactogen a hormone affecting growth and development of the breast in pregnancy. It also has a role in glucose metabolism in pregnancy. This hormone is similar to pituitary human GROWTH HORMONE, although it does not actually promote growth.

placentography radiological visualization of the placenta after injection of a contrast medium.

planned parenthood birth control.

plantar pertaining to the sole of the foot.

plasma a straw-coloured fluid which, with red and white blood cells, makes up the blood. Of the total volume of blood, 55 per cent is made up of plasma. It is 92 per cent water, in which are contained plasma proteins, inorganic salts, foods, gases, waste materials from the cells, and various hormones, secretions and enzymes. These substances are transported to or from the tissues of the body by the plasma.

plasmin an enzyme, FIBRINOLYSIN, which dissolves the fibrin in a thrombus. It is present in blood as plasminogen before it is activated.

Plastibell a presterilized plastic device used for circumcision. The bell is slipped inside the foreskin and a string is tied around it. The foreskin becomes gangrenous and then drops off with the bell.

platelets thrombocytes. Blood platelets are disc-shaped, non-nucleated blood elements with a very fragile membrane; they tend to adhere to uneven or damaged surfaces. They are formed in the red bone marrow and average about 250×10^9 per litre of blood. The functions of platelets are related to coagulation and the clotting of blood. Because of their adhesion and aggregation

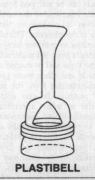

PLASTIBELL

capabilities platelets can occlude small breaks in blood vessels and prevent the escape of blood. *See* Appendix 18.

platypelloid flat. *See* PELVIS.

play group a session of care and activities for pre-school children. It can be organized by any interested person in his/her own home or other premises, but it must be registered by the social services department.

plethora excess of blood.

plethoric having the appearance of plethora, i.e. a florid colouring. Describes the condition usually seen in a baby with a large placental transfusion or in one of the twins with twin-to-twin transfusion syndrome.

pleura the serous membrane lining the thorax and enveloping each lung, the 2 layers enclosing a potential space, the pleural cavity.

pleurisy inflammation of the pleura.

plexus a network of veins or nerves. *Brachial p.* the network of nerves of the neck and axilla. *Solar* or *coeliac p.* the network of nerves and ganglia at the back of the stomach, which supply the abdominal viscera.

pneumonia inflammation of the lung. It may be (*a*) *lobar p.*, usually a pneumococcal infection of one or more lobes of the lung; (*b*) *bronchopneumonia*, in which the bronchioles are affected. A number of bacteria may be responsible, including *Staphylococcus aureus*, streptococcus or *Haemophilis influenzae*; (*c*) *viral*

p. the newborn child is predisposed to pneumonia by the RESPIRATORY DISTRESS SYNDROME. *See* Appendix 17.

pneumothorax accumulation of air or gas in the pleural cavity, resulting in collapse of the lung on the affected side. The condition may occur spontaneously, as in the course of a pulmonary disease, or it may follow trauma to, and perforation of, the chest wall. It may be a complication of vigorous resuscitation, ventilation, CONTINUOUS INFLATING PRESSURE or follow MECONIUM ASPIRATION. *See* Appendix 16. pl. *pneumothoraces.*

Po₂ partial pressure of oxygen. In the blood of an adult it is about 100 mmHg, and of a baby rather lower, about 60–90 mmHg. In a preterm infant there is a danger of RETROLENTAL FIBROPLASIA if it exceeds 100 mmHg. *See also Pco₂.*

podalic version the internal correction of a transverse lie by grasping a foot, thus converting it to a longitudinal lie and breech presentation.

polarity the gradient of the strength of uterine contractions between the fundus (the upper pole where the activity is the strongest) and the lower uterine segment and cervix (the lower pole where contractions are very weak or absent), which brings about dilatation of the cervix.

pole one extremity or end of an organ of the body, e.g. the uterus, or of the fetus.

poliomyelitis infantile paralysis.

Inflammation of the anterior cells of the spinal cord. A virus infection which is a notifiable disease. It affects chiefly young people and can cause such injury to the grey matter that paralysis results. It can be prevented by vaccination.

poly- prefix meaning 'much' or 'many'.

Polybactrin trademark for combination preparations of polymysin, neomycin and bacitracin.

polycystic kidneys a congenital malformation in which the kidneys are enlarged because they contain many cysts. In mild cases the condition may remain undiagnosed, and a woman may have a normal pregnancy, although it predisposes her to urinary tract infection and hypertension. In other cases the baby's kidneys are enlarged at birth and survival is unlikely.

polycythaemia an excess of red blood cells. The newborn child is normally polycythaemic.

polydactyly the existence of supernumerary fingers.

polygraph an apparatus for simultaneously recording several mechanical or electrical impulses, such as blood pressure, pulse, and respiration, and variations in electrical resistance of the skin.

polyhydramnios sometimes used synonymously with HYDRAMNIOS. A demonstrable excess of amniotic fluid. It is associated with maternal diabetes, congenital abnormalities especially of the central nervous system, uniovular twins and a rare tumour of the placenta (CHORIOANGIOMA).

polymorphonuclear possessing multilobed nuclei like most of the white blood cells.

polyneuritis multiple neuritis.

polypus a small pedunculated tumour arising from any mucous surface. *Cervical p.* in the cervical canal. *Fibroid p.* occurs in the uterus and contains fibrous myomatous tissue. *Placental p.* consists of remains of the placenta. pl. *polypi*.

polysaccharide a complex type of carbohydrate, e.g. starch.

polythene a plastic material with a very smooth surface, having a number of uses, e.g. for catheters, tubing, fine oesophageal tubes for feeding preterm infants and disposable syringes.

polyuria an excessive increase in the secretion of urine, due to diuretics or to diabetes.

pons 1. that part of the metencephalon lying between the medulla oblongata and the midbrain, ventral to the cerebellum. 2. any slip of tissue connecting 2 parts of an organ.

popliteal relating to the posterior part of the knee which is described as the *p. fossa* or *p. space.*

pore a minute circular opening on a surface, such as of sweat glands.

port-wine stain naevus flammeus.

portal vein the large vein which carries nutritive material from the digestive tract to the liver. Formed from the gastric, splenic and superior mesenteric veins.

position attitude or posture. *Dor-*

sal p. lying flat on the back.
Genupectoral or *knee–chest p.*
resting on the knees and chest
with arms crossed above the head.
More probably, resting on knees
and elbows. It is the traditional
position to help relieve pressure
on a cord which has prolapsed.
However, if the foot of the bed
can be elevated, and the patient
put into Sims' position, the same
effect is achieved with more comfort and less indignity. *Left lateral
p.* on the left side with right
knee drawn up towards the chin.
Lithotomy p. lying on the back
with thighs raised and knees
supported and held widely apart.
Prone p. lying face down. *Recumbent p.* lying down. *Sims' p.*
Similar to *left lateral*, but almost
on the face, and semi-prone with
the right knee and thigh drawn
up and resting on the bed in front
of the left one. *Trendelenburg p.*
lying on the back on a tilted plane
(usually an operating table at an
angle of 30° to the floor), with the
head lowermost and the shoulders
supported.

position of the fetus the relation
of a particular part of the fetus,
the DENOMINATOR to a particular
part of the mother's pelvis. In
the vertex presentation the
denominator is the occiput. Eight
positions may be described. If
the occiput is directed towards
the symphysis pubis, the position
is direct occipitoanterior; if to the
left or right iliopectineal eminence, it is left or right occipitoanterior; if to the mid-point of
the left or right iliopectineal line,

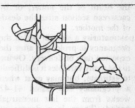

Used for forceps delivery,
perineal repair and many
obstetric operations.
LITHOTOMY POSITION

left or right occipitolateral; if to
the left or right sacroiliac joint,
left or right occipitoposterior; and
if towards the sacrum, direct
occipitoposterior. In practice it
has been found that the head
commonly lies transversely with
the occiput lateral, and thus a
left occipitolateral and a right
occipitolateral position are
described. The breech positions
are similar, but with the sacrum
as the denominator.

**positive end-expiratory pressure
(PEEP)** in mechanical ventilation, a positive airway pressure
maintained until the end of expiration.

posseting regurgitation of a small
amount of milk immediately after
a feed.

post- prefix meaning 'after', e.g.
postnatal clinic.

posterior placed at the back.

posthumous occurring after
death. *P. birth* one occurring after

the death of the father, or by caesarean section after the death of the mother.

postmaturity a state in which the pregnancy is prolonged after the expected date of delivery. Owing to the many variables it is difficult to estimate, but may exist when a pregnancy has lasted 41–42 weeks from the last menstrual period. There is a danger of hypoxia to the fetus. *See* Appendices 9 and 16.

post mortem after death. *P. m. examination* autopsy.

postnatal after childbirth. *P. clinic* an examination centre where the patient can be examined (*postnatally*), preferably 6 weeks following childbirth: (*a*) regarding her general health; (*b*) specifically, to find out the state of the uterus, pelvic floor and vagina.

postnatal period a period not less than 10 and not more than 28 days after the end of labour, during which the continued attendance of a midwife on the mother and baby is mandatory. This is a rule of the United Kingdom Central Council.

postpartum after labour. *P. haemorrhage* and *p. collapse*. *See* Appendix 11.

posture the general attitude of body and limbs.

potassium a metallic element. Symbol K. Forms one of the electrolytes of the blood and tissue fluids and plays an essential role in maintenance of the acid–base and water balance in the body. A proper balance between sodium, calcium and potassium in the blood plasma is necessary for proper cardiac function.

potential existing as a possibility but not in fact. *P. diabetic* a person with normal glucose tolerance but with an increased risk of developing clinical DIABETES, e.g. a woman who has one or both parents as diabetics, or who has given birth to a live or stillborn baby weighing 4.5 kg (10 lb) or more at birth.

Potter's syndrome a congenital condition consisting of renal agenesis and pulmonary hypoplasia. The baby has low-set ears and furrows under the eyes (Potter's facies), and it is commonly associated with only 2 vessels in the umbilical cord. Absence of the kidneys is a rare and fatal condition.

pouch a pocket-like space or cavity. *P. of Douglas* the lowest fold of the peritoneum between the uterus and rectum. *Uterovesical p.* the fold of peritoneum between the uterus and bladder.

Poupart's ligament inguinal ligament. The tendinous lower border of the external oblique muscle of the abdominal wall, which passes from the anterior superior spine of the ilium to the os pubis.

practice the exercise of a profession.

practitioner a person who practises a profession.

prandial pertaining to a meal.

pre- prefix meaning 'before', e.g. prenatal, premature.

precipitate 1. to cause settling in

solid particles of a substance in solution. 2. a deposit of solid particles settled out of a solution. 3. occurring with undue rapidity, as *precipitate labour*. There is a danger to the mother of severe perineal lacerations, and to the child of intracranial trauma as a result of the rapid passage through the birth canal.

preconception care health education and medical examination before conception in order that any problems can be detected and where possible treated, thus promoting optimum health at the time of conception and during the period of organogenesis in the first trimester of pregnancy. It is hoped that such care will reduce the incidence of congenital malformations and improve the mother's health and that of the fetus. Foresight is the organization for the promotion of preconception care in the UK.

precursor something that precedes. In biological processes, a substance from which another, usually more active or mature substance is formed. In clinical medicine, a sign or symptom that heralds another.

pre-diabetes a state which precedes diabetes mellitus, in which the disease is not yet clinically manifested. In pregnancy the diabetes may become evident, or the woman may remain well but give birth to an unusually large child.

predisposition a latent susceptibility to disease which may be activated under certain conditions.

prednisone, prednisolone synthetic preparations with the same action as hormones from the adrenal cortex. These glucocorticoid drugs are used as anti-inflammatory and anti-allergic agents.

pre-eclampsia the precursor of ECLAMPSIA. Now commonly termed pregnancy-induced hypertension. A syndrome with three physical signs which occurs only in pregnancy, usually during the second half. The cause of the arteriolar spasm is still unknown, but it produces the following signs: (*a*) an elevated blood pressure—over 130/80 mmHg is often taken as the significant level, but a rise of 15–20 mmHg above the individual's previous diastolic level is more comprehensive; (*b*) generalized oedema; and (*c*) proteinuria; this is the most serious sign. The diagnosis is usually made when two out of the three signs are present. The disease resolves within 48–72 hours of delivery. In cases where the disease develops before term, unless very severe, the treatment is conservative, allowing the pregnancy to mature as near to 38 weeks as possible, thereby avoiding the risks associated with an immature baby. *See* Appendix 6.

pregnancy the condition of having a developing embryo or fetus within the body; the state from conception to delivery of the fetus. The normal duration is 280 days (40 weeks or 9 months and 7 days) counted from the first day of the last normal menstrual period. The interval from conception to birth—more nearly accurate but less easy to ascertain—averages 265 days. *Ectopic p.* extrauterine pregnancy. This occurs relatively frequently in the fallopian tube and very rarely in the ovary or the abdominal cavity.

pregnancy tests these detect the HUMAN CHORIONIC GONADOTROPHIN (HCG) produced by the embryo 8 days after the first missed period. Immunological laboratory tests, e.g. Gravindex or Pregnosticon, now give 98 per cent accuracy.

pregnanediol a derivative of pregnane, formed by reduction of progesterone and found especially in urine of pregnant women.

pregnant with child; gravid; having a developing embryo or fetus within the uterus.

premature early. *P. baby* one born before 37 completed weeks of pregnancy, and now usually called a preterm baby. It is usually a baby of low birth weight, unless there has been maternal diabetes *see* Appendix 17. *P. labour* labour resulting in the birth of a premature baby. *P. rupture of membranes* rupture of the membranes before the onset of labour.

premedication drugs given prior to a general anaesthetic, e.g. atropine, hyoscine or papaveretum. Opiates, however, are not used before caesarean section to avoid respiratory depression of the baby.

premenstrual preceding menstruation.

premonition a forewarning. *Se* AURA.

prenatal occurring before birth.

preoperative preceding an operation. *P. care* the psychological and physiological preparation of a patient before operation.

prepuce foreskin; a loose fold of skin covering the glans penis.

prescription a formula written by a physician, directing the pharmacist to prepare a drug, or mixture of drugs. NHS prescriptions are free for expectant mothers and mothers who have a child under 12 months old.

presentation that part of the fetus which first enters the pelvis occupying the lower pole of the uterus. Normally cephalic with the vertex presenting, sometimes the breech, and occasionally the face brow or shoulder.

pressor tending to increase blood pressure.

pressure stress or strain, by compression, expansion, pull, thrust or shear. *Arterial p.* the blood pressure in the arteries. Also *see* BLOOD PRESSURE.

pre-term *see* PREMATURE.

prevalence the total number of cases of a specific disease in existence in a given population at a certain time.

preventive serving to avert the occurrence of; prophylactic.

pre-viable before viability. A previable infant is one born alive before the 24th week of pregnancy.

Price precipitation reaction (PPR) a serological test for syphilis.

primary first in order of time or importance.

primary health care medical, midwifery and nursing care provided in the community.

primary health care team the people who provide primary health care in the community. The team is made up of general practitioner, community midwife, community nurse and health visitor. It may also include a social worker. They may be based in a health centre or a general practice area.

primigravida a woman pregnant for the first time.

primipara a woman who has given birth to a viable child, whether alive or stillborn.

primiparous having borne one child.

probability (*P*) a statistical term meaning the likelihood of an association between variables being due to chance.

probe a blunt, malleable instrument for exploring sinus tracks, wounds, cavities or passages.

problem family a family whose way of life does not conform to accepted social standards, with the possible consequences of NON-ACCIDENTAL INJURY (NAI), wife battering and deprivation.

procaine a local anaesthetic; the hydrochloride salt is used in solution for infiltration.

process 1. a prominence or projection, as from a bone. 2. a series of operations or events leading to achievement of a specific result. *Midwifery* or *nursing p.* a systematic, problem-solving approach to

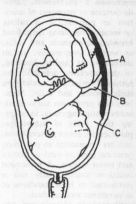

A. *Placenta*; B. *umbilical cord*; C. *liquor amnii*.
NORMAL CEPHALIC PRESENTATION *IN UTERO*

the task of meeting the needs and health care problems of clients.

procidentia complete prolapse of the uterus so that the cervix protrudes through the vulva.

procreation the act of begetting young.

proctalgia pain in the rectum.

proctitis inflammation of the anus or rectum.

proctoscope an instrument for examination of the rectum.

prodromal preceding. Warning of approaching disease, e.g. visual disturbances occurring before ECLAMPSIA.

profession 1. an avowed, public declaration or statement of intention or purpose. 2. a calling or vocation requiring specialized knowledge, methods and skills, as well as preparation, in an institution of higher learning, in the scholarly, scientific and historical principles underlying such methods and skills. Members of a profession are committed to continuing study, to enlarging their body of knowledge, place service above personal gain, and are committed to providing practical services vital to human and social welfare. A profession functions autonomously and is committed to high standards of achievement and conduct.

profibrinolysin plasminogen, the precursor of fibrinolysin.

profile a simple outline, as of the side view of the head or face; by extension, a graph representing quantitatively a set of characteristics determined by tests. A record of achievements developed during a course of study or subsequently.

progeny issue. Descendants.

progesterone the female sex hormone essential to normal life and to maintaining pregnancy. It is produced from the corpus luteum and also the placenta. During the menstrual cycle it is responsible for the secretory changes in the endometrium in preparation for the reception of a fertilized ovum, a slight rise in body temperature at the time of ovulation and premenstrual retention of water and electrolytes. In pregnancy it promotes the formation and maintenance of the decidua, the development of the glandular tissue of the breasts, the relaxation of plain muscle throughout the body and the retention of water and electrolytes in the body tissues.

progestogen any substance having progestational activity.

prognosis a forecast of the course and duration of a disease.

Project 2000 the title of a UKCC Report published in 1986 which proposed major alterations in the process of nurse education. Many of the proposals have since been modified and are now in the process of being implemented. Some of the major recommendations for nurses include a common foundation programme of 18 months followed by a branch programme in either nursing of adults, children, mental illness or mental handicap. In midwifery there are increasing opportunities for the 3 year pre-registration programme and the 18 month post-registration course continues. Where appropriate there is shared learning with nurses. All student nurses and pre-registration student midwives are supernumerary to NHS staffing establishments and receive a bursary.

projectile vomiting see VOMITING.

prolactin a hormone from the anterior lobe of the pituitary gland that stimulates and sustains milk production in postpartum women.

prolapse the descent of an organ

or structure. *P. of the umbilical cord* this is when, following rupture of the membranes, the cord lies in front of the presenting part. The fetus is in great danger of HYPOXIA or ANOXIA when the cord is compressed. Immediate delivery must follow the diagnosis. *P. of rectum* protrusion of the rectal mucosa and, occasionally, of the muscle, through the anal canal to the exterior. *P. of an arm* the fetal arm falls into or through the vagina. A serious complication of uncorrected shoulder presentation. *P. of the uterus* the uterus protrudes into the lower part of the vagina, as a result of the weakening of its supports. Prolapse, unqualified, refers to the descent of one or more of the pelvic structures due to weakness of the pelvic floor. The uterus, vaginal walls, bladder or rectum may be involved.

proliferation rapid multiplication

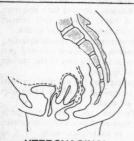

**UTEROVAGINAL
PROLAPSE**

of cells, as may occur in a malignant growth.

prolific rapid production of many offspring.

prolonged labour labour lasting more than 18 hours. *See* Appendix 9.

prolonged pregnancy pregnancy lasting 42 seeks (294 days) or more from the first day of the last normal menstrual period.

promazine (Sparine) a tranquillizer; a phenothiazine derivative. *See* Appendix 19.

promethazine hydrochloride (Phenergan) an antihistamine drug, often allied with pethidine in labour. Also used in the treatment of vomiting in pregnancy; a phenothiazine derivative. *See* Appendix 19.

promontory a projection. The *sacral p.* is an important landmark of the pelvis formed by the projection of the upper border of the first sacral vertebra.

pronation turning downwards. *P. of the hand* the palm is downward.

prone lying face downward.

pronucleus the haploid nucleus of a sex cell.

prophylactic pertaining to prophylaxis.

prophylaxis measures taken to prevent a disease; preventive treatment.

propranolol a β-adrenergic blocking agent used in the treatment of hypertension and some cardiac conditions.

propylthiouracil a thyroid inhibitor used in the treatment of thyrotoxicosis.

prostaglandins a group of substances, first discovered in semen, now known to be present in menstrual blood, amniotic fluid and many other cells. They have an oxytocic effect, so are used to induce abortion before 10 weeks and to ripen the cervix and induce labour.

prostate a gland in the male which surrounds the neck of the bladder and the prostatic urethra. It contributes a secretion to the seminal fluid.

prosthesis the replacement of an absent part by an artificial substitute; an artificial substitute for a missing part. adj. *prosthetic*.

Prostin E a proprietary preparation of prostaglandin E_2. *See* Appendix 9.

protamine sulphate an antidote to heparin overdosage.

protein a material composed of carbon, hydrogen, nitrogen and oxygen. It is the essential constituent of body tissue. Animal sources are meat, fish, milk and eggs; vegetable sources are peas, beans and lentils. During digestion, proteins are broken down into 20 varieties of amino acid. Of these, 8 are essential including PHENYLALANINE and TYROSINE. These are then built up into new cells and used to repair others. Excess amino acids cannot be stored, but are broken down by the liver and excreted in the urine as urea. The proteins in blood plasma are divided in 4 major classes; specific protein carriers, that are involved in the transport of hormones and other substances; acute phase reactants, such as alpha$_1$-antitrypsin or fibrinogen, that are involved in inflammation or in clotting; complement components; and immunoglobulins. Albumin plays an important role in the maintenance of normal distribution of water by exerting osmotic pressure at the capillary membrane. This pressure prevents fluid of the plasma from leaking out of the capillaries and into the space between the tissue cells.

proteinuria any protein, usually albumin, found in the urine.

Proteus a Gram-negative bacteria usually found in faecal and other putrefying matter.

prothrombin a plasma protein synthesized in the liver. It is vital for the blood clotting mechanism as, in the presence of calcium, it forms thrombin when activated by thromboplastin released when tissues are damaged and platelets broken down. The thrombin, with fibrinogen, then forms insoluble fibrin. *P. time* the time, in seconds, required for a specimen of blood brought into contact with thromboplastin, to clot.

prothrombinase thromboplastin.

proton a positively charged particle forming part of the nucleus of an atom.

protoplasm the essential chemical compound of which living cells are made.

Provera trademark for preparations of medroxyprogesterone, a progestational agent. It is an intramuscular contraceptive, effective for 8–12 weeks.

pruritus great irritation of the

skin. It may affect the whole surface of the body, as in certain skin diseases and nervous disorders, or it may be limited in area. *P. vulvae* in pregnancy may be associated with glycosuria or with candidal (monilia) VAGINITIS.

pseudo- prefix meaning 'false'.

pseudocyesis a spurious pregnancy. Subjective manifestation of the symptoms of pregnancy, in the absence of conception.

pseudohermaphroditism apparently having male and female characteristics. More precisely defined as INTERSEX.

pseudomenstruation a blood-stained vaginal discharge which may occur on about the third day of life in baby girls due to withdrawal of maternal oestrogens.

Pseudomonas a Gram-negative, aerobic bacteria, some species of which are pathogenic for plants and vertebrates.

psoas a muscle forming part of the posterior abdominal wall.

psyche the mind, both conscious and unconscious.

psychiatrist a doctor who specializes in psychiatry.

psychiatry study of mental disorders and their treatment.

psychologist one who studies normal and abnormal mental processes, development and behaviour.

psychology the science of the mind and its functions.

psychomotor pertaining to motor effects of cerebral or psychic activity.

psychopath a person with an anti-social personality.

psychoprophylaxis a method of preparation for labour aimed at preventing pain and modifying the perception of painful sensations associated with normal uncomplicated childbirth. Preparation includes education about the process of labour and breathing patterns linked with disassociation and muscular control. This method usually requires intensive practice during the antenatal period.

psychosis a severe mental illness affecting the whole personality. Of organic or emotional origin. It is marked by derangement of the personality and loss of contact with reality, often with delusions, hallucinations, or illusions. adj. *psychotic*.

psychosomatic relating to the mind and the body. *P. disorders* those illnesses in which emotional factors have a profound influence.

psychotherapy any of a number of related techniques for treating mental illness by psychological methods. These techniques are similiar in that they all rely mainly on establishing communication between the therapist and the patient as a means of understanding and modifying the patient's behaviour.

ptosis drooping of the upper eyelid from 3rd nerve paralysis. Dropping downwards of an organ or other structure.

ptyalin an ENZYME in saliva which starts digestion of starches.

ptyalism abnormally increased

salivation. A rare complication of pregnancy.

puberty the age at which the reproductive organs become functionally active. Generally between the 10th and 14th years.

pubes the region over the pubic bones.

pubic pertaining to the pubes, e.g. *p. arch*, the bony arch formed by the junction of the *inferior pubic rami*, forming the anterior part of the pelvic outlet.

pubiotomy cutting through the pubic bone to enable birth to take place.

pubis the anterior portion of the hip bone; called also pubic bone.

public health the field of medicine that is concerned with safeguarding and improving the physical, mental and social well-being of the community as a whole. Environmental aspects are the responsibility of the district local authority, whereas communicable disease control is supervised by the Medical Officer for Environmental Health, from the District Health Authority. Central government formulates national policy and is responsible for international aspects.

pubococcygeus one part of the levator ani muscle. *See* PELVIS.

pubovesical pertaining to the pubis and bladder.

pudenda the external genitalia.

pudendal pertaining to the external genital organs. *P. block* a form of local analgesia induced by injecting a solution of 0.5 or 1 per cent lignocaine around the pudendal nerve.

puerperal pertaining to the puerperium. *P. pyrexia* a rise of temperature in the puerperium *P. psychosis* any psychosis appearing in the puerperium. Pregnancy often acts as a trigger, as can any other major life event. *P. sepsis* infection of the genital tract following childbirth.

puerperium the period following childbirth during which the uterus and other organs and structures are returning to the pregravid state. A period of 6–8 weeks.

pulmonary pertaining to or affecting the lungs. *P. circulation. See* CIRCULATION. *P. embolism. See* EMBOLISM. *P. haemorrhage.* Neonatal death can sometimes be caused by massive haemorrhage into both lungs. *P. infarction* is due to the occlusion of a small blood vessel in the lung by a clot, which causes death of the tissue supplied by that vessel.

pulsation a beating or throbbing.

pulse the local rhythmic expansion of an artery, which can be felt with the finger, corresponding to each contraction of the left ventricle of the heart. It may be felt in any artery sufficiently near the surface of the body. The normal adult rate is about 72 per minute. In childhood it is more rapid, varying from 130 in infants to 80 in older children. *P. pressure* the difference between the diastolic and systolic blood pressures, as measured by the sphygmomanometer.

puncture to pierce. *Lumbar p.* to remove cerebrospinal fluid by puncture between the 3rd and 4th, or 4th and 5th lumbar vertebrae to relieve cerebral pressure, or to obtain cerebrospinal fluid for diagnostic purposes.

PUO pyrexia of unknown origin.

pupil the opening in the centre of the iris through which light enters the eye.

purgative a drug which produces evacuation of the bowels.

purpura haemorrhagica a condition characterized by extravasation of blood in the skin and mucous membranes, causing purple spots and patches. It is sometimes associated with a deficiency of THROMBOCYTES (THROMBOCYTOPENIA).

purulent containing or resembling pus.

pus a thick, semi-liquid substance consisting of dead leucocytes and bacteria, debris of cells and tissue fluids. It results from inflammation caused by invading bacteria which have destroyed the phagocytes and set up local suppuration.

pustule a small, elevated, circumscribed, pus-containing lesion of the skin.

putative supposed, reputed. *P. father* the man believed to be the father of an illegitimate child.

PV *per vaginam.*

pyaemia a condition resulting from invasion of the blood stream by bacteria. Blockage of small blood vessels occurs with resultant formation of abscesses, the development of which causes rigors and high fever.

pyelitis literally inflammation of

the renal pelvis. Usually called PYELONEPHRITIS.

pyelography radiology of the renal pelvis after the injection of radio-opaque contrast medium. *Intravenous p. (IVP)* a water-soluble, iodine-containing contrast medium is injected intravenously and radiographs are exposed as the contrast medium is excreted by the kidneys, and passes down the ureters into the bladder.

pyelonephritis inflammation of the kidneys and ureters, usually caused by ESCHERICHIA COLI. The acute symptoms are severe lumbar pain, hyperpyrexia, often rigors, tachycardia, vomiting and general malaise; the chronic symptoms are backache, vomiting and anaemia, though this type is often symptomless. Either form may occur during pregnancy, usually between 18 and 24 weeks, owing to stasis of urine in the ureters, which have dilated and relaxed under the influence of progesterone, and of pressure from the pregnant uterus, particularly on the right side. Multiplication of bacteria can then take place; asymptomatic bacteriuria often occurs at the start of pregnancy. All women should be screened for bacteriuria early in pregnancy and treated at once if necessary. This urinary tract infection is not uncommon in newborn infants. There are no obvious signs, but the condition may be suspected in any infant who is pale, not feeding well, losing weight and generally not thriving.

pyelonephrosis any disease of the kidney and its pelvis.

pyloric stenosis congenital hypertrophic pyloric stenosis occurs in 3 per 1000 births. In the affected baby the pyloric sphincter becomes thickened, strong and spastic. The stomach enlarges and becomes more powerful from forcing the gastric contents through the narrowed pylorus. Waves of peristalsis can be seen during feeding and the pylorus can be felt as a tumour. Persistent projectile vomiting occurs. These signs rarely occur before 3–4 weeks of age. An antispasmodic drug (e.g. atropine, Eumydrin) may be given with feeds but RAMSTEDT'S OPERATION is often necessary for rapid and complete recovery.

pylorus the opening between the stomach and the duodenum.

pyo- prefix meaning 'pus'.

pyogenic producing 'pus'.

pyometra the condition in which pus is present in the uterus.

pyosalpinx pus in the fallopian tube.

pyretic pertaining to fever.

pyrexia fever; a rise of body temperature above 37.2°C (99°F).

pyridoxine one of the forms of vitamin B_6, chiefly used in the prophylaxis and treatment of vitamin B_6 deficiency.

pyrogen a fever-producing substance, possibly of bacterial origin. Distilled water used for intravenous injection should be pyrogen-free.

pyuria the presence of pus in the urine. The urine is generally cloudy and pus cells will be seen if the urine is examined microscopically.

Q

Q quadrant.

q 1. symbol for the long arm of a chromosome. 2. symbol for the frequency of the rarer allele of a pair.

qd *quaque die* (every day).

qh *quaque hora* (every hour).

qid *quater in die* (4 times a day).

qqh *quaque quarta hora* (every 4 hours).

quadrant 1. one fourth of the circumference of a circle. 2. one of 4 corresponding parts, or quarters, as of the surface of the abdomen or of the field of vision.

quadruplets four children born at the same labour. Formerly very rare; more common since the use of fertility drugs.

quality assurance in the health care field, a pledge to the public by those within the various health disciplines such as midwifery that they will work toward the goal of an optimal achievable degree of excellence in the services rendered to every client. A quality assurance programme takes into acount the need to define that which is to be measured

The development of criteria based on acceptable standards of care and norms of professional behaviour are formulated. The criteria are then used as the 'yardstick' against which actual practice and its results can be evaluated. Evaluation is conducted by a review committee. The ultimate goal is improvement of client care.

quarantine the period during which known infected persons, contacts and suspects are isolated to prevent the spread of infection.

'quickening' the first perceptible fetal movements, felt by the mother at approximately the 18th to 20th week in a primigravid woman and recognized at the 16th to 18th week in the multigravida.

quintuplets five children born at the same labour.

quotient a number obtained by division. *Intelligence q. (IQ)* a numerical expression of intellectual capacity obtained by multiplying the mental age of the subject concerned, ascertained by testing, by 100 and dividing by his/her chronological age.

R

Rx symbol recipe (take); prescription; treatment.

race a class or breed of animals; a group of individuals having certain characteristics in common, owing to a common inheritance.

racemose grape-like. *R. cells* those arranged round a central duct. *R. glands* are compound and lobulated in structure, e.g. salivary glands, cells of the breasts, glands of the cervix.

rachi(o)- word element meaning 'spine'.

rachitic pelvis a flat pelvic brim similar to that of the platypelloid pelvis. This deformity of the pelvic brim is caused by rickets in early childhood.

radial relating to the radius. *R. artery* the artery at the wrist. *R.*

palsy a palsy characterized by wrist drop; it can be seen soon after birth. It usually recovers spontaneously over a varying time.

radical dealing with the root or cause of a disease. *R. cure* one which cures by complete removal of the cause.

radioactive emitting electromagnetic waves, alpha (α), beta (β) or gamma (γ). A radioactive substance may do this naturally, as does radium, or the effect may be produced artificially by bombardment in an atomic pile, e.g. radioactive iodine (^{131}I).

radiograph a picture taken by X-rays.

radiographer a professional health care worker in a diagnostic X-ray department (diagnostic radiographer) or in a radiotherapy department (therapy radiographer).

radiography examination by means of Röntgen or X-rays. This may yield valuable information in pregnancy and labour. *See* Appendix 4.

radioimmunoassay (RIA) a sensitive assay method that can be used for the measurement of minute quantities of specific antibodies or any antigen such as a hormone or drug, against which specific antibodies can be raised. It is a standard method for clinical laboratory measurements of hormones and is also used for therapeutic drug monitoring, drug abuse screening, and other laboratory tests.

radioisotope a radioactive form of an element. A radioisotope consists of unstable atoms that undergo radioactive decay emitting alpha, beta or gamma radiation. Radioisotopes occur naturally, as in the cases of radium and uranium, or may be created artificially.

radio-opaque capable of obstructing the passage of X-rays.

radiotelemetry measurement based on data transmitted by radio waves from the subject to the recording apparatus. Continuous fetal heart monitoring may be carried out by radiotelemetry when the mother is ambulant in labour.

radiotherapy the treatment of disease by ionizing radiation such as X-rays, beta rays and gamma rays; it is mainly used in malignant disease. The source of radiation may be outside the body of the patient or it may be an isotope that has been implanted or instilled into abnormal tissue or a body cavity.

radium a metallic element. Symbol Ra. A metal which has natural RADIOACTIVITY.

Ramstedt's operation Division of a hypertrophied pyloric sphincter to relieve PYLORIC STENOSIS.

ramus a branch, as of the pubic bone which has an upper and lower branch. pl. *rami*.

ranidine an H_2 receptor antagonist which may be given to women in labour prior to general anaesthesia in order to inhibit the production of hydrochloric acid, thereby reducing the risk of Mendelson's syndrome.

rape sexual assault or abuse; criminal forcible sexual intercourse.

raphe a seam or ridge of tissue indicating the juncture of two equal parts, e.g. the median raphe of the perineal body, the anococcygeal raphe.

rapport a term used to describe a satisfactory relationship between two persons, either the doctor and patient, midwife and woman, or the mother with any other person significant to her.

rash a temporary eruption on the skin. *Heat r.* miliaria. *Napkin r.* a cutaneous reaction in an infant, localized in areas ordinarily covered by the napkin. It is due to various primary irritants, such as ammonia in decomposed urine; improperly washed nappies and other contact factors may also be responsible. *Nettle r.* urticaria.

raspberry mark congenital haemangioma.

Rastelli's operation surgical procedure used in the treatment of transposition of the great vessels. The circulation of blood through the heart is diverted to effect adequate oxygenation.

rate the speed or frequency with which an event or circumstance occurs per unit of time, population, or other standard of comparison. *Basal metabolic r. (BMR)* an expression of the rate at which oxygen is utilized in a fasting subject at complete rest as a percentage of a value established as normal for such a subject. *Birth r.* the number of live births in a population in a specified period of time (crude birth rate), for the female population (refined birth rate), or for the female population of childbearing age (true birth rate), usually expressed per year per 1000 of the estimated mid-year population. *Death r.* the number of deaths per stated number of persons (1000 or 10 000, or 100 000) in a certain region in a certain time (crude death rate). The death rate calculated with allowances made for age and sex distribution in the population is termed the standardized death rate. Called also *mortality rate*. *Glomerular filtration r.* an expression of the quantity of glomerular filtrate formed each minute in the nephrons of both kidneys, calculated by measuring the clearance of

specific substances, e.g. insulin or creatinine.

ratio an expression of the quantity of one substance or entity in relation to that of another; the relationship between 2 quantities expressed as the quotient of one divided by the other. *Lecithin-sphingomyelin r.* the ratio of lecithin to sphingomyelin in amniotic fluid.

rationalization an unconscious defence mechanism in which a person finds logical reasons (justification) for his/her behaviour while ignoring the real reasons.

RAWP *see* RESOURCES ALLOCATION WORKING PARTY.

RBC red blood cells; red blood (cell) count.

reabsorption the act or process of absorbing again, as in the absorption by the kidneys of substances (glucose, proteins, sodium, etc.) already secreted into the renal tubules.

reaction counteraction; a response to the application of a stimulus. Evidence of acidity or alkalinity. The pH of a solution.

reagent a substance employed to produce a chemical reaction so as to detect, measure, produce, etc., other substances.

real-time scanner an ULTRASOUND scanner which gives a moving visual display. *See* Appendix 4.

receptor 1. a molecule on the surface or within a cell that recognizes and binds with specific molecules, producing some effect in the cell; e.g. the cell-surface receptors of immunocompetent cells that recognize antigens, complement components, or lymphokines, or those of neurons and target organs that recognize neurotransmitters or hormones. 2. a sensory nerve ending that responds to various stimuli.

recession receding or drawing back. *Rib* or *sternal r.* is commonly seen in the RESPIRATORY DISTRESS SYNDROME of neonates. *See* Appendix 17.

recessive tending to recede. In genetics the opposite of dominant—capable of expression only when borne by both sides of a set of homologous chromosomes, i.e. HOMOZYGOUS and not HETEROZYGOUS.

recipient one who receives, as a blood transfusion, or a tissue or organ graft. *Universal r.* a person thought to be able to receive blood of any 'type' without agglutination of the donor cells.

recombinant 1. a new cell or individual that results from genetic recombination. 2. pertaining or relating to such cells or individuals. *R. DNA technology* the process of taking a gene from one organism and inserting it into the DNA of another; called also gene splicing.

rectal relating to the rectum. *R. examination* digital examination of the rectum or adjacent structures, e.g. during labour, of the cervix uteri and presenting part.

rectocele hernia of the rectum, caused by overstretching of the vaginal wall at childbirth. Treated by posterior colporrhaphy.

rectovaginal pertaining to rectum and vagina. *R. fistula see* FISTULA.

rectovesical pertaining to or communicating with the rectum and bladder.

rectum the lower 15 cm (6 in) of the large intestine extending from the pelvic colon to the anal canal.

recumbent lying down.

recurrent occurring again.

reduction the correction of a fracture, dislocation or hernia.

referred pain that which occurs at a distance from the place of origin, and which is related to the distribution of sensory nerves.

reflex reflected or thrown back. *R. action* an involuntary movement resulting from a stimulus, e.g. the knee jerk, or the withdrawal of a limb from a pinprick. Certain reflexes are present in the mature newborn child, e.g. the sucking,

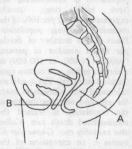

A. *Rectum*; B. *posterior vaginal wall.*
RECTOCELE

swallowing and MORO REFLEXES. *Conditioned r.* one that is not natural but acquired by regular association of a physiological event with an unrelated outside event, e.g. the draught, milk ejection or milk flow reflex that causes the myoepithelial cells in the breast to contract at the sight or sound of the hungry baby, so mobilizing the milk into the lacteal sinuses where it is immediately available to the baby.

regional health authority (RHA) a unit of health administration, of which there are 14 in England, each divided into a varying number of district health authorities (DHA). *See also* Appendix 1.

register an epidemiological term meaning an index on file of all cases with a particular disease or condition in a defined population.

registrar of births, marriages and deaths the official recorder of births, marriages and deaths. In England and Wales, the office comes under the Office of Population and Census surveys, which also regulates and records civil marriages, conducts demographic research and analyses demographic material. Local registry offices are available in most towns. Births should be registered within 6 weeks in England (21 days in Scotland).

regurgitation backward flow, e.g. of food into the mouth from the stomach. Sometimes occurs in newborn babies, when it is associated with weakness of the cardia of the stomach. *Aortic r.* backward flow of blood into the left ventricle when the aortic valve is incompetent. *Mitral r. see* MITRAL. *Gastro-oesophageal r. see* HEARTBURN.

rehabilitation re-education.

Reiter's protein complement fixation (RPCF) a serological test used to aid the diagnosis of syphilis.

relapse the return of a disease, following an apparent recovery.

relaxant causing relaxation; an agent that causes relaxation. *Muscle r.* an agent that either acts at the neuromuscular junction, causing muscle paralysis, and used in anaesthesia, or relieves muscle spasticity and tension by acting on muscle itself, or more commonly on the central nervous system.

relaxation a lessening of tension, as may be observed when muscles slacken after they have contracted. It is important that the patient in labour should rest and relax her muscles between the contractions of labour. Classes may be given to the pregnant woman to prepare her for this. *See also* PSYCHOPROPHYLAXIS.

relaxin a hormone which is thought to cause general 'softening' of the pelvic tissues and joints in the pregnant woman, thereby providing some increase in pelvic capacity.

releasing factor a substance produced in the hypothalamus which causes the anterior pituitary gland to release hormones.

REM rapid eye movement, a phase of sleep associated with dreaming and characterized by rapid movements of the eyes.

renal concerning or affecting the kidney. *R. calculus* stone in the kidney. *R. failure* failure of the renal function, which gives rise to uraemia. *R. threshold* the level of substances in the blood beyond which they are excreted in the urine. Normally the renal threshold for glucose is 10 mmol/l (180 mg/100 ml) and if the blood sugar rises above this level glycosuria results.

renin an enzyme synthesized, stored and secreted by the kidneys; it plays a role in regulation of blood pressure by catalysing the conversion of angiotensinogen to angiotensin I. This, in turn, is converted to angiotensin II which is a powerful vasoconstrictor and also stimulates aldosterone secretion. Aldosterone results in retention of salt and water by the kidneys.

rennin the milk-curdling enzyme found in gastric juice of human infants. Rennin catalyses the conversion of casein from a soluble to insoluble form.

reproduction 1. the process by which a living entity or organism produces a new individual of the same kind. 2. the creation of a similar object or situation; duplication; replication.

reproductive organs, female the ovaries, which produce the ova, or eggs; the uterine tubes; the uterus; the vagina, or birth canal; and the vulva, comprising the external genitalia. The breasts are the secondary sexual characteristics, enclosing the mammary glands. *R. o., male* the external genitalia (the penis, testes and scrotum), accessory glands that secrete special fluids, and the ducts through which these organs and glands are connected to each other, and through which the spermatozoa are ejaculated during coitus.

research an attempt to increase available knowledge by the discovery of new information through systematic scientific enquiry.

resection removal of a part.

residential care (for children) care provided by the local authority social services department, or voluntary organizations registered with the social services department for children up to the age of 18 years. Residential nurseries are provided for the under 5-year-olds, and community homes and hostels for children in care up to the age of 18 years. Boarding out with foster parents is arranged whenever possible.

residual remaining. *R. urine* urine remaining in the bladder after micturition.

resistance the power to overcome. The natural power of the body to withstand and recover from infection or disease. The ability of bacteria to become insensitive to antibiotics, e.g. some staphylococci are resistant to penicillin.

Resources Allocation Working Party (RAWP) was set up to look at the National Health Service resources in different regions, and to make recommendations to reduce any inequalities in allocation.

respiration breathing; the exchange of oxygen and carbon dioxide between the atmosphere and the body cells, including inspiration and expiration, diffusion of oxygen from the pulmonary alveoli to the blood and of carbon dioxide from the blood to the alveoli, and the transport of oxygen to and carbon dioxide from the body cells. *Inspiration* is accomplished by contraction of the external intercostal muscles (which raise the ribs and sternum), and of the diaphragm which descends. In *expiration* the internal intercostal muscles contract, the ribs return to their normal position and the diaphragm relaxes. The normal rate of respiration varies. In neonates it is about 40–50 per minute at rest, and in adults 16. *Artificial r.* the production of respiratory movements by other than natural means.

respiratory distress syndrome (RDS) a condition occurring mainly in preterm babies due to lack of SURFACTANT. It also affects mature babies of diabetic mothers and those born by caesarean section. The onset of respiratory difficulty occurs within 4 hours of birth and the condition gradually worsens.

restitution restoration, putting right. A corrective movement of the fetal head after it is born in the anteroposterior diameter, to right it in relation to the shoulders.

resuscitation restoration from a state of collapse. *See* Appendices 11 and 16.

retardation delay; hindrance; delayed development. *Mental r.* subnormal general intellectual development, associated with impairment either of learning and social adjustment or of maturation, or of both.

retching an involuntary, spasmodic, but ineffectual effort to vomit.

retention holding back. *R. of urine* inability to pass urine from the bladder, which may rarely be due to obstruction or, more commonly in obstetrics, of nervous origin. During labour, as the fetus occupies a large part of the pelvis, there is considerable stretching of the urethra and trigone, which disturbs micturition. In the puerperium both these areas take time to recover. There may be diminished sensation in the bladder and perineal discomfort, coupled with anxiety and lack of privacy, and retention of urine may occur. The woman should be encouraged to empty her bladder within a very few hours of delivery, using various nursing measures. Catheterization should be avoided if possible, as chronic urinary tract infection can occur as a result, leading to renal failure in some cases.

reticular resembling a net.

reticuloendothelial system a network of tissues and cells found throughout the body, especially in the blood, general connective tissue, spleen, liver, lungs, bone marrow and lymph nodes. The very large reticulo-endothelial cells are concerned with blood cell formation and destruction, storage of fatty materials, and metabolism of iron and pigment, and they play a role in inflammation and immunity. Some of the cells are motile, that is, capable of spontaneous motion and phagocytic, i.e. they can ingest and destroy unwanted foreign material. The reticuloendothelial cells of the spleen possess the ability to dispose of disintegrated erythrocytes. The reticuloendothelial cells located in the blood cavities of the liver are called Kupffer cells. These cells, together with the cells of the general connective tissue and bone marrow, are capable of transforming into bile pigment the haemoglobin released by disintegrated erythrocytes.

retina the inner lining of the eyeball formed of nerve cells and fibres, and from which the optic nerve leaves the eyeball and passes to the visual area of the cerebral cortex. The impression of the image is focused upon it.

retinopathy a general term denoting pathological conditions of the retina; they may occur in conjunction with certain systemic disorders, such as hypertension, severe pre-eclampsia or eclampsia, and diabetes. *R. of prematurity* is caused by vasoconstriction of retinal capillaries due to the presence of very high concentrations of oxygen in these blood vessels. This produces the development of an overgrowth of blood vessels in the retina. The vascular proliferation and exudation of blood and serum detaches the retina, and produces scarring and inevitable blindness. Careful monitoring of the newborn and of oxygen tension level is essential because no totally safe dosage of oxygen that will prevent the retinal changes has been found.

retraction drawing back. The process of permanent and progressive shortening of the muscle of the uterus which accompanies contractions during labour (*a*) to dilate the cervix, (*b*) to expel the fetus and (*c*) to separate the placenta and to control bleeding. Over-retraction of the uterus in obstructed labour may cause a *r. ring* to become apparent. *See* BANDL'S RING.

retractor a surgical instrument for drawing apart the edges of a wound to make the deeper structures more accessible.

retro- prefix meaning 'behind' or 'backward', e.g. retroversion of the uterus.

retroflexion a bend backwards; applied to the uterus when the body is bent backwards at an acute angle, the cervix being in its normal position.

retrograde going backwards. *R. pyelography* X-ray of the kidneys and ureters following the injection of a radio-opaque substance into the renal pelvis via the urethra.

retrolental behind the crystalline lens. *R. fibroplasia see* RETINOPATHY OF PREMATURITY.

retroplacental behind the placenta. *R. clot* clot of blood behind the placenta.

retrospection morbid dwelling on memories. Looking back.

retroversion a turning back; applied to the uterus when the whole organ is tilted backwards. cf. RETROFLEXION.

retroverted gravid uterus a pregnant uterus that is tilted backwards. This is a common occurrence, and the uterus almost always becomes spontaneously corrected to an anteverted position. Occasionally the retroversion persists, and a state of INCARCERATION of the retroverted gravid uterus develops, with retention of urine.

retrovirus a large group of RNA viruses, including human T-cell leukaemia viruses, lentiviruses and the causative virus of AIDS, HIV (human immunodeficiency virus).

RGN Registered General Nurse.

Rhesus factor an antigen, the presence or absence of which determines the Rhesus type of human blood as positive or negative. There are three pairs of Rhesus antigens Cc, Dd and Ee. The D antigen is responsible for Rhesus immunity in the majority of cases. A capital letter indicates that the person is Rhesus positive to the factors C, D or E, and a small letter indicates that a person is Rhesus negative to factors c, d or e. About 83% of Caucasians are Rhesus positive and 99–100 per cent of other races. *See* Appendix 17.

rheumatic relating to rheumatism. *R. fever, see* RHEUMATISM.

rheumatism a term used to describe muscular and joint pains, often called fibrositis. *Acute r.* rheumatic fever. An acute fever associated with streptococcal infection and related to chorea and acute tonsillitis. It causes acute rheumatic ENDOCARDITIS, myocarditis and pericarditis and, as SEQUELAE, MITRAL STENOSIS and aortic incompetence may occur. When mild they can be asymptomatic until pregnancy increases the load on the heart. Any pregnant woman who has had rheumatic fever when a child, must have careful assessment of her cardiac condition.

rhinitis inflammation of the mucous membrane of the nose. *Staphylococcal r.* sometimes occurs in the newborn child.

rhomboid of Michaelis a diamond-shaped area at the base of the spine marked by dimpling of the skin. Beneath its superior angle is the spinous process of the 5th lumbar vertebra, and under the lateral angles the posterior superior iliac spines are palpable. Inferiorly is the beginning of the gluteal cleft.

rhythm a measured movement; the recurrence of an action or function at regular intervals. adj. *rhythmic, rhythmical. R. method of family planning* refers to the

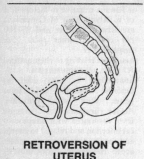

**RETROVERSION OF
UTERUS**

natural methods which include calculating the so-called 'safe' period, taking the temperature daily and observing the mucoid discharge from the vagina, i.e. the Billings' method. *See* Appendix 12.

rib any one of the paired bones, 12 on either side, extending from the thoracic vertebrae toward the median line on the ventral aspect of the trunk, forming the major part of the thoracic skeleton. Called also costal.

riboflavin vitamin B₂, necessary for certain enzymes that catalyse many oxidation–reduction reactions. Found in liver, kidney, heart, brewer's yeast, milk, eggs, greens and enriched cereals.

ribonucleic acid (RNA) the nucleic acid of a cell which translates the 'code' of DEOXYRIBONUCLEIC ACID (DNA) into action.

ribosome a minute granule seen with an electron microscope in the cytoplasm of a cell. Ribosomes are concerned with protein synthesis.

rickets rachitis. A disease of deficient calcification of bone. It results from lack of vitamin D, necessary for the proper absorption of calcium and phosphorus. It leads to characteristic bony deformity of skull, ribs, legs and pelvis. It is preventable, by the administration of vitamin D and by exposure to sunlight or ultraviolet light, and is nowadays uncommon.

rigor a sudden shivering attack in which the temperature usually rises rapidly, remains high for a short time and, following a phase of sweating, declines. It may occur in severe pyelonephritis in pregnancy, or in PUERPERAL SEPTICAEMIA. *R. mortis* the stiffening of the body, occurring soon after death owing to coagulation of the muscle protoplasm.

ritodrine a β₂-adrenergic receptor stimulant used to decrease uterine activity and prolong gestation in the management of preterm labour.

Ritter's disease exfoliative dermatitis. A rare and severe form of PEMPHIGUS NEONATORUM.

RM Registered Midwife.

RNA *see* RIBONUCLEIC ACID.

rockerbottomfeet a feature of certain chromosomal disorders such as Edwards' syndrome (trisomy 18) and Patau's syndrome (trisomy 13) when the infant has prominent heels.

rodent officer an employee of the environmental health department, responsible for control of infestation by rodents.

Rogitine trademark for a preparation of phentolamine, an adrenolytic used to test for the presence of phaechromocytoma.

role a pattern of behaviour developed in response to the demands or expectations of others; the pattern of responses to the persons with whom an individual interacts in a particular situation.

Röntgen rays X-RAYS.

rooming-in the baby remains by the mother's bedside when she is in hospital, rather than being cared for in a nursery. This enables the mother to get to know her baby and strengthens the bond between them as she learns to handle and care for him.

rooting reflex a reflex which can be eliciated in the newborn by stroking the cheek or side of the mouth and in response the baby will turn to the side stimulated and open his mouth ready to suckle.

rotation the turning of a body on its long axis. In midwifery, the turning of the fetal head (or presenting part) for proper orientation to the pelvic axis. It should occur naturally, but if it does not it must be accomplished manually or instrumentally by the obstetrician.

rotator a muscle which causes rotation of any part.

rotavirus a virus which, under the microscope, looks like a wheel. It has been identified in the last 10 years as the single most common cause of acute infantile diarrhoea. Respiratory signs often precede the diarrhoea and vomiting.

Rothera's test a test for the presence of acetone in urine.

roughage indigestible vegetable fibre. Cellulose. It gives bulk to the diet and stimulates peristalsis. Found in bran, cereals, fruit and vegetable fibres.

round ligament see LIGAMENT.

Royal College of Midwives (RCM) founded in 1881 as the professional body concerned with the education and standards of professional practice of midwives. It is the only professional organization solely for midwives. The RCM is now concerned primarily with standards of professional practice, statutory and other post-basic education for midwives and negotiation of conditions of service and salaries. Headquarters: see Appendix 25.

rubella German measles. A mild infective disease causing a faint macular rash on the body and enlargement of the posterior cervical lymph nodes. It is spread by droplets from an infected person 7 days before the rash appears but is of low infectivity. Rubella is uncommon in pregnancy, but the virus crosses the placenta to the fetus and causes abortion, stillbirth or congenital rubella. The incidence of congenital malformations such as cardiac, ear and eye defects, varies according to the period of gestation at which the disease occurs. If in the first month the incidence is 50–60 per cent with multiple defects, and this slowly falls until, in the case of infection in the 16th week, it is about 5 per cent. From this time until the 31st week the fetus may suffer growth retardation and be born with thrombocytopenic purpura. Later in life it may be mentally retarded, physically retarded or deaf. The baby itself may be a source of infection for up to 2 years. For rubella vaccination, *see* Appendix 15. When a woman is exposed to rubella during the first 4 months of pregnancy, serum should be taken to test for immunity to rubella. If this shows immunity and no infection, reassurance can be given to continue the pregnancy. The second serum should be taken 4 weeks later, if the first showed no immunity. Only if this shows evidence of infection should termination be considered.

Rubin test a test for patency of the uterine tubes, made by transuterine inflation with carbon dioxide gas. Called also tubal insufflation.

rugae ridges or creases, e.g. of the mucosa of the stomach, and the squamous epithelium of the vagina.

Rules for Midwives the compliance with the UKCC Midwives Rules is the responsibility of any midwife practising in the United Kingdom whether employed within or without the National Health Service or self-employed. Failure to do so is likely to result in allegation of professional misconduct.

rupture 1. tearing or bursting of a part, as in rupture of an aneurysm, of the membranes during labour or of a tubal pregnancy. *R. of the uterus* may follow obstructed labour, or may occur during pregnancy or labour following previous caesarean section. 2. a term commonly applied to a hernia.

Ryle's tube a thin rubber tube with a weighted end, introduced via the nose into the stomach. It may be used for the withdrawal of gastric contents or for the administration of fluids.

S

S chemical symbol, sulphur.
s second.
Sabine vaccine an oral vaccine against poliomyelitis consisting of three types of live, attenuated polioviruses. It may be given in

a capsule, on a lump of sugar, or by medicine dropper.
sac a pouch-like cavity.
saccharide one of a series of carbohydrates, including the sugars; they are divided into

monosaccharides, disaccharides, trisaccharides, and polysaccharides according to the number of saccharide groups composing them.

sacculation of the uterus a rare complication of incarceration of the retroverted gravid uterus, in which the fundus remains under the sacral promontory, and the anterior wall grows to accommodate the fetus.

sacral relating to the sacrum. *S. promontory* the upper anterior border of the body of the prominent first sacral vertebra.

sacro- concerning the sacrum. *Sacroanterior* and *sacroposterior* the positions that may be encountered in a breech presentation, the sacrum being the denominator.

sacrococcygeal concerning the sacrum and the coccyx. *S. joint* a slightly movable joint of the pelvis, between the sacrum and the coccyx.

sacrocotyloid concerning the sacrum and the acetabulum. *S. diameter* the measurement between the sacral promontory and the nearest point of the iliopectineal eminence on either side of the pelvis. It measures 9.5 cm (3.75 in).

sacroiliac concerning the sacrum and the ilium. *S. joint* or *s. synchondrosis* the slightly movable joint between the sacrum and the ilium.

sacrum a wedge-shaped bone composed of 5 united vertebrae, situated between the lowest lumbar vertebra and the coccyx. It forms the posterior wall of the pelvis.

Saf-T-Coil an intrauterine contraceptive device.

sagittal arrow-shaped. *S. section* an anteroposterior mid-line section. *S. suture* the junction of the parietal bones. A *sagittal* or *third fontanelle* may be noted in the sagittal suture. This condition is sometimes, though not always, associated with DOWN'S SYNDROME.

salbutamol a beta-sympathomimetic drug used to try to suppress premature labour. *See* Appendices 9 and 19.

salicylate any salt or ester of salicylic acid. Aspirin is a salicylate which is used for its analgesic, anti-pyretic and anti-inflammatory effect. The mechanism of most of the effects of aspirin and other salicylates is inhibition of prostaglandin synthesis, thus blocking pyretic and inflammatory processes that are mediated by prostaglandin.

saline containing a salt or salts. *Physiological s.* formerly called *normal s.*, a solution of 0.9% sodium chloride. It is isotonic with blood and may be given intravenously as a temporary means of replacing fluid in shock and haemorrhage, but it is rapidly excreted.

saliva the secretion of the salivary glands, which is poured into the mouth when food is taken. It moistens and dissolves certain substances, and begins carbohydrate digestion by its enzyme ptyalin, the salivary amylase.

salivation the normal flow of saliva. When this is excessive it is referred to as PTYALISM.

Salk vaccine a preparation of killed polioviruses of three types given in a series of intramuscular injections to immunize against poliomyelitis.

Salmonella a genus of bacteria responsible for GASTROENTERITIS.

salpingectomy excision of one or both of the fallopian tubes.

salpingitis inflammation of a fallopian tube.

salpingogram radiological outline of the interior of the fallopian tubes, usually to determine whether they are patent or have some other disorder.

salpinography radiography of the fallopian tubes after intrauterine injection of a radio-opaque medium.

salpingo-oophorectomy removal of a fallopian tube and ovary.

salpingotomy surgical incision of a uterine tube.

salpinx a tube, notably the fallopian tube.

Saluric a proprietary preparation of CHLORTHIAZIDE, a diuretic.

sample a selected group of a population.

saphenous the name given to two superficial veins, the long and the short, which carry blood up the leg from the foot.

sarcoma a highly malignant tumour developed from connective tissue cells and their stroma. *Kaposi's s.* a multifocal, metastasizing, malignant reticulosis principally involving the skin, although visceral lesions may be present. It usually starts on the toes or feet as reddish-blue or brownish soft nodules and tumours. It is viral in origin and is frequently seen in AIDS.

saturated solution a liquid containing the largest amount of a solid which can be dissolved in it without forming a precipitate.

Savlon trademark for combination preparations of chlorhexidine and cetrimide, used as a skin disinfectant.

scalp the layer of tissue covering the cranial bones.

scan an image produced using a moving detector or a sweeping beam of radiation, as in scinti-scanning, B-MODE ULTRASONOG-RAPHY, scanography, or COM-PUTED TOMOGRAPHY.

scanner scintiscanner; called also computed tomography (CT) scanner.

scapula the large flat triangular bone forming the shoulder blade.

schizophrenia a psychosis of unknown cause, but showing hereditary links. The patient feels herself influenced by external forces and suffers delusions and hallucinations. Pregnancy tends to aggravate the condition.

school health service the provision of medical and dental inspection and treatment in schools maintained by local education authorities. The National Health Service Reorganisation Act, 1977 made this service a duty of the DEPARTMENT OF HEALTH. It is now provided by the DISTRICT HEALTH AUTHORITY, see Appendix 1.

Schultze expulsion of the pla-

centa at the end of the third stage of labour the placenta is expelled inverted, the fetal surface appearing first at the vulva. This is commoner than the MATTHEWS DUNCAN EXPULSION; there is less associated bleeding and the placenta was probably lying at a higher level in the uterus.

sciatic relating to the sciatic nerve which runs down the back of the thigh.

sclera the tough, white outer coat of the eyeball, covering approximately the posterior five-sixths of its surface, continuous anteriorly with the cornea and posteriorly with the external sheath of the optic nerve. adj. *scleral*.

sclerema an uncommon disease sometimes seen in newborn babies. It is characterized by hardening of the skin and subcutaneous fat and occurs in HYPOTHERMIA.

sclerosis the hardening of any part from an overgrowth of fibrous and connective tissue, often due to chronic inflammation.

scoliosis abnormal curvature of the spine, most commonly applied to a lateral deviation. *See also* LORDOSIS *and* KYPHOSIS.

scopolamine HYOSCINE.

screening 1. examination of a large number of individuals to disclose certain characteristics, or an unrecognized disease, as phenylketonuria or hypothyroidism in the neonate. 2. fluoroscopy.

Scriver test a biological test used for diagnosing a whole range of inborn errors of metabolism, including phenylketonuria. If the phenylalanine level is found to be above 725 μmol/l treatment for phenylketonuria is necessary.

scrotum the pouch of skin and soft tissues containing the testicles.

scurvy a disease due to a deficiency in vitamin C. It is characterized by weakness, anaemia, and haemorrhage from mucous membranes, purpuric rash, swelling and pain in joints, and ulceration in the mouth. It rapidly improves with a proper diet containing adequate vitamin C.

sebaceous fatty or pertaining to the sebum. *S. glands* are found in the skin, communicating with the hair follicles and secreting sebum.

sebum the fatty secretion of the sebaceous glands.

second degree perineal lacerations *see* PERINEAL LACERATIONS.

second stage of labour the stage of expulsion, lasting from full dilatation of the cervix uteri to complete birth of the child.

secondary second in order of time or importance. *S. postpartum haemorrhage*. See Appendix 11.

secretin a hormone secreted by the mucosa of the duodenum and jejunum when acid chyme enters the intestine; carried by the blood, it stimulates the secretion of pancreatic juice and, to a lesser extent, bile and intestinal secretion.

secretion a substance produced by a gland.

sedative a drug which allays excitement and calms a patient, often helping her to sleep, but not relieving pain.

sedimentation formation of sediment. *S. rate*, *see* ERYTHROCYTE SEDIMENTATION RATE.

segment a section or part. *Upper uterine s.* the upper three-quarters of the uterus, the part which contracts and retracts during labour. *Lower uterine s.* including the cervix. The lowermost quarter of the uterus, which becomes stretched and dilated in the first stage of labour.

segmentation the division of the fertilized ovum into two cells, then four, eight, 16, etc., as it traverses the fallopian tube.

seizure a convulsion or attack of epilepsy.

self-actualization a level of psychological development in which innate potential is realized to the full.

Sellick's manoeuvre the application of backward pressure on the cricoid cartilage in the throat in order to occlude the oesophagus and prevent regurgitation of stomach contents into the pharynx with consequent risk of aspiration into the lungs. The pressure is not released until an endotracheal tube has been inserted and the respiratory tract sealed off.

semen the male secretion of seminal fluid from the prostate gland, and spermatozoa from the testis, produced following ejaculation.

Semmelweiss, Ignaz Philipp *(1818–1865)* Hungarian physician and pioneer of antisepsis in obstetrics.

senna a laxative derived from the cassia plant. A standardized proprietary preparation, Senokot, is much used in pregnancy.

sense a faculty by which the conditions or properties of things are perceived, e.g. hunger, thirst and pain; a sense of equilibrium or well-being and other senses are also distinguished. The five major senses comprise vision, hearing, smell, taste and touch.

sensitive reacting to a stimulus.

sensitization 1. the initial exposure of an individual to a specific antigen, resulting in an immune response. 2. the coating of cells with antibody as a preparatory step in eliciting an immune reaction. 3. the preparation of a tissue or organ by one hormone so that it will respond functionally to the action of another.

sensitized rendered sensitive.

sensory pertaining to sensation. *S. nerve* a peripheral nerve that conducts impulses from a sense organ to the spinal cord or brain; called also afferent nerve.

sepsis infection of the body by pathogenic bacteria. *Puerperal s.* that occurring in the genital tract during the PUERPERIUM.

septic relating to sepsis.

septicaemia the presence and multiplication in the blood of pathogenic bacteria. The signs are a rapid rise of temperature, which is later intermittent, rigors, sweating, and all signs of acute fever. Puerperal sepsis occasionally takes the form of septicaemia. *See also* ENDOTOXIC SHOCK.

septum a division or partition, e.g. that between the right and left ventricles of the heart. One form of congenital heart malformation is characterized by a defect in the interventricular septum.

septuplet one of seven offspring produced at one birth.

sequela a morbid condition following a disease and resulting from it. pl. *sequelae*.

serology the study of antigen–antibody reactions *in vitro*. adj. *serological*.

serrated with saw-like edge, e.g. the bones of fetal skull.

serum clear straw-coloured fluid which is left after blood has clotted. The clear residue of blood, from which the corpuscles and fibrin have been removed. Serum from the blood of a convalescent patient (or animal) may be used to protect another person from the same disease, e.g. in diphtheria or tetanus.

sex 1. the fundamental distinction, found in most species of animals and plants, based on the type of gametes produced by the individual or the category to which the individual fits on the basis of that criteria. Ova, or macrogametes, are produced by the female, and spermatozoa, or microgametes, are produced by the male. The union of these distinctive germ cells results in the production of a new individual in sexual reproduction. 2. to determine the sex of an organism.

sex-linked genes carried on the sex chromosome, usually the X or female chromosome.

sextuplet one of six offspring produced at the same birth.

sexually transmitted diseases (STD) an infectious disease that is usually transmitted by means of sexual intercourse, either by heterosexual or homosexual individuals, or by intimate contact with the genitals, mouth and rectum. STDs include syphilis, GONORRHOEA, human immunodeficiency virus (HIV) infection, herpes genitalis, NON-SPECIFIC URETHRITIS, TRICHOMONIASES, PEDICULOSIS pubis, scabies, genital or venereal WARTS, HEPATITIS B infection and AIDS.

shared care a term used to describe antenatal care carried out by an obstetrician and/or a midwife and a midwife and/or general practitioner. The latter usually carried out the care following the booking until some time in the third trimester.

sheath a tubular case or envelope. A sheath, also known as a condom, can be worn over the erect penis during intercourse to trap the seminal fluid, thereby reducing the incidence of pregnancy. The use of a spermicidal preparation with sheaths increases their reliability up to about 97%.

Sheehan's syndrome hypopituitarism. This uncommonly occurs following severe and prolonged shock after ABRUPTIO PLACENTAE and POSTPARTUM HAEMORRHAGE, where there is necrosis of the anterior pituitary, giving rise to AMENORRHOEA, genital atrophy and premature senility.

Shirodkar operation an operation

to prevent abortion resulting from cervical incompetence. The internal os is closed by means of a nylon suture which is removed shortly before term, or earlier if labour should begin. Now commonly known as cervical cerclage.

shingles HERPES ZOSTER.

shock collapse due to acute peripheral circulatory failure, resulting usually from severe trauma or haemorrhage. *See* Appendix 11.

shoulder presentation the state which develops when labour begins with the fetus lying obliquely and this lie is not corrected. The shoulder is driven down into the maternal pelvis, and labour becomes obstructed. This may occur during the second stage of a twin labour, after the birth of the first child.

'show' a term used to denote the blood-stained discharge at the onset of labour which comes from the cervical canal plug, the operculum.

shunt 1. to turn to one side; to divert; to bypass. 2. a passage or anastomosis between two natural channels, especially blood vessels, either by natural means or operation.

SI units the units of measurement generally accepted for all scientific and technical uses. Together they make up the International System of Units. The abbreviation SI, from the French Système International d'Unités, is used in all languages. *See* Appendix 20.

Siamese twins identical (monozygotic) twins joined together at birth. The connection may be slight or extensive. It involves skin and usually muscles or cartilage of a limited region, such as the head, chest or hip. The twins may share a single organ, such as an intestine, or parts of the spine. Where possible the twins are separated by surgery soon after birth.

sibling one of two or more children having the same parents.

sickle cell disease a severe type of anaemia found in the West African and West Indian races. *See* Appendix 6.

SIDS sudden infant death syndrome.

silver nitrate $AgNO_3$. A crystalline salt. Used in solid form as a caustic for reducing excessive granulation tissue.

Silverman–Anderson score a system for evaluation of breathing performance of preterm infants. It consists of five items: 1. chest retraction as compared with abdominal retraction during inspiration; 2. retraction of the lower intercostal muscles; 3. xiphoid retraction; 4. flaring of the nares with inspiration; and 5. expiratory grunt. Each of the five is graded 0, 1 or 2. A sum of these factors yields the score. Adequate ventilation is indicated by a 0, severe respiratory distress is indicated by a score of 10.

Simmonds' disease underactivity of the whole PITUITARY GLAND (HYPOPITUITARISM), so affecting the total endocrine system. It may follow SHEEHAN'S SYNDROME.

Sims' position *see* POSITION.

Sims' speculum *see* Appendix 10.

sinciput the brow. That part of the skull between the coronal suture and the orbital ridges.

Singer's test a blood test to distinguish fetal from maternal blood.

sinoatrial node a collection of specialized muscle fibres in the wall of the right atrium where the rhythm of cardiac contraction is usually established; also called pacemaker of the heart.

sinus a cavity. A general anatomical term for all cavities in the cranial bones or the dilated channels for venous blood also found in the cranium. *See* INTRACRANIAL MEMBRANES.

skeleton the bone structure of the body, which supports and protects the organs and soft tissues.

Skene's ducts the largest of the female urethral glands, which open within the urethral orifice; they are regarded as homologous with the prostate.

skull the bony structure of the head enclosing and protecting the brain. The fetal skull is considered in three parts, the vault, the base and the face. The bones of the base and face are firmly united and, therefore, incompressible. The vault is made up of two frontal bones, two parietal bones, two temporal bones and one occipital bone. At birth the vault is not fully ossified and thus there are membranous spaces between the bones called sutures. Where three or more sutures meet the membranous space is called a fontanelle. During labour there is considerable pressure on the fetal skull and moulding takes place whereby the bones overlap the sutures.

slough a mass of dead tissue either in or which separates from the adjacent tissue.

small for gestational age baby a baby who is smaller or lighter than expected for its gestational age. The definition varies: some authorities include those below the 10th PERCENTILE and some below the 5th percentile. *See* Appendix 17.

smear a specimen of superficial cells, e.g. from the vagina or cervix, which, when examined microscopically, gives information about the level of hormones or early malignant disease.

smoking the act of drawing into the mouth and puffing out the smoke of tobacco contained in a cigarette, pipe or cigar. Smoking is harmful in pregnancy because carbon monoxide reduces oxygen transport and nicotine causes vasoconstriction of arterioles. The result is a diminished supply of food and oxygen to the fetus. Fetal growth and development may therefore be retarded.

snuffles the noisy breathing and nasal catarrh noted in infants with CONGENITAL SYPHILIS.

social class a classification, by the Registrar General, of persons by their occupation from I to V: I, professions; II, intermediate; III, skilled workers; IV, semi-skilled; V, unskilled.

social fund payments made on a discretionary basis to low income families whose needs cannot be met from regular weekly benefits. The maternity grant and death grant are paid from the social fund to low income families receiving income support and family credit. It also provides help for emergency situations, although such payments are recoverable.

social services services provided by the community to meet certain individual needs. It excludes those provided for profit.

social services department a department of the local authority, set up in 1971 following the Local Authority Social Services Act, 1970. Its purpose is to coordinate the social services. It has a responsibility to children and young persons, the elderly, the mentally and physically handicapped, the socially inadequate, and the unsupported parent. It has the power to delegate some areas to voluntary organizations. It may also act as an adoption agency.

social worker a specially trained and qualified person to assess social need and provide the necessary resources.

sociology the scientific study of relationships and phenomena.

sodium symbol Na. A metallic element widely distributed in nature, and forming an important constituent of animal tissues. Sodium is the major cation, i.e. positively charged ion, of the extracellular fluid (ELF) and thus determines the osmolality of the ECF. The serum sodium level is normally about 140 MEq/l. If the sodium level and osmolality fall, osmoreceptors in the hypothalamus are stimulated and cause the release of an antidiuretic hormone (ADH) from the posterior lobe of the pituitary gland. ADH increases the absorption of water in the collecting ducts in the kidneys so that water is conserved while sodium and other electrolytes are excreted in the urine. If the sodium level and osmolality rises, neurons in the thirst centre in the hypothalamus are stimulated and the thirsty person drinks enough fluid to restore the osmolality of the ECF to the normal level. A decrease in serum sodium concentration below normal levels can occur in a variety of conditions associated with fluid volume deficit such as diarrhoea and vomiting, acute or chronic renal failure and in diuretic therapy. An increase in serum sodium concentration above normal levels (HYPERNATRAEMIA) occurs when insensible water loss is not replaced by drinking, and in the newborn when artificial feeds are made up incorrectly with too high a concentration of milk powder. *S. bicarbonate* is used to reverse metabolic ACIDAEMIA following hypoxia to the tissues. It is used in varying strengths, 8.4 or 5%, the more concentrated used where fluid levels are critical, as in the neonate. *S. citrate* a substance added to donor blood to prevent clotting.

soft chancre a venereal ulcer, not due to syphilis. The infecting organism is *Haemophilus ducreyi* (Ducrey's bacillus).

soft palate the fleshy structure at the back of the mouth which, together with the hard palate, forms the roof of the mouth. From the middle of the free border of the soft palate hangs the uvula. In swallowing the soft palate is drawn upward against the back of the pharynx, and prevents food and fluids from entering the nasal passage while they pass through the throat.

solute a substance dissolved in a solution.

solvent a liquid which dissolves, or has the power to dissolve.

somatic relating to the body as opposed to the mind.

somatome 1. an appliance for cutting the body of a fetus. 2. a somite.

somatotrophin growth hormone. adj. *somatotrophic.*

somite one of the paired segments along the neural tube of the vertebrate embryo, formed by transverse subdivision of the thickened mesodeum next to the mid-plane, that develop into the vertebral column and muscles of the body.

sonar a term for ULTRASOUND in medical diagnosis. *See* Appendix 4.

sonogram a record or display obtained by ultrasonic scanning.

sonography ultrasonography. adj. *sonographic.*

soporific causing sleep.

sordes brown crusts which form on the teeth and lips of unconscious patients, or those suffering from acute or prolonged fevers. The result of neglecting mouth hygiene.

sore buttocks a non-specific term generally referring to perianal excoriation which is commonly associated with frequent loose stools. It is more likely to occur in babies who are artificially fed. Other causes include infrequent changing of the napkin, poor hygiene, loose frequent stools, incorrect laundering of napkins, diet (extra sugar) and infection such as candidiasis. Treatment includes good hygiene, exposure of the buttocks to the air and investigations of feeding, laundering napkins and for infection. *See* NAPKIN RASH.

souffle a soft blowing sound heard on auscultation of the abdomen in pregnancy. *Uterine s.* is due to the blood passing through the uterine arteries of the mother, particularly over the placental site. It is synchronous with the maternal pulse.

soya milk used as a milk substitute for babies who cannot tolerate constituents of breast or cow's milk such as lactose. There are now soya-based milk substitutes prepared specifically for infant formulae. They contain only vegetable fats.

Spalding's sign gross overlapping of the fetal cranial bones, seen on abdominal radiograph. It indicates that intrauterine death has occurred several days previously.

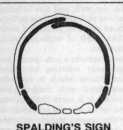

SPALDING'S SIGN

spasm a sudden involuntary muscle contraction.

spastic pertaining to spasm. The term is used to describe special types of increased tone in muscles which results from brain or spinal cord injury. It is also used as a term for CEREBRAL PALSY.

specific gravity the weight of a substance compared with that of an equal volume of another substance, e.g. the specific gravity of water is taken to be 1000. That of other substances such as urine (1010–1020) or blood (1055) may thus be compared.

specular reflection reflecting as from a surface. A term used in ULTRASOUND to describe an interface which gives a strong reflection or echo, e.g. the fetal skull.

speculum an instrument used to open up a cavity, normally not visible, to enable a hidden structure to be inspected. pl. specula. *See* Appendix 10.

Spencer Wells a variety of artery forceps.

sperm the male reproductive cell; spermatozoon.

spermatic pertaining to the spermatozoa or to semen. *S. cord* the structure extending from the abdominal inguinal ring to the testis, comprising the pampiniform plexus, nerves, ductus deferens, testicular artery and other vessels.

spermatogenesis the development of mature spermatozoa from spermatogenia.

spermatozoa (pl.) the male generative cells which form the essential part of semen. The normal count of cells is 50 million per ml. sing. *spermatozoon.*

spermicide an agent that destroys spermatozoa. Often used as a cream or paste applied to vaginal or cervical caps, as vagitories or as foam.

sphenoid wedge-shaped. *S. bone* forms part of the base of the skull.

spherocyte a small, globular completely haemoglobinated erythrocyte without the usual central pallor; characteristically found in hereditary spherocytosis but also in acquired haemolytic anaemia.

spherocytosis the presence of spherocytes in the blood.

sphincter a ring-shaped muscle, contraction of which closes a natural orifice.

sphingomyelin a complex molecule of protein and fatty acid which is used as a standard to measure the ratio of LECITHIN in the liquor.

sphygmomanometer an instrument used to measure arterial blood pressure.

spina bifida a condition in which the arches at the back of the spine are incomplete. Sometimes there is only a bony gap (*spina bifida occulta*) but sometimes the spinal cord is exposed. When there is a sac over the spinal cord it is called a MENINGOCELE or, if nerves are exposed or involved in the sac, a MYELOMENINGOCELE (*see* Figure).

spinal relating to the spine. *S. cord, see* CORD.

spine 1. the vertebral column. 2. a sharp process of bone.

spirit an alcoholic solution of a volatile substance, or an alcohol itself.

Spirochaeta a group of micro-organisms with a flexible, spiral filament, e.g. *Treponema pallidum*, the cause of SYPHILIS.

spirograph an apparatus for measuring and recording respiratory movements.

spirometer an instrument for measuring air taken into and expelled from the lungs.

splanchnic pertaining to viscera.

spleen a very vascular lymphoid organ, situated in the left hypochondrium under the border of the stomach. The framework of the organ consists of fibrous trabeculae with pulp in the spaces. the functions are (*a*) formation of erythrocytes in fetal life only; (*b*) production of lymphocytes throughout life; (*c*) control of red cell breakdown and excretion of the resulting products; and (*d*) formation of ANTIBODIES.

splenomegaly enlargement of the spleen.

splint a piece of wood or metal used to support, and possibly to immobilize, an injured limb.

spondylolisthesis a forward displacement of the 5th lumbar vertebra on the first sacral segment. This narrows the true conjugate by the formation of a false promontory, and is a rare cause of DYSTOCIA.

spondylosis ankylosis of a vertebral joint; also, a general term for degenerative changes in the spine.

spontaneous occurring naturally with no external aid. *S. evolution, see* EVOLUTION. *S. version* the change of the fetus from one lie to another with no obstetrical interference.

sporadic scattered or discontinuous. Applied to isolated cases of a disease which occurs in various and scattered places.

spore the reproductive element of certain plants, fungi and bacteria. Tetanus bacilli are spore-bearing, and the spores are resistant to high temperatures and strong antiseptics, and thus difficult to kill, as they can remain dormant for years.

spurious labour false labour. *See* LABOUR.

squamous scaly or plate-like. *S. bone* the thin part of the temporal bone which articulates with the parietal bone. *S. epithelium* thin-celled skin, e.g. the lining of the vagina.

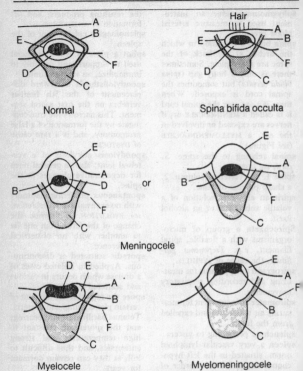

Normal

Spina bifida occulta

Meningocele

Myelocele

Myelomeningocele

A. *Skin*; B. *arch of vertebra*; C. *body of vertebra*; D. *spinal cord*; E. *meninges*; F. *spinal nerve*.

NORMAL SPINAL COLUMN AND SPINA BIFIDA

squatting a position with the hips and knees flexed, the buttocks resting on the heels; partial or a full squatting position may be adopted by the parturient at delivery.

standard deviation (σ) a measure of the dispersion of a random variable: the square root of the average squared deviation from the mean. For data that have a normal distribution about 68 per cent of the data points fall within one standard deviation from the mean and about 95 per cent fall within two standard deviations.

Staphylococcus a genus of pyogenic bacteria which, under the microscope, appear grouped together in small masses like bunches of grapes. Staphylococci cause skin infections, including PEMPHIGUS NEONATORUM, MASTITIS and, sometimes, PUERPERAL SEPSIS. *S. aureus* or *S. pyogenes* is coagulase-positive, can cause severe infections and, in hospital, may be resistant to antibiotic drugs. *S. albus* is a skin COMMENSAL but may also cause urinary tract infection.

stasis stagnation or stoppage. *Intestinal s.* sluggish movement of the muscles of the bowel wall, causing constipation. *S. of urine*, which occurs in pregnancy, predisposes to urinary tract infection. *See* PYELONEPHRITIS.

station the location of the presenting part of the fetus in the birth canal, designated as −5 to −1 according to the number of centimetres the part is above an imaginary plane passing through the ischial spines, 0 when at the plane, and +1 to +5 according to the number of centimetres the part is below the plane.

statistics 1. numerical facts pertaining to a particular subject or body of objects. 2. the science dealing with the collection, tabulation and analysis of numerical facts.

status condition, state. *S. epilepticus* rapid succession of epileptic spasms without intervals of consciousness; brain damage may result.

statutory bodies the statutory control of the practice of midwives is the responsibility of the United Kingdom Central Council for Nursing, Midwifery and Health Visiting (UKCC) and four National Boards for Nursing, Midwifery and Health Visiting, one in each of the four countries of the UK. These five bodies are called statutory bodies as they are established in accordance with the Nurses, Midwives and Health Visitors Act, 1979. *See* Appendix 22.

Stein–Leventhal syndrome a condition in which either AMENORRHOEA or OLIGO-MENORRHOEA occurs, associated with hirsutism and infertility. Enlarged cystic ovaries are often found, from which excessive male hormones may be produced.

Stemetil trademark for preparations of prochlorperazine, a major tranquilliser and anti-emetic.

stenosis narrowing or contraction of a channel or opening. *Aortic s.*

narrowing of the aortic valve of the heart due to scar tissue resulting from inflammation. *Mitral s.* of the mitral orifice from the same cause. *Pyloric s.* due generally to congenital hypertrophy.

stercobilin a bile pigment derivative formed by air oxidation of stercobilinogen; it is a brown–orange–red pigmentation contributing to the colour of faeces and urine.

sterile 1. barren; incapable of producing young. 2. free from micro-organisms.

sterilize 1. to make sterile by operation, e.g. ligation of the fallopian tubes. 2. to render sterile dressings, instruments, etc. *See* Appendix 12.

sterilizer an apparatus in which objects can be sterilized.

sternum a plate of bone forming the middle of the anterior wall of the thorax and articulating with the clavicles and the cartilages of the first seven ribs. At 36 weeks gestation the uterine fundus normally reaches the xiphoid process at the lower end of the body of the sternum.

steroids substances of a particular chemical structure of carbon and hydrogen and including sex hormones, adrenocortical hormones, cholesterol and bile acids.

stethoscope an instrument used to auscultate sounds within the body, e.g. of heart, lungs. *Binaural s.* branches into two flexible tubes, one for each ear of the examiner. *Fetal* or *monaural s.* a metal trumpet-shaped instrument which can be placed on the abdomen over the fetal shoulders to hear the heart sounds. Sometimes called Pinard's stethoscope.

stilboestrol a synthetic OESTROGEN.

stilette a wire for keeping clear the lumen of hollow structures such as needles. A fine probe.

stillbirth a baby which has issued forth from its mother after the 24th week of pregnancy and has not, at any time after being completely expelled from its mother, breathed or shown any sign of life. adj. *stillborn*.

stillbirth certificate a certificate issued by a registered medical practitioner or a registered midwife who was present at the birth, or examined the body. It is a statutory duty to give it to the qualified informant (usually the father or mother) so that the registration of birth can be made and a Certificate of Burial or Cremation be issued to them. The midwife normally only completes the certificate if no arrangements for maternity care have been made with a medical practitioner. In cases where there has been an inquest, the coroner will issue the order for burial.

stomach the dilated portion of the alimentary canal between the oesophagus and the duodenum, just below the diaphragm. Its wall consists of four coats: serous, muscular, submucous and mucous. The gastric juice contains the enzymes PEPSIN and RENNIN, and HYDROCHLORIC ACID.

stomatitis inflammation of the lining of the mouth.

stool a motion or discharge from the bowel. The stool of the new-born child is at first meconium, then gradually changes to a soft bright yellow stool.

strabismus deviation of the eye that the patient cannot overcome; the visual axes assume a position relative to each other different from that required by the physiological conditions; called also squint.

strawberry mark congenital haemangioma.

Streptococcus a genus of bacteria occurring in a chain-like formation. Streptococci may be haemolytic or non-haemolytic, and aerobic or anaerobic. The beta-haemolytic streptococcus of Lancefield group A (*Streptococcus pyogenes*) is the cause of scarlet fever, severe tonsillitis and can cause severe PUERPERAL SEPSIS. Puerperal sepsis may also be caused by anaerobic streptococci.

streptokinase an enzyme produced by streptococci that catalyses the conversion of plasminogen to plasmin. Streptokinase, when administered as a thrombolytic, requires careful usage to avoid haemorrhage. It is also capable of producing severe antigenic reactions upon readministration.

stress undue strain exerted upon mind or body. Strain liable to cause impairment of mental or physical function. The body's reaction to emergency stress is set off by the adrenal medulla which pours adrenaline into the blood stream. This causes a rise in heart rate, blood pressure and blood glucose, and dilatation of the blood vessels in the muscles to give them immediate use of this energy. In cases of continuing stress the glands continue to produce a steady supply of hormones that apparently increase the body's resistance. Psychological situations can have the same effect. The diseases most often associated with a stressful environment are coronary artery disease and 'heart attack', high blood pressure and cancer.

striae gravidarum the marks due to skin stretching, which are seen on the abdomen, and to some extent on the breasts and thighs, during and after pregnancy. They occur first as reddish marks, and later fade to a silvery white colour.

Stroganoff's treatment a method of treating severe PRE-ECLAMPSIA, described by the Russian obstetrician Stroganoff in 1911, where the patient was kept quiet in a darkened room to reduce external stimuli and sedated with morphine and chloral hydrate. The darkened room may still be used but with a different drug regimen.

styptic an astringent which, applied locally, arrests haemorrhage.

sub- prefix meaning 'under' or 'below'.

subarachnoid below the arachnoid. *S. space* the space between the arachnoid and the pia mater, in which the cerebrospinal fluid circulates. *S. haemorrhage* haemorrhage into this space.

subclavian beneath the clavicle. *S. artery* the main artery to the arm.

subcutaneous beneath the skin, e.g. subcutaneous injection.

subdural under the dura mater. *S. haemorrhage* bleeding under the dura mater. One form of intracranial haemorrhage seen in the neonate, often as the result of a traumatic delivery. A subdural tap is sometimes used to withdraw blood to relieve the pressure.

subfertility a state of less than normal fertility.

subinvolution incomplete or delayed return of the uterus to its pre-gravid size during the puerperium, usually due to retained products of conception and infection.

subluxation partial dislocation.

submucous beneath the mucous membrane.

subnormal below normal.

subtotal hysterectomy *see* HYSTERECTOMY.

succenturiate additional or accessory. *S. placenta*, *see* PLACENTA.

sudden infant death syndrome (SIDS) the sudden and unexpected death of an apparently healthy infant, typically occurring between the ages of 3 weeks and 5 months, and not explained by careful post-mortem studies. They are often found dead in the cot, hence the popular name 'cot deaths'. Sometimes the baby has had a slight cold, but more often

there have been no symptoms. It is more common in babies born before term and less common in breast-fed babies. The incidence is about 6 per 1000 live births. The prone position, tobacco smoke and overheating have recently been found to increase the risk of cot death, so should be avoided.

sugar a class of carbohydrates which includes monosaccharides such as glucose, fructose and galactose, and disaccharides such as sucrose (cane sugar) and lactose (the sugar in milk). The sugar in the blood is glucose.

sulcus a groove or furrow, as between the cotyledons of a placenta.

sulphonamides a group of chemotherapeutic drugs much used in the treatment of bacterial infections. They are given orally and are often effective in the treatment of infections with streptococci, gonococci, *E. coli* and other bacteria, although some of these organisms are now resistant.

super- prefix meaning 'over' or 'above'.

superego a part of the psyche derived from both the ID and the EGO, which acts, largely unconsciously, as a monitor over the ego. It is that part of the personality concerned with social standards, ethics and conscience.

superfecundation the fertilization of two ova from the same ovulation by spermatozoa from two different individuals.

superfetation fertilization of an

ovum occurring during the course of pregnancy.

supervisor of midwives the UKCC Midwives Rules 1991 state that a supervisor of midwives is a person appointed in accordance with Section 16(3) of the Nurses, Midwives and Health Visitors Act, 1979, by a local supervising authority to exercise supervision over midwives in its area. The supervisor shall be a registered midwife with a minimum of 3 years experience as a practising midwife, not less than one year of which shall have been in the 2 years immediately preceding the appointment, or shall be eligible to practise and shall undertake any further midwifery experience as may be required by the relevant board. Midwives appointed as supervisors of midwives are required to attend a course of instruction within 12 months of appointment unless they have completed such a course within 3 years of appointment. Subsequently they are required to undertake further instruction at intervals of not more than 5 years.

supination turning upwards. *S. of hand* the palm is upward. cf. PRONATION.

supine lying on the back. *S. hypotensive syndrome* hypotension occurring from pressure of the gravid uterus on the inferior vena cava, thus reducing the venous return and the cardiac output. It may happen when a woman in late pregnancy lies in the dorsal position, and can be aggravated by EPIDURAL ANALGESIA.

supplement something added to supply a deficiency.

supplementary of the nature of a supplement. *S. feed* a feed given to an infant instead of or in addition to a breast feed. cf. COMPLEMENTARY.

supply order form the official authorization, provided by the supervisor of midwives, to a practising midwife to enable her to obtain a supply of PETHIDINE. *See* Appendix 19.

suppository a solid cone-shaped medicated compound to be introduced into the rectum, either to cause a bowel action (e.g. glycerine or bisacodyl suppositories) or to administer drugs, particularly analgesics (e.g. Anusol suppository for painful haemorrhoids). Medicated suppositories may also be introduced into the vagina or urethra.

suppression complete cessation of a secretion. Lactation is suppressed in cases where breast-feeding is not desired or contra-indicated. It may be achieved naturally, i.e. by not removing the milk, or with the use of drugs such as bromocriptine which inhibits the release of prolactin from the pituitary gland.

suppuration the formation or discharge of pus.

supra- prefix meaning 'above'.

suprapubic above the pubic bones.

suprarenal above the kidney. *S. glands* two small triangular endocrine glands, one above each kidney. They secrete ADRENALINE and NORADRENALINE from the medulla, and a number of hormones from the cortex.

surfactant a LECITHIN found in the lungs, which helps the alveoli to remain open. Babies who suffer from the RESPIRATORY DISTRESS SYNDROME do not have enough of this substance. This may be predicted by estimating the LECITHIN/SPHINGOMYELIN RATIO before delivery. *See* Appendix 17.

surrogate a substitute. *S. mother* a woman who carries a child for another with the intention that the child be handed over after birth.

survey a systematic collection of information, not forming part of a scientific epidemiological study.

suture 1. a stitch or series of stitches used to close a wound. 2. the fibrous joint where the opposed bony surfaces are very closely united by thin connective tissue, permitting movement only in the neonate. For details, *see* FETAL SKULL.

symmetrical cortical necrosis a rare complication of severe concealed ABRUPTIO PLACENTAE where there is destruction of large areas of the cortex of both kidneys due to internal spasm of the renal cortical arteries. Impaired renal function or death from renal failure may follow. *See also* TUBULAR NECROSIS.

sympathetic exhibiting sympathy.

sympathetic nervous system that part of the autonomic system which, when stimulated, prepares the body for emergency or flight. The pulse rate increases, the blood pressure rises, the pupils are dilated, while peristalsis is slowed.

symphysiotomy division of the symphysis pubis, a method of facilitating delivery in cases of disproportion, used: (*a*) where caesarean section is not practicable; (*b*) to avoid delivering a woman too many times by caesarean section; and (*c*) in regions where the midwifery services are inadequate, to avoid leaving a woman with a scar in her uterus.

symphysis a joint where the bone surfaces are joined by fibrocartilage and movement is very slight. *S. pubis* the fibrocartilaginous junction of the two pubic bones.

symptom any evidence of a disease or condition observed by the patient herself. Thus AMENORRHOEA and certain breast changes are symptoms of pregnancy. To be distinguished clearly from a sign, which is any feature observed by the doctor or midwife.

syn- prefix meaning 'together'.

synapse the junction between the processes of two neurons or between a neuron and an effector organ, where neural impulses are transmitted by chemical means. The impulse causes the release of a neurotransmitter, e.g. acetylcholine or noradrenaline, from the presynaptic membrane of the oxon terminal.

synclitism the state when the fetal head enters the pelvic brim with both parietal eminences at the same level. *See* ASYNCLITISM.

syncope fainting. Loss of consciousness, due to cerebral anaemia.

syncytium, syncytiotrophoblast the outlet layer of the TROPHOBLAST which does not have cell boundaries but scattered nuclei in the protoplasm. This layer persists throughout pregnancy covering the CHORIONIC VILLI, unlike the CYTOTROPHOBLAST cells.

syndactyly webbed fingers or toes.

syndrome a group of symptoms and signs typical of a distinctive disease, and of that disease only.

synthesis the joining together of substances, either naturally or artificially. Substances thus built up artificially, e.g. stilboestrol, are termed synthetic.

synthetic chemical, an artificially formed compound.

Syntocinon a proprietary preparation of synthetic OXYTOCIN. *See* Appendix 19.

Syntometrine an oxytocic drug containing 0.5 mg ergometrine and 5 units of Syntocinon which is commonly administered to the mother intramuscularly with the birth of the anterior shoulder of the fetus.

syphilis a contagious venereal disease, caused by *Treponema pallidum*. It may be *congenital* or *acquired*. The acquired type is manifested in four stages: *Primary* incubation, 2–6 weeks, when the specific primary chancre appears, usually on the vulva, followed by enlargement of the regional lymph glands. The sore is painless and heals quickly, hence this phase could easily be overlooked. *Secondary* this develops a few weeks later with rashes, condylomata around the anus and vulva, and general enlargement of the lymph glands. This stage is highly infectious. It varies considerably, and in a number of cases the symptoms do not appear, or are very slight; the patient, however, is not cured, but has *latent* syphilis. *Tertiary* may appear years later. Characterized by gummatous tumours in various tissues. *Quaternary* lesions are: tabes dorsalis, general paralysis of the insane, etc. *Treponema* can cross the placenta and cause abortion or stillbirth, or the baby may be born with *congenital syphilis*. Signs are: a brownish-red rash on the buttocks, sores about the mouth and rhinitis with discharge from the nose (snuffles). Later the 'saddle' nose, Hutchinson's teeth, deafness or impaired vision may occur. Screening of all pregnant women for syphilis is vital, as prompt treatment can prevent congenital syphilis. The Wassermann reaction (WR) and Kahn tests may give positive results which then need testing more specifically with *Treponema pallidum* haemaglutination (TPHA) test, *Treponema* immobilization test (TPI) and venereal disease research laboratory (VDRL) test. All tests, except the VDRL, may give false positives with YAWS, malaria and glandular fever. Treatment with large doses of penicillin is effective. The mother can be cured and the child will be healthy, but it is wise to treat her in any further pregnancies, as congenital syphilis may occur unexpectedly.

syringocele a cavity containing herniation of the spinal cord through the bony defect in spina bifida.

syringomyelocele hernial protrusion of the spinal cord through the bony defect in a spina bifida, the mass containing a cavity connected with the central canal of the spinal cord.

Système International d'Unités (SI units) the international system for measurement in science, industry and general use. It was agreed in 1960, and it is now illegal in the United Kingdom to prescribe or dispense drugs in any other units. *See* Appendix 20.

systemic pertaining to or affecting the body as a whole.

systole the contraction of the heart. cf. DIASTOLE. *Ventricular s.* the contraction of the ventricles, by which the blood is pumped into the aorta and pulmonary arteries.

systolic pertaining to systole. *S. murmur* an abnormal sound produced during systole, in heart affections. *S. pressure, see* BLOOD PRESSURE. *S. sound* the dull sound of the heart in ventricular systole, caused by its movement against the chest wall.

T

T cell a lymphocyte which is derived from the thymus and is responsible for cell-mediated immunity.

TAB a vaccine which gives some protection against typhoid fever, paratyphoid A and paratyphoid B. *TABT* protects against tetanus in addition.

taboo any of the negative traditions and behaviours generally regarded as harmful to social welfare and sometimes health.

tachycardia abnormally rapid action of the heart and pulse rate.

tachypnoea abnormally rapid respirations, as sometimes seen in the newborn child in RESPIRATORY DISTRESS SYNDROME. *See also* Appendix 17.

tactile pertaining to touch.

taking up of cervix the effacement of the cervical canal early in labour. *See* DILATATION.

talipes clubfoot. A congenital deformity in which the foot has developed at an abnormal angle to the leg. The cause is not fully understood. In some cases, notably in patients with OLIGOHYDRAMNIOS the child has been cramped *in utero* and is born with mild position talipes. In *t. equinus* the toes point downwards and in

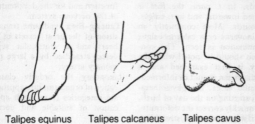

Talipes equinus   Talipes calcaneus   Talipes cavus

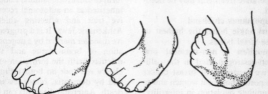

Talipes varus   Talipes equinovarus   Talipes calcaneovarus

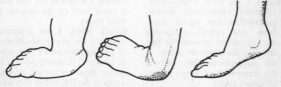

Talipes valgus   Talipes calcaneovalgus   Talipes equinovalgus

TALIPES

t. calcaneus the heel is downwards. In *t. varus* the foot is turned inwards, and in *t. valgus*, outwards. Most commonly an equinovarus or a calcaneovalgus combination is seen. The condition should be noted when the baby is first examined and a paediatrician should be informed. In mild cases, the physiotherapist, starting on the day of birth, can quickly correct the deformity, but if it is more severe, stretching, massage, or splinting or even operative treatment may be needed.

talipomanus clubhand.

talus ankle bone; the highest of the tarsal bones.

tamoxifen a non-steroidal oral anti-oestrogen used in the palliative treatment of breast cancer in postmenopausal women and to stimulate ovulation in infertility.

tampon a gauze plug with a long tape. Commonly introduced into the vagina during repair of episiotomy or perineal laceration.

tarsus 1. the seven bones—talus, calcaneus, navicular, medial, intermediate and lateral cuneiform, and cuboid—composing the articulation between the foot and leg; the ankle or instep. 2. the cartilaginous plate forming the framework of either (upper or lower) eyelid.

taurine a crystallized acid from the bile; found also in small quantities in lung and muscle tissue. Taurine is present in high quantities in breast milk and is necessary for the conjugation of bile acids in the first week of life until glycine takes over the function and for the development of the nervous system.

Taussig–Bing syndrome transposition of the great vessels of the heart and a ventricular septal defect straddled by a large pulmonary artery.

taxonomy the orderly classification of organisms into appropriate categories (taxa) with application of suitable and correct names.

Tay–Sachs disease the infantile form of amaurotic familial idiocy, inherited as an autosomal recessive trait and affecting chiefly Ashkenazic Jews. It is a progressive disorder marked by a degeneration of brain tissue and the maculas (with the formation of a cherry red spot on both retinas) and by dementia, blindness and death. Antenatal diagnosis can be made at 14 weeks of pregnancy. An absence of the enzyme hexosaminidase A indicates conclusively that the fetus has Tay–Sachs disease. Carriers of the trait have a lower level of the enzyme in their blood.

Tecota Mark 6 an apparatus designed for the administration of trichlorethylene for pain relief in labour. Trichlorethylene is no longer approved for use by midwives in the UK unless they have medical supervision, but is still used in some overseas countries.

teething eruption of the teeth through the gums. The average baby cuts his first tooth between the 6th and 9th months. The full set of 20 baby teeth erupt gradually over a period of up to about 30 months; usually two teeth, one on each side of the jaw, appear at a time.

telemeter to transmit readings of an instrument by radio waves.

telemetry the record of fetal heart beats and uterine contractions by remote control, so that the mother is able to walk about during labour.

temazepam (Normison) a hypnotic drug. *See also* Appendix 19.

temperature that degree of heat of a substance or body as measured by a thermometer. *Normal t.* of the human body = 36°–37°C (97°–98.4°F). It varies slightly during the day, and in women it is higher during the second half of the menstrual cycle. It indicates the balance between heat production and heat loss. A thermometer inserted under the tongue or into the rectum will register slightly higher than when placed in the axilla or groin. *See* PYREXIA *and* FEVER.

temporal pertaining to the side of the head. *T. bone* an irregular bone of the skull, the squamous part of which forms part of the vault.

tendon a cord or band of strong white fibrous tissue that connects a muscle to a bone. When the muscle contracts, it pulls the tendon, which moves the bone.

TENS transcutaneous electrical nerve stimulation. It is used for pain relief in labour.

tension 1. the act of stretching or the state of being stretched. 2.

the pressure or concentration of a gas. *See* P_{O_2} *and* P_{CO_2}.

tentorium cerebelli a septum of dura mater, separating the cerebral hemispheres from the cerebellum. *See* INTRACRANIAL MEMBRANES.

tepid slightly warm; 32°–37°C (90°–98°F).

ter in die **(tid)** three times a day.

teras a malformed fetus or infant. adj. *teratic*.

teratogen an agent or influence that causes physical defects in the developing embryo. adj. *teratogenic*.

teratoma a congenital tumour containing teeth, hair and cells of other tissues not normally found in the place where it is situated.

term when pregnancy has lasted for 280 days or 40 weeks counted from the time of the first day of the last normal menstrual period.

termination of pregnancy (TOP) an abortion which is induced, legally or illegally.

tertiary third. *T. syphilis. See* SYPHILIS.

test 1. an examination or trial. 2. a significant chemical reaction. 3. a reagent. *Agglutination t.* one whose results depend on agglutination of bacteria or other cells; used in diagnosing certain infectious diseases and rheumatoid arthritis, the cross-matching of blood and in pregnancy tests. In the latter tests no agglutination indicates a positive pregnancy test, whereas when agglutination occurs the result is negative. *Complement-fixation t's* tests that utilize antigen–antibody reaction and result in haemolysis to determine the presence of various organisms in the blood. *Concentration t.* a test of renal function based on the patient's ability to concentrate urine. *Creatinine clearance t.* a test for renal function based on the rate at which ingested creatinine is filtered through the renal glomeruli. *Early pregnancy t.* a do-it-yourself immunological test for pregnancy, performed as early as 9 days after menstruation was expected. *Glucose tolerance t.* a metabolic test of carbohydrate tolerance used to diagnose diabetes mellitus. *Glycosylated haemoglobin t.* measurement of the percentage of haemoglobin A_1 (HbA_1) molecules which helps to assess diabetic control. HbA_1 is a type of adult haemoglobin where one part of the beta chain has been combined with glucose, and increases in diabetes, especially when the blood glucose control is poor. *Histamine t.* following a rapid intravenous injection of histamine phosphate, the blood pressure normally falls, but in patients with phaechromocytoma, after the fall, there is a marked rise in blood pressure. *Pregnancy t's* laboratory procedures for early determination of pregnancy. *Sickling t.* a method to demonstrate haemoglobin S and the sickling phenomenon in erythrocytes, performed by reducing the oxygen concentration to which the red cells are exposed. Treponema pallidum *haemagglutination (TPHA)t.*, Treponema pallidum *immobilization (TPI)t.* serological tests related directly to the causative organism, used in the diagnosis of syphilis. *VDRL t.* a slide flocculation test for syphilis designed by the Venereal Disease Research Laboratory, USA.

test weighing a method of determining the amount of breast milk taken by weighing the baby before and after the feed without changing any of its clothes, so that the difference equals the feed. Sometimes called test feeding. With successful demand feeding, there should be no need for this scheme.

testicles, testes the two glands in the scrotum which produce spermatozoa and male sex hormones. *Undescended t.* when the organ remains in the pelvis or inguinal canal.

testosterone the hormone produced by the testes which stimulates the development of male characteristics.

tetanic relating to tetanus. *T. spasms* occur in strychnine poisoning.

tetanus a disease due to the *Clostridium tetani*, an anaerobe found in cultivated soil and manure, and therefore likely to infect accidental wounds. In persons thus exposed to the infection, tetanus antitoxin will confer passive immunity.

tetany a condition resulting from calcium deficiency, alkalaemia or impaired function of the parathyroid glands. The chief sign is tonic contraction of the muscles of the hands and feet (carpopedal spasm) with hypersensitivity of other muscles. It is sometimes seen in newborn babies who have been artificially fed. They have low calcium concentrations in the blood. See also HYPOCALCAEMIA.

tetracycline an antibiotic substance that is effective against many different micro-organisms.

tetradactyly the presence of four digits on the hand or foot.

tetralogy a group or series of four. *Fallot's t.* a congenital defect of the heart that combines four structural anomalies: pulmonary stenosis; ventricular septal defect; dextroposition of the aorta, in which the aortic opening overrides the septum and receives blood from both the right and left ventricles; and right ventricular hypertrophy. Surgical correction is required whenever possible.

thalamus that part of the brain at the base of the cerebrum. Most sensory impulses pass from the body to the thalamus and are transmitted to the cortex and forebrain.

thalassaemia Cooley's anaemia. A severe type of anaemia. See ANAEMIA *and* Appendix 6.

thalidomide a sedative and hypnotic drug which, when used in early pregnancy caused serious developmental deformities, mainly of one or more limbs.

theophylline a respiratory stimulant given to reduce the incidence of apnoeic attacks in the small preterm infant. It has no known long-term side-effects.

therapeutic abortion *see* ABORTION.

therapy treatment. *Chemotherapy* treatment with chemical drugs.

thermometer an instrument for measuring temperature. *Clinical t.* a special type used to measure and record the body temperature.

thiamine vitamin B₁; a component of the B complex group of vitamins, found in various foodstuffs and present in the free state in blood plasma and cerebrospinal fluid. Deficiency results in neurological symptoms, cardiovascular dysfunction, oedema, and reduced intestinal motility.

thiaziole any of a group of benzothiadiazinesulphonamide derivatives, typified by chlorothiazide, that act as diuretics by inhibiting the reabsorption of sodium in the proximal renal tubule and stimulating chloride excretion, with resultant increase in excretion of water.

thiopentone (Pentothal) a barbiturate, given intravenously to induce general anaesthesia. *See* Appendix 19.

third degree perineal laceration *see* PERINEAL LACERATIONS.

third stage of labour the period from the birth of the child to complete expulsion of the placenta and membranes.

thoracic relating to the thorax. *T. duct* the large lymphatic vessel situated in the thorax along the spine. It opens into the left subclavian vein.

thorax the chest; cavity containing the heart, lungs, bronchi and oesophagus. It is bounded by the diaphragm below, the sternum in front and the dorsal vertebrae behind, and is enclosed by the ribs as a protective framework.

threshold the level that must be reached for an effect to be produced, as the degree of intensity of stimulus which just produces a sensation.

thrill a tremor or vibration elicited by tapping the wall of a cavity containing fluid, e.g. a pregnant uterus with POLYHYDRAMNIOS.

thrombectomy surgical removal of a clot from a blood vessel.

thrombin a substance formed in the blood by the action of thromboplastin on PROTHROMBIN in the presence of calcium. The thrombin then converts the plasma protein fibrinogen into fibrin which, with the cells, forms a clot.

thrombocyte a blood platelet. *See* Appendix 18.

thrombocythaemia an increase in the number of circulating platelets.

thrombocytopenia an uncommon condition of deficiency of PLATELETS, sometimes seen in the newborn child especially of a mother with purpura, and characterized by purpuric haemorrhages. It usually clears up spontaneously. It also occurs in congenital RUBELLA.

thromboembolism obstruction of a blood vessel with thrombotic material carried by the blood from the site of origin to plug another vessel.

thrombokinase activated clotting factor X.

thrombolysis dissolution of a thrombus.

thrombophlebitis inflammation of a vein, with clot formation. The clot tends to be adherent to the wall of the vein, and rarely separates, so that the danger of EMBOLISM is small. *Femoral t.* may occur following labour as an extension of pelvic infection. cf. PHLEBOTHROMBOSIS.

thromboplastin a substance liberated by injured tissue and platelets. *See* THROMBIN *and* PROTHROMBIN.

thrombosis the formation of a thrombus. *Coronary t.* formation of a clot in a coronary vessel, by which the heart muscle is deprived of blood according to the size of the vessel blocked. If the thrombus detaches itself from the wall and is carried along by the bloodstream, the clot is called an embolus. The condition is known as EMBOLISM.

thrombus a stationary blood clot produced by coagulation of the blood, usually in a vein, and often the result of PHLEBITIS.

thrush a condition in which whitish spots form on the mucous membrane of the mouth, due to the fungus *Candida albicans*. In babies it may be transferred from the vulva of a woman with candidal (monilial) vaginitis during vaginal delivery. If untreated the infection will spread to other parts of the infant's neonatal tract. An erythemateus napkin rash with small, white-headed pustules is usually due to *Candida albicans*. In artificially fed infants it may spread quickly, as it is killed only by autoclaving and not by other methods of sterilization. The treatment is to give antibiotics and fungicidal drugs such as nystatin. *See* Appendices 17 and 19.

thymus a gland situated between the lungs and above the heart. It grows until puberty and then gradually involutes. The cortex contains many small T lymphocytes which play a part in the immunological reactions of the body.

thyroid gland an endocrine gland situated in the neck in front of the trachea. Its secretions, thyroxine and triiodothyronine, control metabolism. Overactivity causes thyrotoxicosis, and underactivity myxoedema. Infants whose thyroid secretions are defective are cretins.

thyrotoxic marked by toxic (excessive) activity of the thyroid.

thyrotrophin a hormone secreted by the anterior lobe of the anterior pituitary gland that stimulates the thyroid gland. Also called thyroid-stimulating hormone (TSH).

thyroxine a hormone of the thyroid gland that contains iodine and is a derivative of the amino acid TYROSINE. Thyroxine affects the metabolic rate (oxygen consumption); growth and development; metabolism of carbohydrates, fats proteins, electrolytes and water; vitamin requirements; reproduction; and resistance to infection. Thyroxine can be extracted from animals or produced synthetically and is prescribed for HYPOTHYROIDISM and for some types of GOITRE.

tidal volume the amount of gas passing into and out of the lungs in each respiratory cycle.

tissue a mass of cells or fibres uniting to perform a particular function in the body. *Connective t.* there are many types: adipose (fatty), areolar (elastic supporting), bone, blood and cartilage. *Brown adipose t., brown fat t.* a thermogenic type of adipose tissue containing a dark pigment, and arising during embryonic life in specific areas such as between the shoulder blades, behind the sternum, in the neck and around the kidneys and suprarenal glands. It is utilized by the newborn for the production of heat, as required. *Epithelial t.* covers all inner and outer body surfaces. Some varieties are ciliated (e.g. the lining of the fallopian tubes), some columnar (e.g. the lining of the cervical canal) and some squamous (e.g. the lining of the vagina). *Erectile t.* spongy tissue that expands and becomes hard when filled with blood. *Granulation t.* material formed in repair of wounds and soft tissue, consisting of connective tissue cells and ingrowing young capillaries; it ultimately forms fibrous tissue; a scar; *Muscular t.* the three types are striated (skeletal or voluntary), unstriated (plain or involuntary) and cardiac (striated but involuntary). *Nervous t.* this consists of nerve cells and their processes. *Subcutaneous t.* the layer of loose connective tissue directly under the skin.

tissue fluid the fluid in the tissue

spaces between the cells, sometimes called extracellular fluid. A demonstrable excess constitutes OEDEMA.

titre the amount of a substance, e.g. an antibody, in the blood. It is estimated by finding the amount of it needed to correspond with a known amount of another substance.

toco-, toko- word element meaning 'childbirth', 'labour'.

tocograph an instrument for measuring the pattern and pressure of uterine contraction.

tocolytic drugs drugs used to arrest threatened preterm labour; ritodrine hydrochloride (Yutopar); salbutamol (Ventolin).

tomography any method that produces images of single tissue planes. *Computed t.* (*CT*) a radiological imaging modality that uses computer processing of X-ray photons detected by a detector bank after passing through the patient. The image generated is a representation of tissue densities within a 'slice', 1–10 mm thick, through the patient's body. Called also COMPUTERIZED AXIAL TOMOGRAPHY (CAT). *Ultrasonic t.* the ultrasonographic visualization of a cross-section of a predetermined plane of the body; see B-mode ULTRASONOGRAPHY.

tone the normal degree of tension, e.g. in a muscle.

tongue tie shortening of the frenulum, a band of tissue which anchors the tongue to the floor of the mouth. It does not usually interfere with feeding.

tonic contraction of the uterus this may be *general*, where the uterus is in a state of powerful continuous contraction, leading to anoxia of the fetus, or *local*, a ring of tonic contraction called a *constriction ring*. It forms most commonly round the fetal neck, so preventing progress in labour. Deep anaesthesia is usually required to give relaxation, although inhaling amyl nitrite may sometimes help.

tonus muscle tone.

TORCH infections include TOXOPLASMOSIS, RUBELLA, CYTOMEGALOVIRUS and HERPES.

torsion twisting. May occur in the pedicle of a cyst which produces venous congestion in the cyst and consequent gangrene—a possible complication of ovarian cyst.

torticollis a contracted state of the cervical muscles, producing torsion of the neck. The deformity may be congenital, hysterical, or due to pressure on the accessory nerve, inflammation of the glands of the neck, or to muscle spasm.

tourniquet an instrument applied to a limb to arrest bleeding or to make a vein more prominent.

toxaemia poisoning of the blood by the absorption of toxins, once thought to be responsible for PRE-ECLAMPSIA.

toxic poisonous, relating to a poison.

toxin a poison, particularly that produced by pathogenic bacteria. Bacterial toxins do not produce symptoms until after a variable period of incubation while the microbes multiply sufficiently to overwhelm the leukocytes and other types of antibodies. Toxins cause antitoxins to form in the body, thus providing a means of establishing immunity to certain diseases.

toxoid toxin which has been rendered non-toxic but which retains its protective qualities. APT (alum-precipitated toxoid), used in diphtheria immunization, is such a preparation.

Toxoplasma a genus of protozoa which acts as parasites. They cause TOXOPLASMOSIS.

toxoplasmosis infection with *Toxoplasma*, causing a glandular-fever-like syndrome. When it occurs during pregnancy the fetus may become infected and as a result have hydrocephalus, intracranial calcification, splenomegaly, anaemia, jaundice and retinal damage.

trachea the windpipe; a cartilaginous tube lined with ciliated epithelium, extending from the lower part of the larynx to the bronchi.

trachelorraphy operation for the repair of a lacerated cervix.

tracheo-oesophageal fistula a congenital defect in which there is an opening between the trachea and the lower oesophagus. *See also* OESOPHAGEAL ATRESIA.

tracheostomy creation of an opening into the trachea through the neck, with insertion of an indwelling tube, undertaken in an emergency to restore the airway in acute obstruction, or to improve the airway and aspirate secretions.

trait a characteristic behaviour pattern. *Sickle cell t.* a tendency for red cells to sickle, without accompanying anaemia, found when an individual is HETEROZYGOUS for the condition.

tranquillizers drugs which allay anxiety and calm the patient. Valuable for women who begin labour in great fear and anxiety. Chlorpromazine and promethazine are examples.

transactional analysis a theory of personality structure and a psychotherapeutic method originated by Dr Eric Berne. The personality is viewed as consisting of three ego states; the Parent, the Adult, and the Child. The word transaction refers to the communication that takes place between two people, e.g. when a stimulus from the ego state of one person elicits a response from the ego state of another person. In a successful or complementary transaction the stimulus and response are between the same ego states; i.e. Parent–Parent and Adult–Adult. In unsuccessful transactions one person is speaking from one ego state, but gets a response from a different ego state. Analysis refers to an investigation into the feelings and behaviour patterns that are demonstrated during the transaction.

transcutaneous blood gas monitors the application of a probe to the baby's skin which is heated to a temperature of 44°C and enables measurements of Po_2 and Pco_2 to be made. Accuracy depends on the quality of the peripheral circulation, thus trans-cutaneous blood gas monitoring is usually used in conjunction with intermittent arterial sampling.

transcutaneous electrical nerve stimulation (TENS) a procedure in which mild electrical stimulation is applied by electrodes in contact with the skin over a painful area. TENS stimulates the large myelinated nerve fibres and relieves pain in line with the gate control theory. It also causes the release of endogenous opiates or endorphins in the cerebro-spinal fluid, and this reduces the perception of pain. When used for pain relief in labour, four electrodes are placed parallel and close to the spine between T10 and T11 and in the sacral area between S2 and S4. Pain relief is controlled by the mother who is able to increase the degree of stimulation during a contraction, and is able to be ambulant if she wishes. The UKCC has recently approved the use of TENS by midwives on their own responsibility, provided they have been instructed in its use.

transducer a device which transforms one form of energy into another. The one used in ULTRASOUND contains ceramic crystal moulded into a disc. This transforms vibrations from electrical charges into waves of ultrasound of a certain frequency. *See* Appendix 4.

transferase an enzyme that catalyses the transfer, from one molecule to another, of a chemical group that does not exist in free state during the transfer.

transferrin a serum globulin that binds and transports iron.

transfusion the direct administration into the blood stream of blood or other solutions to increase the blood volume. *Exchange t.* repeated small withdrawals and replacement of blood to alter the constituents but not the blood volume, e.g. in haemolytic disease of the newborn it is used to decrease the amount of bilirubin. Sometimes called replacement transfusion. *Feto-maternal t.* from fetus to mother via the placenta. Also called transplacental transfusion (TPT). *See* Appendix 17.

transillumination the passage of a strong light through a body structure, to permit inspection by an observer on the opposite side.

translocation in GENETICS, the shifting of part of one CHROMOSOME on to another.

transmigration wandering. *External t.* the passage of an ovum from its ovary to the fallopian tube on the opposite side.

transplacental through the placenta.

transport movement of materials in biological systems, particularly into and out of cells and across epithelial layers. *Active t.* movement of materials across cell membranes and epithelial layers resulting directly from expenditure of metabolic energy.

transposition a cross-placement. *T. of the great vessels* the pulmonary artery arises from the left ventricle instead of the right, so that poorly oxygenated blood leaves the right ventricle by the aorta. Life can only be maintained if there is a patent ductus or if an atrioseptal shunt is created.

transudate any fluid which passes through a membrane, e.g. the vaginal fluid. In contrast to an exudate, it has a high fluid content and low protein and cellular content.

transvaginal through the vagina.

transverse arrest occurs when fetal head is deflexed and is arrested above the level of the ischial spines with the sagittal suture in the transverse diameter of the pelvis.

transverse lie a condition in which the longitudinal axis of the child lies across that of the mother's uterus. If it is not corrected before, or very shortly after the onset of labour, it can result in a SHOULDER PRESENTATION and obstructed labour. *See* Appendix 9.

transvestite a person, usually a male, who experiences a habitual and strongly persistent desire to dress as a member of the opposite sex.

trauma injury.

traumatic caused by injury.

travail labour, childbirth.

Trendelenburg position *see* POSITION.

Treponema pallidum the SPIROCHAETE causing syphilis.

trial of labour this is conducted to see if normal vaginal delivery

is possible despite the fact that the head is not engaged, owing to a slight degree of cephalopelvic disproportion. It should only be carried out in a well equipped hospital on a young, healthy NULLIPARA. If good contractions occur, the head may flex more and descend with moulding through the pelvic brim, the joints of which relax a little in the process. A normal delivery should then result from the successful trial. Should the observer performing the vaginal examinations note a lack of progress in the descent of the head and in dilatation of the cervix, in spite of good contractions, or any sign of fetal or maternal distress, the trial of labour should be ended quickly by caesarean section.

trichomoniasis, *Trichomonas vaginalis* one of the commonest sexually transmitted diseases caused by *Trichomonas vaginalis*, an oval flagellate protozoon. The infection causes a thin and watery, or yellow-green and frothy vaginal discharge, vulval pruritis and inflammation. The usual treatment is metronidazole 200 mg daily for 10 days. The partner should be treated at the same time to avoid reinfection.

triglyceride a compound consisting of three molecules of fatty acids bound with one molecule of glycerol; a neutral fat that is the usual storage form of lipids in animals.

trigone a triangular area. *T. of the bladder* the triangular non-elastic area forming the base of the

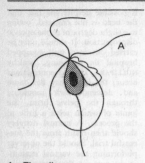

A. *Flagellum.*
**TRICHOMONAS
VAGINALIS**

bladder, between the ureteric openings and the urethral orifice. It is embedded in the anterior vaginal wall, and so, when this is distended during labour, its functions may be disturbed.

trimester a period of 3 months.

tripartite placenta a placenta divided into three lobes, each with a cord leaving it which join to form one cord a short distance from the lobes.

triple vaccine a combined dose of diphtheria, tetanus and pertussis immunization. *See* Appendix 15.

triplets three children carried in the uterus at once and born at one labour. Incidence formerly about 1 in 6400 births; now, as a result of treatment of subfertility, more common.

trisomy an additional chromosome with one particular pair. *Trisomy*

21 has the extra chromosome with the 21st pair and occurs in DOWN'S SYNDROME. *Trisomy 18* (EDWARD'S SYNDROME; *trisomy 13* (PATAU'S SYNDROME)

trochanter one of two prominences below the neck of the femur. *Greater t.* that on the outer side. *Lesser t.* the one on the inner side.

trophoblast the outer covering of the blastocyst, from which the placenta and chorion develop.

trophoblastic tissue SYNCYTIO-TROPHOBLAST and CYTOTROPHO-BLAST.

true conjugate *see* CONJUGATE.

trypsin a powerful pancreatic enzyme which continues protein digestion to form amino acids.

tubal ligation ligation of the uterine tubes, a method of sterilization. Laparoscopic sterilization using diathermy, or the application of potentially removable clips to the uterine tubes are alternative methods commonly undertaken.

tubal mole a mass of blood clot retained in the fallopian tube after a tubal pregnancy.

tubal pregnancy a pregnancy embedded in the lining of the fallopian tube.

tube feeding administration of liquid (and for adults semi-solid foods) through a nasogastric, gastrostomy, or enterostomy tube. A common method of feeding for the preterm infant who easily tires when suckling and has immature swallowing and gag reflexes.

tuberculosis a specific infection caused by *Mycobacterium tubercu-*

losis. Occurs commonly in the lung, but any part of the body may be affected.

uberosity an expanded portion of bone, or protuberance, e.g. the ischial tuberosities between which is measured the transverse diameter of the pelvic outlet.

ubular necrosis (acute) 1. when protein is deposited in the collecting and distal convoluted renal tubules, as with an incompatible blood transfusion or septic abortion, the epithelium is damaged and urine dammed back, thus preventing further activity of the GLOMERULUS. It may clear in 7–14 days. 2. if the proximal convoluted tubule becomes ischaemic or bacterial toxins are released, the epithelium may necrose with death of the tubule. The kidney may recover its function in 10–30 days if there is only partial necrosis.

ubule a microscopic tube forming one part of the nephron.

umour a growth or swelling.

unica a coat. *T. albuginea* a dense layer of connective tissue below the germinal epithelium of the ovary.

unnel a passageway through a solid body with open ends. *Carpal t.* the osseofibrous tunnel for the median nerve and the flexor tendons. Carpal tunnel syndrome occurs when the median nerve becomes compressed and results in pain and tingling paraesthesia in the fingers and hand, sometimes extending to the elbow. It is a fairly common disorder of pregnancy due to oedema causing compression of the median nerve.

Turner's syndrome a congenital defect in which the person has 45 instead of 46 chromosomes. Only one sex chromosome (X) is present, described as XO, so the individual appears female with a normal vagina, uterus and fallopian tubes but, as the ovaries do not function, AMENORRHOEA and sterility occur. Webbing of the neck may also be evident.

twins two infants developing in the uterus together from one or two ova. *Binovular, dizygotic* or *fraternal t.* those developed from two separate ova fertilized by two spermatozoa. There are two complete pregnancies in the uterus, i.e. two fetuses, two placentae, two chorions, two amnions. The infants may be of the same or different sexes, and as like or unlike each other as any two members of a family. *Uniovular, monozygotic* or *identical t.* Twins developed from the fertilization of a single ovum. The embryonic cell mass has divided into two identical halves, each of which has developed into a fetus. Thus there are two fetuses and two amniotic membranes, but only one placenta and one chorion. The babies are of the same sex, and alike in all characteristics. Rarely, incomplete division of the embryonic cell mass gives rise to conjoined, or Siamese, twins.

tympanic of or pertaining to the tympanum. *T. membrane* a thin, semi-transparent membrane that stretches across the ear canal separating the tympanum (middle ear) from the external meatus (outer ear); called also eardrum.

typing a method of measuring the degree of organ, solid tissue or blood compatibility between two individuals in which specific histocompatibility antigens, e.g. those present on leukocytes or erythrocytes, are detected by means of suitable isoimmune antisera.

tyrosine a naturally occurring amino-acid present in most proteins; it is a product of phenylalanine metabolism and a precursor for melanin, catecholamines, and thyroid hormones.

U

UKCC United Kingdom Central Council for Nursing, Midwifery and Health Visiting. *See* Appendix 22.

ulcer a lesion of the free surface of the skin or mucous membrane, caused by trauma, infection, pressure or nerve injury.

ultrasonic beyond the audible range; relating to sound waves having a frequency of more than 20 000 cycles per second.

ultrasonogram an echo picture obtained from using ULTRASOUND.

ultrasonography a radiological technique in which deep structures of the body are visualized by recording the reflections (echoes) of ultrasonic waves directed into the tissues. In diagnostic ultrasonography, the ultrasonic waves are produced by electrically stimulating a crystal called a transducer. As the beam strikes an interface or boundary between tissues of varying density some of the sound waves are reflected back to the transducer as echoes. The echoes are then converted into electrical impulses that are displayed as a television image, presenting a visual display of the tissues under examination. Ultrasonography is used widely in obstetrics to evaluate fetal size and maturity, placental localization, to diagnose fetal abnormalities and uterine tumours, and other pelvic masses. *A-mode u., B-mode u., Doppler u., real-time u., see* Appendix 4.

ultrasound sound at frequencies above the upper limit of normal hearing, i.e. greater than about 20 000 Hz (cycles per second); used in medicine in the technique of ULTRASONOGRAPHY.

umbilical relating to the umbilicus. *U. hernia* a protrusion of intestine through the umbilicus, usually slight but occasionally severe. *See* EXOMPHALOS.

umbilical cord the cord which connects the fetus and the placenta. It is usually 50–60 cm

(20–24 in) long, has a spiral twist and consists of two umbilical arteries carrying deoxygenated blood and one umbilical vein carrying oxygenated blood, surrounded by Wharton's jelly and covered by amnion. *Presentation of the u.c.* the cord lies below the presenting part, the membranes being intact. *Prolapse of the u.c.* the cord lies in advance of the presenting part, the membranes being ruptured. There is grave danger of pressure on the vessels of the cord and consequent fetal anoxia. The cause is a high or an ill-fitting presenting part, which allows a loop of cord to slip past. The principles in the treatment of this emergency are: (*a*) to lessen the pressure on the cord

PROLAPSE OF THE UMBILICAL CORD

by any possible means, and permit the fetal oxygen supply to be maintained, and (*b*) to deliver the woman as quickly as possible. Soon after birth the umbilical cord is clamped and cut. A stump of about 2.5 cm is left attached to the baby's umbilicus and this dies and separates naturally by a process of dry, aseptic necrosis within 5–7 days.

umbilicus the navel; the scar in the abdomen marking the point at which the umbilical cord was attached.

unconscious 1. insensible; incapable of responding to sensory stimuli. 2. that part of the mental activity which includes primitive or repressed wishes, concealed from consciousness by the psychological censor.

uni- a prefix meaning 'one'.

unicellular consisting of one cell.

unilateral on one side only.

uniovular from one ovum. *See* TWINS.

United Kingdom Central Council (UKCC) for Nursing, Midwifery and Health Visiting a statutory body set up as a result of the 1979 Nurses, Midwives, and Health Visitors Act. *UKCC Code of Practice for Midwives, UKCC Code of professional conduct for the nurse, midwife and health visitor, UKCC Handbook of Midwives Rules, see* Appendix 2.

unstable lie when the lie of the fetus changes from one examination to another after 36 weeks gestation.

unsupported mother a mother without a partner to support her;

a one-parent family. The mother may be unmarried, separated, divorced or widowed.

urachus a fibrous band uniting the apex of the bladder to the umbilicus. It is a remnant of a canal present in the fetus.

uraemia the condition of renal failure in which the blood urea is very high. It is characterized by headache, vertigo, vomiting and convulsions; coma may ensue. It may complicate nephritis, concealed ABRUPTIO PLACENTAE or ECLAMPSIA.

urea the end product of protein metabolism, which is excreted in the urine. *Blood u.* the amount of urea present in the blood; normally 2.5–5.8 mmol/l (15–35 mg/100 ml) but in pregnancy usually 2.3–5.0 mmol/l (14–30 mg/100 ml).

ureter one of the two fibromuscular tubes which convey urine from the kidney to the bladder. They become dilated during pregnancy as PROGESTERONE relaxes the smooth muscle, leading to stasis of urine and multiplication of micro-organisms. *See* PYELONEPHRITIS.

ureteric relating to the ureter. *U. catheter* a fine catheter for insertion via the ureter into the pelvis of the kidney, either for drainage or for retrograde PYELOGRAPHY.

ureterovesical pertaining to a ureter and the vagina.

ureterovesical fistula an abnormal passage between a ureter and the vagina; a rare complication of prolonged or obstructed labour when the tissue of the ureter becomes devitalized due to prolonged pressure by the fetal head.

urethra the canal through which the urine is discharged from the bladder. The male urethra is 20–22.5 cm (8–9 in) long, the female urethra 3.7 cm (1.5 in).

urethral relating to the urethra.

urethritis inflammation of the urethra. *Non-specific u.* a sexually transmitted disease, occurring in the male, the cause of which has not yet been identified.

uric pertaining to the urine. *U. acid* the end product of purine metabolism or oxidation in the body. It is present in the blood in a concentration of about 0.13–0.42 mmol/l and is excreted in the urine in amounts of slightly less than 1 g per day.

urinalysis analysis of the urine as an aid in the diagnosis of disease. In pregnancy the urine is regularly tested for the presence of protein, glucose and ketones. Blood and pus may also be detected in cases of infection.

urinary relating to urine.

urination micturition.

urine the fluid secreted by the kidneys, and excreted from the urinary bladder in micturition. The reaction is normally about pH 6. It consists of water (96 per cent) in which are dissolved waste products of metabolism such as UREA and CREATININE, and other substances including sodium chloride and phosphates, but not normally glucose.

urinometer a glass instrument having a graduated stem weighted with a mercury bulb, used for measuring the specific gravity of urine.

urticaria a vascular reaction of the skin marked by transient appearance of slightly elevated patches which are redder or paler than the surrounding skin and often accompanied by severe itching; called also nettle rash. The cause may be certain foods, infection, or emotional stress.

uterine pertaining to the uterus. *U. souffle,* see SOUFFLE. *U. tubes,* FALLOPIAN TUBES.

uteroplacental pertaining to the uterus and placenta.

uterosacral pertaining to the uterus and sacrum. *U. ligaments* two ligaments which pass backward from the cervix to the sacrum, encircling the rectum. These ligaments help to maintain the uterus in a position of anteversion.

uterosalpingography radiography of the uterus and uterine tubes; hysterosalpingography.

uterotomy hysterotomy; incision of the uterus.

uterovesical referring to the uterus and bladder. *U. pouch* the fold of peritoneum between these two organs.

uterus the womb; a pear-shaped, hollow, muscular organ situated in the pelvic cavity between the bladder and the rectum, and supported by the parametrium. It is about 7.5 cm (3 in) long, 5 cm (2 in) at the widest part, and may be divided into two parts, the corpus, or body, which in the adult virgin uterus is the upper two-thirds, and the cervix, or neck, the lower third. The uppermost part, between the cornua, is termed the fundus, and the constriction between the corpus and cervix is described as the isthmus. The cavity of the body of the uterus is a triangular slit, communicating at the cornua with the fallopian tubes, and at the internal os with the cervix. The body of the uterus has a mucous membrane lining of ENDOMETRIUM which is shed about every 28 days. Should an ovum be fertilized, it embeds after 8 days and develops within the uterine cavity. The MYOMETRIUM, which is composed of interlacing spiral muscle fibres, hypertrophies, so growing to accommodate the fetus. *Bicornuate u.* a type of congenital malfor-

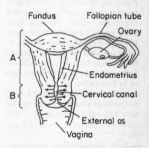

A. *Body of uterus*; B. *cervix.*
UTERUS AND APPENDAGES

mation in which the uterus has two horns. *U. didelphys* a double uterus resulting from the failure of the two sides to unite during development. *U. unicornus* a uterus with only one horn, the other being underdeveloped.

uvula a small, fleshy mass hanging from the soft palate above the root of the tongue.

V

vaccinate to inoculate with a vaccine in order to procure immunity to a disease. *See* IMMUNITY.

vaccination 1. usually inoculation with the vaccinia virus in order to protect against smallpox. It was given routinely during the second year and again between the ages of 8 and 12 years. 2. where specified, the injection of a particular bacterial vaccine. *See* BACILLE CALMETTE–GUÉRIN, TAB *and* Appendix 15.

vaccine a suspension of killed organisms in normal saline. *Attenuated v.* one prepared from living organisms which, through long cultivation, have lost their virulence. *Bacille Calmette–Guérin v.* an attenuated bovine bacillus to give protection from tuberculosis. *Salk v.* one prepared from a strain of poliomyelitis virus.

vacuum aspiration a method used to perform abortions during the first 3 months of pregnancy; also used to remove a hydatidiform mole.

vacuum extractor an apparatus, introduced first in Sweden, for use in suitable cases as an alternative to delivery by obstetric forceps. A metal cup is attached by suction to the fetal scalp, and gentle traction, synchronizing with the uterine contractions, is exerted. *See* Appendix 10.

vagal pertaining to the vagal nerve.

vagina the canal lined with squamous epithelium which leads from the vulva to the cervix uteri. It form a part of the birth canal. The anterior wall, 6.5–7.5 cm (2.5–3 in) in length has the urethra and bladder base embedded in it. The posterior wall, 9–10 cm (3.5–4 in) long, is in contact with the perineal body, the rectum and the pouch of Douglas. The lateral walls are in contact with the levator ani muscles.

vaginal pertaining to, or through, the vagina. *V. bleeding, see* Appendices 6 and 11. *V. discharge, see* DISCHARGE. *V. examination or examination per vaginam* a means of assessing factors of pregnancy, labour and puerperium and gynaecological conditions by palpation with one or two fingers in the vagina.

vaginismus painful spasms of the muscles of the vagina.

vaginitis inflammation of the vagina. In pregnancy it is commonly due to infection with the fungus *Candida albicans*. This causes considerable irritation and is usually treated with NYSTATIN pessaries or rarely by swabbing with 0.5 per cent aqueous gentian violet solution. Vaginitis due to *Trichomonas vaginalis* is also common. It is characterized by a frothy, intensely irritant, greenish discharge. The woman and her sexual partner are treated with metronidazole (Flagyl).

vagus the 10th cranial nerve, a parasympathetic nerve having a wide distribution in the body and supplying the heart, lungs, liver and part of the alimentary tract.

Valium trademark for a preparation of diazepam, an anxiolytic and skeletal muscle relaxant.

Valsava manoeuvre increase of intrathoracic pressure by forcible exhalation against the closed glottis. Infants with respiratory distress adopt a partial Valsava manoeuvre by grunting, thereby maintaining a positive pressure in the chest even during exhalation, i.e. a POSITIVE END-EXPIRATORY PRESSURE (PEEP).

value a measure of worth or efficiency; a quantitative measurement of the activity, concentration, etc., of specific substances. *Normal v's* a range in concentration of specific substances found in normal healthy tissues, secretions, etc.

valve a membranous fold in a canal or passage that prevents backward flow of material passing through it.

valvotomy a surgical operation to

increase the lumen of a narrowed valve, e.g. mitral valvotomy to relieve MITRAL STENOSIS.

valvuloplasty plastic repair of a valve, especially a valve of the heart.

vanillylmandelic acid an excretory product of the catecholamines, used as a test for adrenaline metabolism.

variable in epidemiology any measurement that can have different values. *Dependent v.* a variable which is dependent on the effect of other variables in an epidemiological study. *Independent v.* a variable not influenced by other variables in an epidemiological study but which may be the cause of alterations in these variables.

variance a measure of the variation seen in a set of data.

varicella chickenpox.

varicose swollen or dilated. *V. veins* abnormally distended and tortuous veins, usually those of the leg, due to inefficient valves which permit some back- or cross-flow of blood, particularly in the communicating veins between the superficial and deep veins. They may appear or become troublesome for the first time during pregnancy, when high progesterone levels relax the vessel walls, so permitting further stasis and inefficient venous return. The woman is advised to walk about, so that muscle contractions can aid the venous return, rather than to stand still with the legs crossed or dependent. Resting with the legs elevated above the level of the heart or wearing elastic tights or stockings, put on before getting out of bed, should be encouraged. After delivery the condition improves. Sometimes injections to sclerose the inefficient portions of the vein are carried out during pregnancy, but more often this is left until afterwards, when the condition may also be treated operatively.

variola smallpox.

varix an enlarged tortuous vein, artery, or lymphatic vessel. pl. *varices*.

vas a vessel. pl. *vasa*. *V. deferens* the tube through which the spermatozoa pass from the testis to be stored in the seminal vesicle to become part of the semen. *V. previa* vessels in front of the presenting part. A rare condition of velamentous insertion of the umbilical cord, usually with a degree of placenta previa, in which the vessels in the membranes are lying in front of the presenting part. When the membranes rupture there is risk of compression of, or even haemorrhage from, these vessels, and, accordingly, hypoxia or haemorrhage to the child.

vasa praevia the presentation, in front of the fetal head during labour, of the blood vessels of the umbilical cord where they enter the placenta in a velamentous insertion of the cord. When the membranes rupture, bleeding from these vessels may occur causing severe fetal distress.

vascular relating to, or consisting largely of, vessels.

vasectomy removal of a portion of the VAS DEFERENS through a small incision in the scrotum so that the semen is free of spermatozoa after about 4 months. Other methods of contraception should be continued until three consecutive semen specimens have been clear.

vasoconstrictor causing contraction of blood vessels.

vasodepressor 1. having the effect of lowering the blood pressure through reduction in peripheral resistance. 2. an agent that causes vasodepression.

vasodilator causing dilatation of blood vessels.

vasomotor controlling the muscles of blood vessels, both dilator and constrictor.

vasopressin a pressor agent produced in the pituitary gland. Also known as antidiuretic hormone.

vasopressor 1. stimulating contraction of the muscular tissue of the capillaries and arteries. 2. a vasopressor agent.

vault the part of the fetal skull (excluding the base and face), which contains the cerebral hemispheres. It is made up of the two frontal, two parietal, two temporal and one occipital bone. These bones are separated by membranous sutures which allow moulding of the fetal skull in labour and growth of the brain. *V. cap* a contraceptive device; a bowl-shaped cap which is attached to the vaginal vault by suction to prevent spermatozoa entering the cervix and the subsequent risk of pregnancy. It should be used in conjunction with a spermicidal agent to increase its effectiveness. *V. of the vagina* the upper part of the vagina into which the cervix protrudes.

VDRL Venereal Disease Research Laboratory.

vegan a vegetarian who excludes from his/her diet all foods of animal origin.

vegetarian a person who eats only food of vegetable origin. *V. diet* one in which no meat is eaten. A *lacto-vegetarian* diet prohibits the intake of meat, poultry, fish and eggs. An *ovo-lacto-vegetarian* diet allows all foods from plants plus eggs, milk and other dairy products. An *ovo-vegetarian* diet allows eggs and foods of plant origin, but prohibits all animal and dairy products.

vein a vessel carrying blood from the capillaries back to the heart. It has thin walls and a lining endothelium from which the venous valves are formed.

velamentous like a veil. *V. insertion of the umbilical cord* a placenta in which the umbilical cord vessels divide before reaching the placenta. *See also* VASA PREVIA.

vena cava one of the two trunk veins which return the venous blood from the upper and lower parts of the body, respectively, to the right atrium of the heart.

venepuncture the puncture of a vein, usually to obtain blood or administer a drug.

venereal concerning or resulting

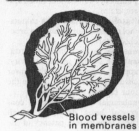

Blood vessels in membranes

VELAMENTOUS INSERTION OF CORD

from sexual intercourse. *V. diseases* SYPHILIS, GONORRHOEA and SOFT CHANCRE.

venesection opening a vein and withdrawing blood to relieve congestion.

ventilation 1. providing fresh air in a room or building. 2. the process of exchange of air between the lungs and ambient air. Pulmonary ventilation refers to the total exchange whereas alveolar ventilation refers to the ventilation of the alveoli where gas exchange with the blood takes place. *Intermittent positive-pressure v. (IPPV)* mechanical ventilation by a machine designed to deliver breathing gas until equilibrium is established between the patient's lungs and the VENTILATOR.

ventilator an apparatus designed to qualify the air that is breathed through it or to either intermittently or continuously control pulmonary ventilation; called also respirator.

Ventolin trademark for a salbutamol metered-dose inhaler; a bronchodilator.

ventouse *see* VACUUM EXTRACTOR.

ventricle a small pouch or cavity; applied especially to the lower chambers of the heart, and to the four cavities of the brain.

ventricular septal defect a congenital heart defect in which there is persistent patency of the ventricular septum which allows a flow of blood directly from one ventricle to the other, thereby bypassing the pulmonary circulation and causing cyanosis because of oxygen deficiency.

ventrosuspension an operation. At LAPAROTOMY or laparoscopy the round ligaments are shortened to help antevert a RETROVERTED UTERUS.

venule a minute vein.

vernix caseosa the greasy substance which covers the fetus *in utero*. It is a secretion from the sebaceous glands, together with desquamated cells, which appears at about 30–32 weeks, is abundant at 36–37 weeks, and may remain until or even past full term.

version turning the fetus *in utero*, to alter a lie or presentation to one which is more favourable. *Cephalic v.* turning the child to make the head present. *External v.* turning the child by manipulation through the abdominal wall. *Internal v.* inserting the hand into the uterus, turning the child with one hand in the uterus

and the other on the abdomen. *Podalic v.* turning the child to make the breech present. In practice, external cephalic version is fairly frequently carried out about the 34th week of pregnancy in a case of breech presentation, since vertex delivery is so much more favourable to the child than breech delivery. Internal version is seldom performed, as with good antenatal care the necessity seldom arises. Occasionally, an internal podalic version (followed by a breech extraction) may be performed when a multigravid woman is in labour with an oblique lie of the fetus or in the event of an oblique lie of a second twin.

vertebrae the irregular bones forming the spinal column. They are divided into 7 cervical, 12 dorsal, 5 lumbar, 5 sacral (sacrum) and 4 coccygeal (coccyx) bones. sing. *vertebra.*

vertex an area of the head bounded by the anterior and posterior fontanelles, and laterally by the parietal eminences. *V. presentation* the fetus is so flexed that the vertex lies over the internal os, and is the first part to appear at the vulva.

vertigo giddiness, a temporary dizzy sensation, with loss of equilibrium.

vesica a bladder; usually referring to the urinary bladder; *See* ECTOPIA VESICAE.

vesical relating to the bladder.

vesicle a blister or small sac usually containing fluid.

vesicovaginal pertaining to the

bladder and vagina. *V. fistula* an abnormal opening between the bladder and the vagina; a rare complication of prolonged or obstructed labour when the tissues of the bladder are devitalized by prolonged pressure of the fetal head.

vesicular relating to, or containing, vesicles. *V. mole* HYDATIDIFORM MOLE.

vestibule an entrance. The part of the vulva lying between the labia minora.

vestige a remnant of a structure that functioned in a previous stage of species or individual development. adj. vestigal.

viable capable of independent life. A term applied to the fetus after 24 weeks of intrauterine life.

vicarious 1. substituted for another; used when one organ functions instead of another. 2. occurring in circumstances where not normally expected. *V. liability* a situation in which the employer is vicariously liable for the torts of the employee during the course of his employment, e.g. a health authority is vicariously liable for the torts of a midwife during the course of her employment.

villi fine hair-like processes projecting from a surface. *Chorionic v.* branched processes which develop on the trophoblast, and which dip into the maternal blood of the placental site. *See* PLACENTA *and* CHORIONIC VILLI. *Intestinal v.* minute projections on the intestinal mucosa. Each villus has a blood capillary and a lacteal. They are the sites of absorption of fluids and nutrients.

viraemia the presence of viruses in the blood.

viral caused by or having the nature of a virus.

virgin a girl or woman who has not had sexual intercourse.

virus small infective agent which can only grow and reproduce in living cells, and can only be seen with the electron microscope. They are complex and often difficult to culture. They cause, amongst many other diseases: smallpox, poliomyelitis, influenza, rabies, measles and rubella. Viruses cross the placenta and can cause fetal abnormalities, especially during the first trimester of pregnancy.

viscera internal organs in the body cavities, e.g. heart, liver, uterus.

viscid sticky and glutinous.

visual analogue scale a method of quantifying subjective feelings such as pain, sedation, etc. Consists of a line 10 cm long, one end of the line indicating absence of the feeling, e.g. pain, and the other extreme sensation or pain. The individual marks a point along the line which represents the pain or other sensation he or she is feeling at that time. The distance from the left-hand end of the line to the point is measured and represents a numerical assessment of the pain or other sensation.

vital relating to or necessary to life. *V. statistics* the records kept of births and deaths among the population, including the causes of death, and the factors which seem to influence their rise and fall. *See* Appendix 20.

vitamins essential food substances, minute quantities of which are essential to nutrition and health. Vitamins A, D, E and K are fat-soluble, and B and C water-soluble. *Vitamin A* found in fish liver oils, cream, milk and egg yolk and in vegetables such as carrots, spinach and watercress. Deficiency causes night blindness, failure of growth and lack of resistance to infection. *Vitamin B* this group consists of a number of substances. (*a*) Thiamine (aneurine vitamin B_1) is found in the husks of cereals and yeasts. Deficiency results in neurological symptoms, cardiovascular dysfunction, oedema and reduced intestinal motility. (*b*) Nicotinic acid (niacin) is found in liver, kidney and yeast. Deficiency causes pellagra, where gastrointestinal, skin and mental disturbances occur. (*c*) Riboflavin (B_2) is found in liver, kidney, heart, brewer's yeast, milk, eggs, greens and enriched cereals. Deficiency causes inflammation of the tongue and seborrhoeic dermatitis. (*d*) Cyanocobalamin (B_{12}) and folic acid are both essential for red cell formation. If there is a deficiency, as may occur due to fetal demands in pregnancy, megaloblastic or macrocytic ANAEMIA may develop. (*e*) Pantothenic acid, pyridoxine (B_6) and biotin are also part of the B complex. *Vitamin C* ascorbic acid. Found in fresh fruits, especially citrus, blackcurrants, tomatoes and rosehips. Deficiency causes scurvy and delays the healing of wounds, probably due to slow formation of collagen. *Vitamin D* found in similar animal sources to vitamin A, but can also be manufactured by skin exposed to sunlight. It is essential for the absorption of calcium and phosphorus. Deficiency causes rickets, osteomalacia and NEONATAL HYPOCALCAEMIA. Both vitamins are especially necessary during pregnancy and lactation. *Vitamin E* deficiency leads to sterility in rats, but the function in man is not known. *Vitamin K* necessary for the formation of PROTHROMBIN. It is found in spinach, cabbage, cauliflower and oats. It is also synthesized in intestine by bacteria. Deficiency rarely occurs except when the gut is sterile, i.e. when taking a broad-spectrum antibiotic or if HAEMORRHAGIC DISEASE occurs in the first days of life.

VMA vanillylmandelic acid.

volt the unit of electromotive force (EMF).

volvulus torsion of a loop of intestine, causing obstruction with or without strangulation.

vomiting expulsion of the contents of the stomach through the mouth. *V. of blood* HAEMATEMESIS. *V. in the newborn* This is very common and has many causes. (*a*) Bile-stained vomit without the passage of meconium indicates intestinal obstruction; the sooner after delivery the higher the site. (*b*) Blood-stained vomit may be due to maternal blood swallowed at delivery or ingested from cracked nipples, or to the infant's own blood in cases of HAEMOR-RHAGIC DISEASE. Maternal and infant blood may be differentiated by SINGER'S TEST. (c) Milk may be vomited owing to various infections (including infections of the urinary tract, GASTROENTER-ITIS and MENINGITIS), to a relaxed cardia, to feeding problems or to raised intracranial pressure. V. in pregnancy (a) 'morning sickness' occurs between the 4th and 12th week in 50–60 per cent of pregnancies and is characterized by nausea, sometimes accompanied by vomiting, occurring on rising in the morning, but often at other times. There have been many theories as to the cause, but none is as yet proved. (b) HYPEREMESIS GRAVIDARUM. (c) Intercurrent vomiting in pregnancy is often due to PYELONEPHRITIS, other infections and diseases of the gastrointestinal tract and other severe illnesses. The midwife should consult a doctor about any patient who has persistent vomiting after the 14th week of pregnancy or who, at any time, has KETONURIA. Projectile v. this occurs in hypertrophic PYLORIC STENOSIS.

vomitus material vomited.

vulsellum see FORCEPS and Appendix 10.

vulva the external female genital organs.

vulvectomy excision of the vulva.

vulvitis inflammation of the vulva.

W

'waiter's tip' a characteristic position of forearm and hand with ERB'S PARALYSIS.

warfarin an anticoagulant drug which crosses the placenta so, if used, is confined to the weeks 16–36. See Appendix 19.

warts an epidermal tumour of viral origin. Genital w. spread in pregnancy and may cover the vulva, perineum and anal regions. They can be treated effectively with podophyllin applied locally.

Wassermann reaction a serological test used in the diagnosis of SYPHILIS.

WBC white blood cell (leukocyte); white blood (cell) count.

weaning detaching or alienating from an accustomed habit or enjoyment. In infant feeding it can be from breast to bottle or cup feeding, from bottle to cup feeding or, more commonly from any type of milk feed to solid food.

webbed connected by a membrane or strand of tissue.

wedlock the state of being married.

weight gain during pregnancy the normal weight gain is about

10–12 kg (24–26 lb), though there are appreciable variations. It is accounted for as follows: full-term fetus 3.4 kg (7.5 lb), placenta 0.7 kg (1.5 lb), liquor amnii 1 kg (2.2 lb), uterus 1 kg (2.2 lb), blood 1.4 kg (3 lb), breasts 1 kg (2.2 lb) and a considerable increase in tissue fluid and fat and protein deposition. The weight gain is about 2.5 kg (5.5 lb) in the first 20 weeks and 10 kg (22 lb) in the last 20 weeks, so a weekly gain of more than 0.5 kg (1lb) may indicate occult OEDEMA which occurs as an early sign of PRE-ECLAMPSIA. *W. g. in babies, see* Appendix 13.

welfare foods nutritious foods sold in clinics at non-profit-making prices.

well woman clinic a 'prophylactic' clinic available to screen women for breast and cervical cancer, anaemia, diabetes and hypertension.

Wernicke's encephalopathy acute haemorrhagic encephalitis, occurring occasionally in severe HYPEREMESIS GRAVIDARUM.

Wertheim's operation *see* HYSTERECTOMY.

wet-nurse a woman who breast feeds infants other than her own.

Wharton's jelly connective tissue of the umbilical cord.

whey the fluid part of milk, separated from the curd after the addition of rennet. It is easily digested, as the casein and fat have been removed.

white asphyxia a term formerly used to describe a baby with a low APGAR SCORE where the skin is white due to circulatory collapse. Now called severe asphyxia. *See* ASPHYXIA NEONATORUM.

white leg *see* PHLEGMASIA ALBA DOLENS.

white matter, white substance the white nervous tissue, constituting the conducting portion of the brain and spinal cord, composed mostly of myelinated nerve fibres. Grey matter or substance is the term used to describe the tissues composed of unmyelinated fibres.

WHO World Health Organisation.

whooping cough *see* PERTUSSIS.

Widal reaction a blood test used in the diagnosis of typhoid and paratyphoid fevers.

Wilson–Mikity syndrome BRONCHOPULMONARY DYSPLASIA, which is a condition occurring in babies who have been ventilated for long periods or have needed prolonged oxygen therapy. *See* Appendix 17.

wolffian bodies two small organs in the embryo, which are the primitive kidneys.

womb the uterus.

Woolwich shell a plastic or glass appliance worn over the breast, with the hole on the flat side over the flat or slightly retracted nipple to encourage it to become more prominent, coupled with the pressure on the surrounding areola. It is worn inside a well-fitting brassière during pregnancy, first for an hour a day then for gradually increasing lengths of time. Now rarely used.

World Health Organisation (WHO) the specialized agency of the United Nations that is concerned with health on an inter-

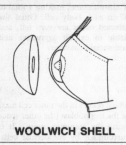

WOOLWICH SHELL

national level. One of its present campaigns is Safe Motherhood for all by the year 2000, since the maternal mortality rate is still very high in many developing countries.

wound a bodily injury caused by physical means, with disruption of the normal continuity of structures. In healing of a wound by first intention, restoration of tissue continuity occurs directly, without granulation; in healing by second intention, wound repair following tissue loss is accomplished by closure of the wound with granulation tissue; healing by third intention occurs when a wound is initially unable to close owing to contamination, and is closed 4–5 days after the injury.

Wrigleys forceps obstetric forceps used for very low forceps deliveries, the aftercoming head of the breech, or at caesarean section.

X

X chromosome one of the two sex chromosomes, the other being Y. Female cells carry two X chromosomes (XX) and male cells one X and one Y chromosome (XY). During maturation of the ovum and spermatozoon, one of these is cast off. At fertilization the two remaining determine the sex of the child: X and X, a girl, X and Y, a boy. *See also* TURNER'S SYNDROME *and* KLINEFELTER'S SYNDROME.

X-linked transmitted by genes on the X chromosome; sex-linked.

xiphisternum XIPHOID PROCESS.

xiphoid process a small cartilaginous process at the lower end of the sternum. Also termed xiphisternum and ensiform cartilage. One of the landmarks to which the FUNDUS UTERI is related in the latter weeks of pregnancy.

X-rays RÖNTGEN RAYS. Electromagnetic waves of short wavelength which are capable of penetrating many substances, such as paper, wood and flesh, but are absorbed by lead, platinum or bone.

XO symbol for the karyotype observed in most cases of TURNER'S SYNDROME, in which there is only one sex chromosome, an X chromosome.

Xylocaine a proprietary preparation of lignocaine used for local anaesthesia. *See* Appendices 10 and 19.

XYY syndrome a rare condition in males in which there is an extra Y chromosome, making a total of 47 in each body cell. Often the affected males are very tall, and liable to exhibit aggressive and anti-social behaviour.

Y

Y chromosome one of the two sex chromosomes, which, united with x is found in the cells of males.

yaws a non-venereal treponemal infection found widely in tropical areas. Local lesions resemble those of SYPHILIS and serological tests for syphilis are positive.

yeast a species of fungi which reproduce by budding. They produce fermentation in malt and fruit juices, producing alcohol, as in beer and wine. THRUSH is due to infection by the yeast-like fungus *Candida albicans.*

yolk sac one of the two spaces which occurs in the inner cell mass of the trophoblast (the other space being the amniotic cavity). It is surrounded by entodermal cells, whereas the amniotic cavity is surrounded by ectodermal cells and between the two is an intervening layer of mesoderm. The embryo is formed from the area where the three tissues, ectoderm, mesoderm and entoderm lie in apposition.

Yutopar trademark for ritodrine hydrochloride; used in selected cases to inhibit preterm labour.

Z

zero the symbol 0. Nought. The point in any thermometric scale at which the measuring of temperature starts. In the Celsius thermometer, zero is the melting point of ice. In the Fahrenheit thermometer, zero is 32° below the melting of ice. *See* FAHRENHEIT *and* CELSIUS.

zinc a trace element that is the component of several enzymes. It is found in red meat, shellfish, liver, peas, lentils, beans and rice. A severe deficiency of zinc can retard growth in children, cause a low sperm count in men and retard wound healing.

zona pellucida the transparent, non-cellular, secreted layer surrounding an OVUM. SPERM release the enzymes which allow penetration of the zona pellucida but only one will enter the ovum at the time of fertilization.

Zovirax trademark for preparations of acyclovir, an anti-viral agent.

zygote the fertilized OVUM prior to SEGMENTATION.

APPENDICES

APPENDIX 1

The National Health Service

The National Health Service Act was passed in 1946 and implemented in 1948. It followed the publication of a report published in 1942 by a committee set up to review social insurance and certain allied subjects under the chairmanship of Sir William Beveridge. One of the main recommendations of the Beveridge report was the provision of a comprehensive health service and this was designed by Aneurin Bevan, Minister of Health in the post-war government.

Structure of the National Health Service (NHS)

The health service was divided into three parts, known as the tripartite structure, and was under the Ministry of Health. The hospital and specialist services were provided by regional hospital boards, their hospital management committees and boards of governors of the teaching hospitals; the general medical services by executive councils; and the remainder of the community services by the local health authorities, namely the county councils and the county borough councils. These services, all provided without charge, were supported by massive legislation giving insurance cover and allowances (*see* Figure 1).

This welfare state pattern developed rapidly, with enormous improvements in standards of health, and impressive advances in health curative and preventive medicine. Midwives, apart from a small number in independent practice or in the private sector, were now employed in the NHS in hospitals or the community. All mothers and babies also now had free access to a doctor, the general practitioner in the community and an obstetrician in hospital. As a result the midwives role began to change as the care of mothers and babies became increasingly medically dominated, and the problem of duplication of care began to arise.

There were also problems with the tripartite structure of the NHS, mainly financial and administration. Communications between the three divisions were often poor and services duplicated or even triplicated. In 1959 the Cranbrook Committee, reviewing possible unification of the maternity services, recommended the continuation of the three-part structure, but with better collaboration and liaison at all levels—a decision which evoked a good measure of adverse criticism. By the late 1960s it was clearly apparent that unification of the entire NHS was necessary to enable the service to develop and fulfil its role more effectively.

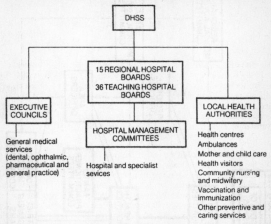

Figure 1. National Health Structure Before Reorganization in 1974.

The NHS Reorganization Act, 1973

The NHS Reorganization Act of 1973 was implemented in 1974 and unified the three parts of the health service under a single management structure, as is shown in Figure 2. The service had a three-tier structure: the Department of Health and Social Security, 14 regional health authorities and 90 area health authorities. For operational purposes most of the areas were divided into districts (*see* Figure 3). The Regional Health Authority (RHA) became the Local Supervising Authority for midwives.

The Health Services Act, 1980

A Royal Commission set up to examine the NHS published its report in 1979. It recommended simplifying the lines of communication and responsibility for the health service at local level. The government accepted these recommendations and in 1979 published a consultative document entitled 'Patients first'.

As a result of the consultation, The National Health Services Act,

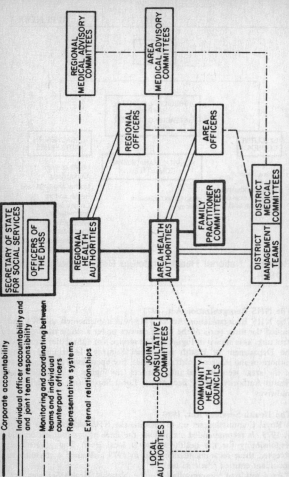

Figure 2 Framework of the NHS 1974–1982 Organizational Structure in England

Corporate accountability

Individual officer accountability and
and joint team responsibility

Monitoring and coordinating between
teams and individual
counterpart officers

Representative systems

External relationships

SECRETARY OF STATE
FOR SOCIAL SERVICES

OFFICERS OF
THE DHSS

REGIONAL
MEDICAL ADVISORY
COMMITTEES

AREA
MEDICAL ADVISORY
COMMITTEES

REGIONAL
OFFICERS

AREA
OFFICERS

REGIONAL HEALTH
AUTHORITIES

AREA HEALTH
AUTHORITIES

FAMILY
PRACTITIONER
COMMITTEES

DISTRICT MEDICAL
COMMITTEES

DISTRICT
MANAGEMENT
TEAMS

JOINT
CONSULTATIVE
COMMITTEES

COMMUNITY
HEALTH COUNCILS

LOCAL
AUTHORITIES

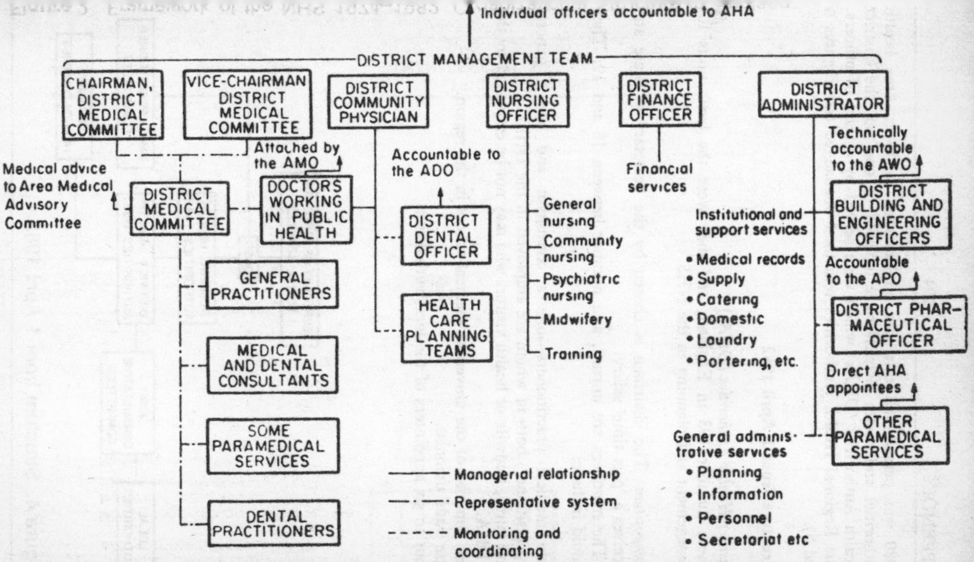

Figure 3. Framework of the NHS 1974–1982. District Organization.

Individual officers accountable to AHA

— DISTRICT MANAGEMENT TEAM —

DISTRICT ADMINISTRATOR

DISTRICT FINANCE OFFICER

DISTRICT NURSING OFFICER

DISTRICT COMMUNITY PHYSICIAN

Accountable to the ADO

DISTRICT BUILDING AND ENGINEERING OFFICERS — Technically accountable to the AWO

DISTRICT PHARMACEUTICAL OFFICER — Accountable to the APO

OTHER PARAMEDICAL SERVICES — Direct AHA appointees

Financial services

General nursing
Community nursing
Psychiatric nursing
Midwifery
Training

Institutional and support services
• Medical records
• Supply
• Catering
• Domestic
• Laundry
• Portering, etc.

General administrative services
• Planning
• Information
• Personnel
• Secretariat etc

Chairman, DISTRICT MEDICAL COMMITTEE

Vice-Chairman DISTRICT MEDICAL COMMITTEE

DISTRICT MEDICAL COMMITTEE

Attached by the AMO

DISTRICT DENTAL OFFICER

HEALTH CARE PLANNING TEAMS

Medical advice to Area Medical Advisory Committee

DOCTORS WORKING IN PUBLIC HEALTH

GENERAL PRACTITIONERS

MEDICAL AND DENTAL CONSULTANTS

SOME PARAMEDICAL SERVICES

DENTAL PRACTITIONERS

——— Managerial relationship
– – – Representative system
········ Monitoring and coordinating

1980 was passed and this was implemented in 1982. Area health authorities and health districts were replaced by one tier, the District Health Authorities (DHAs) which were served by a team of officers. The Regional Health Authorities remained unchanged (*see* Figures 4 and 5).

Structure from 1 April 1982

District Health Authorities (DHAs)
These number 193 in England, and they were the basic units for management and planning in the NHS.

Composition: The chairman is chosen by the Secretary of State and receives a 'part time' salary.

The members are unpaid, and number between 16 and 19. They should include:

Two medical practitioners—one a consultant and one a general practitioner, both of whom are employed in the DHA.
One nurse, midwife or health visitor, who may not be employed by the DHA.
One nominee of the university medical school in the region.
One trade unionist.
Four to six appointees of the local authorities.

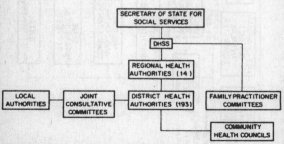

Figure 4. Structure from 1 April 1982.

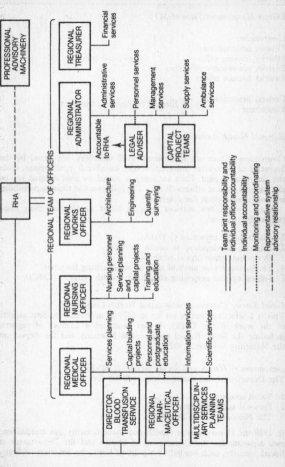

Figure 5. Framework of NHS Regional Health Authority Organization 1974.

Key elements within the figure:

PROFESSIONAL ADVISORY MACHINERY

RHA

REGIONAL TEAM OF OFFICERS

REGIONAL MEDICAL OFFICER
— Services planning
— Capital building projects
— Personnel and postgraduate education
— Information services
— Scientific services

REGIONAL NURSING OFFICER
— Nursing personnel
— Service planning and capital projects
— Training and education

REGIONAL WORKS OFFICER
— Architecture
— Engineering
— Quantity surveying

REGIONAL ADMINISTRATOR
Accountable to RHA
— Administrative services
— Personnel services
— Management services
— Supply services
— Ambulance services

REGIONAL TREASURER
— Financial services

LEGAL ADVISER

CAPITAL PROJECT TEAMS

DIRECTOR, BLOOD TRANSFUSION SERVICE

REGIONAL PHARMACEUTICAL OFFICER

MULTIDISCIPLINARY SERVICES PLANNING TEAMS

——— Team joint responsibility and individual officer accountability
——— Individual accountability
········· Monitoring and coordinating
– – – Representative system advisory relationship

District Management Team (DMT)

Composition:
District administrator
District nursing officer
District community physician
District finance officer
} Appointed officers

General practitioner
Consultant
} Elected by district colleagues

Regional Health Authorities

Composition: There are approximately 20 members, appointed by the Secretary of State after consultation with interested organizations. Only the chairman is paid. Each authority is served by paid officials led by the regional team of officers (RTO). The full team and their responsibilities can be seen from the diagram.

Apart from a few services such as blood transfusion, their main responsibilities are:

1. Allocation of resources to DHAs.
2. Planning development of health services.
3. Designing major capital projects.
4. Employing senior medical staff in non-teaching hospitals.
5. Setting up and reviewing community health councils (CHCs).

Social Service Committee (now called Health Committee)
This is a select committee set up in 1979 to investigate various aspects of the work of the DHSS. It has produced a number of reports, including the Short Report on Perinatal Mortality and the Report on the Maternity Services, 1992.

Department of Health and Social Security (DHSS)
The Department had national responsibility for:

1. Social security.
2. Personal social services.
3. The National Health Service

In 1988 the Department of Health and Social Security was divided into two departments, the Department of Health and the Department of Social Security, each headed by a political head, the Secretary of State.

The Department of Health has national responsibility for the National Health Service and the Department of Social Security for the personal social services and social security.

The 'Griffiths Report', 1983

In 1983 a NHS Management Inquiry Team, headed by Sir Roy Griffiths, was established to examine and give advice on the effective use and management of manpower and related resources in the NHS. Their recommendations were published in October 1983 and led to widespread changes in the management of the NHS at all levels.

Changes at the Department of Health (then the DHSS)

1. A *Health Services Supervisory Board* was established to:

determine the overall objectives of the NHS;
to approve the overall budget and resource allocations;
to make strategic decisions;
to monitor performance.

2. A *NHS Management Board* was also set up under the direction of the Supervisory Board. Its main responsibilities are:

to plan implementation of the policies approved by the Supervisory Board;
to give leadership to the management of the NHS;
to control performance;
to achieve consistency and drive.

Changes at Regional and District Authority level

The findings of the Inquiry highlighted the lack of a clearly defined general management function throughout the NHS, thus *general managers* were appointed at both regional and district level throughout the service. The general managers have responsibility for: planning, implementing and control of performance. Greater freedom was given for health authorities to organize the management structure at both district and regional level, thus different patterns have emerged to suit local situations.

Units of Management

Each Health District is divided into Units of Management, and each Unit is headed by a Unit General Manager. Midwives have endeavoured to maintain an integrated midwifery service by supporting Units of Midwifery which include both hospital and community services, but in many instances the midwifery service has been included in a Unit with other specialties. The Unit General Manager's main responsibilities are to plan the management structure of the Unit and to plan for day to day decisions.

Introduction of Resource Management

The resource management initiative was launched by the Department of Health in 1986 when six experimental projects were set up. Now over half the large (average 500 beds) general hospitals in England and Wales have started the process. The aim of resource management is to ensure that hospital and community-based groups providing health care institute devolved management arrangements, such as clinical directorates, which fully involve clinical and management staff. This should result in better, more effective and efficient use of available resources, thereby benefitting the patients.

With the introduction of resource management in the NHS, *clinical directorates* have been established within many Units of Management. Each clinical directorate manages a speciality such as obstetrics and gynaecology and is headed by a director who is usually a medical practitioner, and he or she is assisted by a senior nurse or midwife and a business manager. In some cases the senior nurse or midwife has also taken on the role of business manager. Budgets are devolved down to directorate level.

A key process of resource management is the formulation of a business planning cycle which is based on detailed information and is capable of quickly adjusting the resources to meet changing demands.

Information systems include:

1. Patient administration system (PAS) which holds all the biographical details of each patient centrally, thus it was accessible to all departments and prevents duplication of effort.
2. Operational systems (OS) which record the care or services the patient receives from all departments in the hospital. Departments may also build into their systems an indicator of the quality of service provided (Stewart, 1989).
3. Case mix database (CMD) is the combination of all the data from the PAS and OS (called feeder systems) which forms a comprehensive set of information about all the treatments and services provided for each patient during an episode of care. This information has many uses, for example, to develop 'normal' care profiles for different groups, analysis and comparisons of various treatment regimes, to produce comparative costings for different treatments and so on. It can also be used as part of the medical audit process.

National Health Service and Community Care Act, 1990

The major reforms of the NHS proposed in the White Paper 'Working for Patients' and enacted in the NHS and Community Care Act, 1990 started to be introduced in April 1991.

Self-governing trusts (SGTs)

One of the major changes is the establishment of NHS trusts. These are hospitals or other establishments or facilities which assume responsibility for their own ownership and management, i.e. they 'opt out' of direct NHS control. Trust status has to be approved by the Secretary of State and in April 1991 the first 57 SGTs were established. A further wave of SGTs have been approved for April 1992. Each trust has a Board of Directors (both executive and non-executive directors) and a Chairman approved by the Secretary of State.

Directly-managed units (DMU)

The management of hospitals and community health services which have not 'opted out' (i.e. become SGTs) has been devolved to unit level.

Internal market and contracts

The function of health authorities (HAs) has changed from that of managing institutions and community care services to purchasing for populations. In order to achieve this the HAs are required to:

1. Identify the total health needs of their resident population.
2. Plan how to meet these needs.
3. Secure the best and most effective services possible.

HAs are able to *purchase* these services from a range of different *providers* within or outside their own district, or from SGTs or the private sector. The provision of health services is therefore being negotiated between purchasers and providers, on the basis of quality, quantity and cost. Contracts will obviously be placed with those who can offer the best and most cost-effective service, thereby increasing their income so that they have the resources to further develop their services.

Fund-holding practices

General practitioners (GPs) may apply to the relevant Regional Health Authority (RHA) for recognition as a fund-holding practice. Those granted this status receive an alloted sum each year from the RHA. Fund-holding practices purchase services for their patients from providers. An increasing number of GPs are now applying for recognition as fund-holding practices.

References and further reading

Department of Health and Social Security (1983) *National Health Service Management Inquiry. (Griffiths Report)*. HMSO: London.

Health Committee, Second Report (1992) *Maternity Services* Vol. 1. Chaired by Mr Nicholas Winterton. HMSO: London.

Ministry of Health (1959) *Report of the Maternity Services Committee. (Cranbrook Report)*. HMSO: London.

Stewart D (1989) Resource management made easy. *Nursing Standard* **34**:3.

Social Insurance and Allied Services (1942) *Report by Sir William Beveridge (Beveridge Report)*. HMSO: London.

Social Services Committee Session (1979–1980) Perinatal and Neonatal Mortality. Vol. 1. Chaired by Mrs Renee Short. HMSO: London. HC 663-1.

APPENDIX 2

The Practice and Education of the Midwife and other Health Care Professionals

The title of midwife is an ancient one and means 'with woman'. Biblical references to midwives have always been to their honour. Through the centuries midwives had little or no instruction in their work, learning their skills by working alongside experienced midwives, or practising with no prior instruction at all. In the sixteenth century legislation required midwives to apply to the bishop for a licence to practise and their application had to be supported by character references. Midwives were honoured and respected members of the community but their reputation deteriorated, as is depicted by Charles Dickens in his drunken and disreputable characters, Sairey Gamp and Betsey Pug.

In Great Britain, during the seventeenth and eighteenth centuries, there were a few attempts—mostly unsuccessful—to train midwives and to obtain for them some kind of state recognition, but it was not until the latter part of the nineteenth century that any real progress was made. The 30 years from 1872 saw the London Obstetrical Society's training and examination in midwifery, the General Medical Council's efforts to gain state recognition for the profession and the formation in 1881 of the Midwives Institute, now the Royal College of Midwives.

At this time various public-spirited people obtained the introduction of a number of Bills to Parliament. Eight were unsuccessful; the ninth, passed in 1902, brought about the formation of the Central Midwives Board and only then was midwifery organized on a national basis with state certification. The midwife in those days was a lone worker in the health field, attending women in labour and in the lying-in period—antenatal care was to come later—and calling a doctor only when serious complications arose.

The Central Midwives Board, set up 1902, was the body which governed midwifery practice in the United Kingdom until the Nurses, Midwives and Health Visitors Act, 1979 was implemented in 1983 (see Appendix 22).

The following amended definition of a midwife was adopted by the International Confederation of Midwives, the International Federation of Gynaecologists and Obstetricians and the World Health Organisation in 1990, 1991 and 1992 respectively.

The definition of a midwife

'A midwife is a person who, having been regularly admitted to a midwifery educational programme, duly recognised in the country in which it is located, has successfully completed the prescribed course of studies in midwifery and has acquired the requisite qualifications to be registered and/or legally licensed to practise midwifery.

She must be able to give the necessary supervision, care and advice to women during pregnancy, labour and the postpartum period, to conduct deliveries on her own responsibility and to care for the newborn and the infant. This care includes preventative measures, the detection of abnormal conditions in mother and child, the procurement of medical assistance and the execution of emergency measures in the absence of medical help. She has an important task in health counselling and education, not only for the women, but also within the family and the community. The work should involve antenatal education and preparation for parenthood and extends to certain areas of gynaecology, family planning and child care. She may practise in hospitals, clinics, health units, domiciliary conditions or in any other service.'

The activities of a midwife are defined in the European Community Midwives Directive 80/155/EEC Article 4 as follows.

'Member States shall ensure that midwives are at least entitled to take up and pursue the following activities:

1. to provide sound family planning information and advice;
2. to diagnose pregnancies and monitor normal pregnancies; to carry out examinations necessary for the monitoring of the development of normal pregnancies;
3. to prescribe or advise on the examinations necessary for the earliest possible diagnosis of pregnancies at risk;
4. to provide a programme of parenthood preparation and a complete preparation for childbirth including advice on hygiene and nutrition;
5. to care for and assist the mother during labour and to monitor the condition of the fetus in utero by the appropriate clinical and technical means;
6. to conduct spontaneous deliveries including where required an episiotomy and in urgent cases a breech delivery;
7. to recognise the warning signs of abnormality in the mother or infant which necessitate referral to a doctor and to assist the latter where appropriate; to take the necessary emergency measures in the doctor's absence,* in particular the manual removal of the placenta, possibly followed by manual examination of the uterus;

---

* In present day practice in the Unitied Kingdom the midwife should not normally find herself in a position where medical aid is not available for such a grave emergency measure as manual removal of the placenta (UKCC, 1991).

8. to examine and care for the new-born infant; to take all initiatives which are necessary in case of need and to carry out where necessary immediate resuscitation;

9. to care for and monitor the progress of the mother in the postnatal period and to give all necessary advice to the mother on infant care to enable her to ensure the optimum progress of the new-born infant;

10. to carry out the treatment prescribed by a doctor;

11. to maintain all necessary records.'

Midwifery education and training

Midwifery training came under statutory control in 1902, consequent upon the passing of the first Midwives Act. As its inception the training lasted only 3 months but was doubled to 6 months in 1916, and further increased over the years until, in 1981, the EEC Midwives' Directives brought about the 18 months training (termed post-registration) for registered general nurses (RGNs) and 3 year programmes (called pre-registration) for all other entrants.

Major changes in initial midwifery education have taken place in recent years, especially since the publication of new proposals for nurse education in 'Project 2000, A New Preparation for Practice in 1986' (UKCC, 1986). Although midwives rejected some of the recommendations, such as joining the common foundation programme and being a branch of nursing, they agreed to others, including shared learning with other professional groups in appropriate subjects and the development of more 3 year programmes. By the mid 1980s there was only one 3 year midwifery programme in the UK, but now over 20 have been validated. All are at diploma or degree level and the students have supernumerary status and therefore receive a bursary rather than a salary. The 18 month midwifery education programmes for RGNs continue and by 1994 are required to be at diploma level, and some will be at degree level. Joint professional and academic validation is required for all midwifery education programmes, the National Boards being responsible for professional validation and an Institute of Higher Education for academic validation.

Another major change of the late 1980s is the amalgamation of Schools of Midwifery to form Colleges of Midwifery, or to become part of Colleges of Nursing and Midwifery, or Colleges of Health Care Studies. In the latter case other professional groups such as physiotherapists and radiographers may be part of the College. All these Colleges have links with an Institute of Higher Education and, in some parts of the country, midwifery and nurse education have become fully integrated into the higher education system.

The curriculum for initial midwifery education now includes more in-depth study of the behavioural and biological sciences and research-based practice. Students are encouraged to take responsibility for their own learning and to develop their analytical, critical and reflective skills both in theory and practice. The length of clinical placements in the community has been extended because that is where most ante- and postnatal care now takes place, but whether in the hospital or community setting, all students have a midwife mentor to guide and support them.

The outcomes of programmes of education leading to admission to Part 10 (midwife) of the register which are stated in the Midwives' Rules (UKCC, 1991) are listed below:

1. The content of programmes of education shall be such as the Council may from time to time require.
2. Programmes of education shall be designed to prepare the student to assume on registration the responsibilities and accountability for their practice as a midwife.
3. Such programmes of education shall:
   (a) meet the requirements of the Midwives' Directive;
   (b) be provided at an approved educational institution; and
   (c) enable the student midwife to accept responsibility for [his or] her personal professional development and to apply [his or] her knowledge and skill in meeting the need of individuals and groups throughout the antenatal, intranatal and postnatal periods and shall include enabling the student to achieve the following outcomes:
      (i) the appreciation of the influence of social, political and cultural factors in relation to health care and advising on the promotion of health;
      (ii) the recognition of common factors which contribute to, and those which adversely affect, the physical, emotional and social well-being of the mother and baby, and the taking of appropriate action;
      (iii) the ability to assess, plan, implement and evaluate care within the sphere of practice of a midwife to meet the physical, emotional, social, spiritual and educational needs of the mother and baby and the family;
      (iv) the ability to take action on their own responsibility, including the initiation of the action of other disciplines, and to seek assistance when required;
      (v) the ability to interpret and undertake care prescribed by a registered medical practitioner;
      (vi) the use of appropriate and effective communication skills with mothers and their families, with colleagues and with those in other disciplines;

(vii) the use of relevant literature and research to inform the practice of midwifery;

(viii) the ability to function effectively in a multi-professional team with an understanding of the role of all members of the team;

(ix) an understanding of the requirements of legislation relevant to the practice of midwifery;

(x) an understanding of the ethical issues relating to midwifery practice and the responsibilities which these impose on the midwife's professional practice;

(xi) the assignment of the midwife of appropriate duties to others and the supervision and monitoring of such assigned duties.

Continuing education of the midwife

Once registered, midwives are expected to take responsibility for assessing their own educational needs and for continuing their own professional education. This includes regular reading of appropriate journals, research reports and other professional documents, as well as attending study days, conferences and courses.

Refresher courses

All midwives are required to complete a course of instruction or provide evidence of appropriate professional education approved by a Board every 5 years (UKCC, 1991). This may be:

1. A planned study period of 1 week.
2. Accumulated studies (7 days in 5 years).
3. Planned practical experience (2 weeks).

These courses are to be accredited on the Credit Accumulation and Transfer Scheme (CATS) to enable a midwife to accrue credits towards a degree.

Post-registration Education and Practice Project (PREPP)

In October 1990, the UKCC published the PREPP Report which makes several recommendations about the continuing education of practitioners, one of them being that all practitioners (i.e. nurses, midwives and health visitors) should have a minimum of 5 study days every 3 years. Another recommendation is that all practitioners should record their professional development in a personal professional profile. Some of the other recommendations such as return to practice programmes and notification of practice are already a requirement for midwives, although midwives notify their intention to practise annually and this is to continue, whereas for other practitioners it will be 3 yearly. A period of support for all newly registered practitioners by a preceptor is in the process of being introduced in many clinical areas.

Diploma in Professional Studies in Midwifery/Advanced Diploma in Midwifery

From 1991, the Diploma in Professional Studies in Midwifery (DPSM) replaces the Advanced Diploma in Midwifery (ADM). The taught DPSM extends over a period of 1 academic year and accrues 120 points at level two on the CATS scheme. The distance learning course is part-time over 2 years.

Degree courses

An increasing number of degree courses for midwives is now available, including a Masters Degree in Advanced Midwifery Practice offered by the Royal College of Midwives and the University of Surrey.

Other courses for midwives

These include:

1. Teaching and Assessing in Clinical Practice. ENB course 997. This course aims to help midwives to teach and assess learners more effectively.
2. Education for Family-Centred Care. This course is to enable midwives to teach parents in preparation for parenthood.
3. Special and Intensive Care of the Newborn. ENB course 405.
4. Family Planning in Society. ENB course 901.
5. Counselling courses.
6. Research courses.

Many of the above courses are approved as refresher courses by the National Board. An increasing number of other courses are also available now.

ENB Higher Award for nurses, midwives and health visitors

In 1990, the ENB announced a new framework for continuing professional education and Higher Award for nurses, midwives and health visitors which is to be introduced in April 1992. Practitioners who wish to participate in this scheme will be required to index with the ENB. They will then complete a modular programme of professional development linked to increasing expertise in 10 key areas, gaining credits on the CATS scheme as they proceed. Those who complete all modules successfully, integrating all 10 key characteristics in professional practice, will gain the Higher Award which will equate to a minimum of a first degree.

Midwives' Rules and Code of Practice

The Midwives' Rules (UKCC, 1991) are approved and made by the UKCC, and are framed in accordance with the recommendations of the Council's Midwifery Committee, following wide consultation. They are legally expressed in the form of Statutory Instruments. The Midwife's Code of Practice (UKCC, 1991) is complementary to the Midwives' Practice Rules and provides guidance to all midwives in relation to their professional practice. The Midwives' Rules and Code of Practice apply to midwives practising in all parts of the UK. They are separate documents and are available from the UKCC.

The UKCC Code of Professional Conduct for the nurse, midwife and health visitor also applies to the midwife and is supplemented by other UKCC documents with which the midwife should be familiar, for example, 'Exercising Accountability' (UKCC, 1989). The Midwife's Code of Practice clearly states that 'Each midwife as a practitioner of midwifery is accountable for [his or] her own practice in whatever environment [he or] she practices. Guidance on the interpretation of the concept of accountability is provided in the document 'Exercising Accountability'.

Local Supervising Authorities and Supervisors of Midwives

In the first Midwives Act of 1902, Local Supervising Authorities (LSAs) were appointed to supervise the practice of midwives. At that time the LSAs were local government bodies but, in the reorganization of the NHS in 1974, the Regional Health Authorities (RHAs) in England, District Health Authorities (DHAs) (formerly Area Health Authorities) in Wales, Health Boards in Scotland, and Health and Social Services Boards in Northern Ireland became the LSAs. The National Boards are required to provide the LSAs with advice and guidance.

The LSAs are responsible for appointing Supervisors of Midwives who should develop a relationship as supportive colleague, counsellor and advisor to the midwife.

Supervisors of midwives

1. A person to be appointed in accordance with Section 16(3) of the Act by a local supervising authority to exercise supervision over midwives in its area shall be a registered midwife and either:

   (a) shall have had 3 years experience as a practising midwife not less than 1 year of which shall have been in the 2 years immediately preceding the appointment; or

    (b) shall be eligible to practise and shall undertake any further midwifery experience as may be required by the relevant Board.

2. A person to be appointed a supervisor of midwives shall:
    (a) undertake a course of instruction within 12 months of appointment; or
    (b) have completed such a course not more than 3 years prior to appointment;

    and shall undertake to receive further instruction at intervals of not more than 5 years.

3. In sub-paragraph (2) of this rule a course means a course approved by a Board for the instruction of a person in the duties of a supervisor of midwives. (UKCC, 1991)

A midwife should contact her supervisor of midwives on all matters as required by the Midwives' Rules. The Supervisor of Midwives monitors the practice of the midwives within her sphere of responsibility in order to improve standards of practice and care.

European Economic Community 1980

The official journal of the European Communities published on 11 February 1980, L33, volume 23, contains the Midwifery Directives (signed in January 1980) which were implemented in January 1983. The purpose of these is to aid freedom of movement of midwives between EEC member states. In order to achieve mutual recognition of formal qualifications, certain changes had to be made and, even with the UK 18-month programme for general nurses, midwives need a certificate of 1 year's satisfactory professional practice after qualification. They will then—provided they are nationals of a member state, and have documents showing good character—be recognized.

    Those who are not general trained nurses, must take a 3-year full-time course for recognition. If they do not possess educational qualifications equivalent to university admission, they will, in addition to their qualification, need a certificate on completion of 2 years' satisfactory professional practice.

Other health care professionals

Health visitor
A health visitor is a registered general nurse who has undergone a further year's training and obtained a Certificate or Diploma for Health Visiting. Multidisciplinary courses for health visitors and other community staff are now being introduced in many areas. The health visitor's role is preventive, and can be described under four broad headings:

1. The prevention of mental, physical and emotional ill-health and all their consequences.
2. The early detection of ill-health and surveillance of high-risk groups.
3. The recognition of need and mobilization of resources.
4. Health education.

Health visitors work either attached to a group practice or in a geographic area. They have a special responsibility towards families where there are young children, and take over the care of new babies from the midwife. Around the 10th day after birth health visitors will make their first visit to the home. The mother will be advised of the child health clinic facilities, and any feeding problems will be discussed. In some areas the hand-over from midwife to health visitor is done at this time. It is customary to obtain consent for the child to participate in the immunization programme, and the health visitor may examine the baby. Unless further home visits are indicated, the child is seen subsequently at the child health clinic.

At the other end of the scale, the health visitor's work includes regular visits to the elderly and the housebound. He or she also has a supportive role towards the mentally or physically handicapped, and to those families with special problems.

District nurse

District nurses are either registered general nurses or enrolled nurses, preferably with the District Nursing Certificate, who provide nursing services to people in their own homes. They work either in a geographic area or attached to a group practice.

Much of their work is concerned with the elderly, but they also provide a valuable follow-up for surgical patients, often enabling them to return home earlier. In midwifery the district nurse occasionally takes over where there is some infection, the midwife retaining his or her statutory responsibility.

Practice nurses

Practice nurses are employed by general practitioners (GPs) and provide nursing services within the GP's surgery or health centre. Only practice nurses, who are registered midwives and have notified their intention to practice are eligible to provide midwifery care.

Proposals for the future of community education and practice

In 1991 the UKCC published a Report on 'Proposals for the Future of Community Education and Practice'. The report identifies community health care nursing as a unified discipline to include such groups as health visitors, community nurses, occupational health nurses and practice nurses. It proposes a common community education programme for the above groups which would include a choice of modules to equip the community health care nurse to work in differing environments. Already in some areas core curricula have been developed for community programmes. At the time of writing this report is still under discussion.

General practitioner services

General practitioners are responsible for the provision of a 24-hour service for the treatment of illness. Their contract with the Family Health Services Authority requires them to provide: 'all necessary and appropriate personal medical services of the type usually provided by general medical practitioners . . . to their patients'.

Some general practitioners work alone, others work in group practices and the rest work from health centres. In the last there may be as many as 12 doctors engaged in practice. Many general practitioners use some form of deputizing service to cover the night hours.

To register with a general practitioner the person takes their medical card to the chosen surgery, and, provided there is room on the list, he or she will be accepted. Should there be any difficulty in registering with a doctor, an application is made to the Family Health Services Authority. The will allocate the person to a practice with a vacancy.

With the increase in group practice there is a trend towards the various members of the partnership specializing in that branch of general practice which particularly interests them, e.g. maternity, paediatrics, geriatrics.

In order to be classified as a general practitioner obstetrician (GPO), additional experience or qualification in obstetrics is required. GPOs are entitled to provide maternity services to anyone who applies to them, and they are prefixed 'M' in the family practitioner list.

Since the National Health Service and Community Care Act of 1990, an increasing number of GPs hold their own budget and are the purchasers of services for their patients.

References

UKCC (1984) *Code of Professional Conduct for the Nurse, Midwife and Health Visitor*. UKCC: London.

UKCC (1986) *Project 2000, A New Preparation for Practice*. UKCC: London.

UKCC (1989) *Exercising Accountability*. UKCC: London.

UKCC (1990) *Post-Registration Education and Practice Project*. UKCC: London.

UKCC (1991) *A Midwife's Code of Practice*. UKCC: London.

UKCC (1991) *Midwives Rules*. UKCC: London.
UKCC (1991) *Proposals for the Future of Community Education and Practice*. UKCC: London.

APPENDIX 3

Preconception and Antenatal Care

Preconception care

The importance of couples being in good health at the time of conception is now widely accepted. The critical time of fetal development is during the first 8 to 10 weeks of pregnancy, yet few women receive midwifery or medical care at this time. Fetal abnormalities occur in 2.5% of all live births. With good preconception care it is hoped to reduce this figure and prevent other problems such as intrauterine growth retardation and preterm labour.

Couples can obtain preconception care from their general practitioner, at clinics run by the health authority, or at private clinics offered by Foresight, an association for the promotion of preconception care. They are advised to attend about 6 months before planning to conceive.

Medical screening includes a detailed personal, medical, family and reproductive history, including lifestyle, dietary and smoking habits, and consumpton of alcohol and drugs. A full medical examination is performed, including a gynaecological examination on the woman and cervical smear. Investigations include full urinalysis and blood tests for rubella antibodies, haemoglobin level, haemoglobinopathies, syphilis and HIV antibodies, the latter being offered to those in high-risk groups. Hair and drinking water analysis may be carried out to test for concentrations of toxic metals. Occasionally semen analysis and stool tests for suspected infestation are also required. Women with medical problems should be referred to an appropriate physician before pregnancy and couples with known familial disorders are offered genetic counselling.

Midwives have an important role in taking the full and detailed history, collecting the specimens required for investigations and promoting health education. Dietary advice is particularly important since Smithels *et al.* (1980) reported a reduction in neural tube defects in babies whose mothers had been prescribed periconception vitamin supplementation.

Antenatal care

Aims

1. Maintenance and improvement of health in pregnancy.
2. Early detection of any deviations from the normal and prompt treatment.
3. Preparation for labour, thereby empowering the woman and her partner to achieve a pleasurable, fulfilling experience of childbirth.

4. Promotion of breast feeding in a sensitive manner and building up the woman's confidence in her ability to feed.
5. The birth of a live, mature and healthy baby who soon becomes happily integrated into the family.
6. Health education on a wide range of relevant topics, including family planning.

The expectant mother is encouraged to contact her midwife or doctor early in the pregnancy to start antenatal care. After confirmation of the pregnancy and an initial examination, the possible patterns of antenatal care and place of confinement are discussed.

Patterns of antenatal care and place of confinement
1. Community care from midwife and/or general practitioner (GP), with delivery at home, or in a GP unit, or in a consultant unit with the community midwife accompanying the woman into hospital and caring for her in labour and at delivery. This is called the Domino scheme.
2. Shared care between community and hospital staff. The community midwife and GP carry out most of the antenatal care, but the woman also attends the hospital antenatal clinic to be seen by obstetricians and midwives on two or three occasions, and is booked for hospital confinement. The recently published Health Committee Report on the Maternity Services (House of Commons, 1992) recommends that the present system of shared care should be abandoned because hospitals are not the appropriate place for healthy women.
3. All antenatal care is carried out by midwives and obstetricians in a consultant maternity unit and the woman is booked for hospital delivery.

In an increasing number of districts, the consultant obstetricians are going out to community antenatal clinics, rather than requiring women to travel to hospital clinics. If complications arise when a woman is being cared for in the community she is referred to a consultant obstetrician. Efforts are being made to improve continuity of care by ensuring that the woman sees a midwife whom she knows at each antenatal visit and, where possible, in labour and the postnatal period.

The mother and her partner should be given sufficient information to enable them to make an informed choice about the place of confinement. A sub-committee of the then Department of Health and Social Security's Standing Maternity and Midwifery Advisory Committee, under the chairmanship of Sir John Peel, recommended in 1970 that facilities should be provided to allow 100% hospital delivery because it was considered safer for mother and child. Now, in the early 1990s, that objective has been obtained since over 99% of women have hospital deliveries, but the view that delivery in hospital is safer is being increasingly challenged (Tew, 1990). The Health Committee Report on the Maternity Services (House of Commons, 1992) states that hospital deliveries can no longer be justified on grounds of safety.

Women advised to have a hospital delivery on medical grounds include those suffering from serious medical conditions such as anaemia, heart disease and diabetes mellitus; women with a history of severe obstetric complications which are likely to recur, and those with complications in the present pregnancy such as pre-eclampsia, malpresentation, twins and those in whom Rhesus incompatibility may be anticipated.

All 'high-risk' women (i.e. the above) should be delivered in well-equipped and adequately staffed maternity hospitals, where experienced obstetricians and paediatricians are readily available and where ultrasound and laboratory investigations, and blood transfusions can be quickly undertaken.

A healthy woman who is under 35 years old should be able to have her baby at home if she chooses.

The wide range of women being advised to have hospital deliveries nowadays is being challenged, and some healthy primigravidae and others who have a strong desire to have a home birth are refuting medical advice. If there are no GPs prepared to take responsibility for a woman having a home confinement, the midwife should discuss the situation with her Supervisor of Midwives, and agree and record appropriate arrangements to provide advice and support when necessary (UKCC, 1991). Emergency obstetric units (so-called 'flying squads') now have such a small role in most areas that many have been disbanded.

Frequency of antenatal examinations

With a normal pregnancy the mother usually visits an antenatal clinic at monthly intervals until the 28th week of pregnancy, then fortnightly until the 36th week and subsequently weekly until labour begins. In the event of any complication, either more frequent visits may be paid or admission to hospital may become necessary.

The routine frequency of visits is at present under scrutiny, as it is questionable whether well women with no complications need such frequent antenatal examinations, whereas those identified as being at risk of developing complications may require closer surveillance.

History

At the booking interview a detailed history is obtained, preferably by the midwife in the woman's own home, but if this is not possible, at the first clinic visit, where a full medical examination is also carried out. The midwife uses her communication skills to put the woman at ease, develop a good relationship and establish a dialogue. The pregnant woman should then feel that the midwife is concerned with her as a person and not just as a clinical case, and therefore will benefit from all the available facilities.

Social history In order to consider the woman holistically, the expectant mother's response to her pregnancy and that of her partner and family is assessed. In addition, information on marital status, housing, employment and any serious financial problems enables the midwife to offer help and make appropriate referrals, if required.

The present pregnancy. The date of the first day of the last normal menstrual period is ascertained and the expected date of delivery is calculated by counting forwards 9 calendar months and 7 days (40 weeks). Normal symptoms of pregnancy are noted, minor disorders are discussed and any necessary advice is given.

Previous obstetric history. This includes details of all normal confinements, including the weights of the babies. Also noted are any abnormal events such as miscarriage, preterm labour, difficult or prolonged labour, forceps delivery, caesarian section, stillbirth, neonatal death, the subsequent health of the mother and child, and method of infant feeding, including any breast-feeding problems, the purpose being to identify 'at risk' factors and prevent a recurrence where possible.

Medical history. A record should be made of any potentially serious illness, such as scarlet fever, rheumatic fever, any cardiac, pulmonary or renal disease, diabetes mellitus, rubella or mental illness; of previous operations, especially those of a gynaecological nature; of accidents; and of blood transfusions and their dates. Allergic conditions, especially asthma, eczema and hay fever should be noted.

Family history. This should note the incidence of twins or of any familial disease (e.g. diabetes, hypertension, tuberculosis).

First examination

The woman is weighed and her height measured. Her urine is tested for protein, glucose and ketones and a mid-stream specimen sent to the laboratory for bacteriological examination to detect asymptomatic bacteriuria because if untreated, this may lead to pyelonephritis.

A full physical examination is carried out. This includes observations of her colour; her teeth, throat and tonsils; the breasts and nipples; the abdomen (after the 12th week of pregnancy when the uterus is usually palpable); the vulva; the legs and feet. The doctor examines the heart and lungs, and may make a pelvic examination. In the early weeks the latter confirms the probable duration of the pregnancy, and excludes pelvic tumours. A cervical smear may be obtained for routine cytology. A blood test is carried out, ABO group, Rhesus type and haemoglobin value being ascertained. The Venereal Disease Research Laboratory (VDRL) test and treponema pallidum haemagglutination adherence (TPHA) test are usually used to detect syphilis. West African and West Indian women should have, additionally, a sickling test. Screening for rubella and other antibodies is important in all women. Alpha-fetoprotein (AFP) levels in the blood may be measured to detect open neural tube defects at approximately 16 weeks' gestation.

Most mothers are found to be completely healthy.

Subsequent visits

At every visit the woman should see a midwife whom she knows. She is asked how she feels, and is given an opportunity to discuss any symptoms about which she may be worried. She may only need reassuring that all is well, or the condition may require investigation and treatment.

At every visit a careful examination is made to detect any evidence of pre-eclampsia. The blood pressure is recorded, the urine tested for protein, and the woman is weighed and examined to discover any oedema. The clinical sign of oedema is swelling which pits on pressure; occult oedema (fluid retention not clinically apparent) is recognized by an unusually great increase in weight. Any sign of pregnancy induced hypertension should be reported immediately to a doctor.

Further haemoglobin estimations are undertaken at intervals of 4–6 weeks. From the 32nd week the lie and presentation of the fetus become important. A breech presentation or an oblique lie should now be referred to a doctor for investigation and correction.

After the 36th to 38th week the fetal head engages in a primigravida or can be made to engage on pressure, indicating that the pelvic brim is adequate in size. In most cases the pelvis is perfectly adequate. In a few in which cephalopelvic disproportion is suspected or diagnosed, suitable management can be planned.

The majority of women proceed through their pregnancies with no major complications and are able to anticipate a straightforward labour and the birth of a healthy, normal baby.

Emotional factors in pregnancy

There has been much criticism about antenatal care being so technical that many women claim their feelings are frequently ignored. Anxieties and disorders, so important to the sufferer, receive little or no attention, the emphasis being on the various tests which are carried out. Kitzinger

(1987) estimates that 'the whole system of prenatal care works efficiently for only 10% of women: that is half of the 20% who are at risk of an abnormal pregnancy. Duplication of care by obstetrician and midwife is another problem (Robinson, 1985), but this situation is gradually improving as midwives take responsibility for the antenatal care of women with normal pregnancies, leaving obstetricians more time for those with problems. Midwives are increasingly organizing themselves into teams with a caseload of women to whom they give individualized care throughout pregnancy, labour and the postnatal period. Seeing the same midwife at each antenatal visit promotes a closer relationship between mother and midwife and enables anxieties of a very wide nature to be expressed, discussed and, it is hoped, resolved.

A woman's first pregnancy is a momentous event in her life. Even when she is eagerly looking forward to the baby, she experiences doubts and fears, and her emotions may be labile. These are amplified where there is a lack of support, financial concern, marital disharmony or housing problems. Unsupported mothers have very difficult decisions to make about the child's future. Their instincts to keep and bring up their babies may be overwhelmed by financial insecurity (*see* Appendix 5).

Where a previous pregnancy and labour have occurred, there may be other anxieties. These relate to their past experiences, some of which could have been traumatic. These can be documented for consideration by the midwife giving care in labour.

All this may appear time-consuming at a busy clinic, but it is rewarding in the mother's increased confidence and freedom from anxiety, and it may help her towards an easier labour.

Antenatal education

Advice and education in preparation for labour and for parenthood form an important part of the antenatal care which a women and her husband/partner receive. Most clinics issue booklets setting out general advice, but the greatest benefit is gained through group teaching.

Antenatal classes should be of a simple and informal type, preferably in small groups of eight or ten parents. It is important to identify the needs and expectations of parents attending the classes and to plan each session to meet their particular needs (Perkins, 1980). Most of the women attending these classes are primigravid, but an increasing number of health districts are now offering antenatal classes for special groups such as teenagers, multigravida and those from ethnic minorities. The total number of classes will vary from one hospital or clinic to another, 6–8 being usual. Classes are given principally by midwives, with valuable help from health visitors, physiotherapists and sometimes obstetricians. The following subjects are usually discussed.

Pregnancy. General information is given about normal pregnancy and the minor disorders which may arise (see below), together with a simple explanation of the changes in the body and, in particular, of the growth of the uterus and the development of the fetus. Information and advice is given about good nutrition in pregnancy, and the possible problems associated with smoking, drugs and a high intake of alcohol. Other topics which the parents may wish to discuss include special antenatal investigations, certain complications of pregnancy and emotional problems which may be of concern.

Labour. Labour is discussed in some detail, focusing particularly on the aspects which are of concern to the couples attending the classes. The stages of labour are explained in simple terms and illustrated by charts, films or diagrams showing dilatation of the cervix and then the birth of the child and placenta. Discussion includes the various positions the woman may choose to adopt in labour and the many ways in which pain may be relieved. The woman is thus well prepared and can make informed choices about possible positions and methods of pain relief. The midwife explains the observations and examinations carried out in labour and, on a tour of the delivery suite, can show couples the complex and possibly intimidating apparatus which is sometimes used. Most couples appreciate some discussion on topics such as induction and augmentation of labour and on operative procedures which include episiotomy, forceps delivery, vacuum extraction and caesarean section. Throughout the sessions, discussion is encouraged, information given and questions answered, thereby increasing understanding and confidence. The woman and her partner are then better prepared to discuss decisions related to their care in labour and have a greater sense of autonomy and control. They are encouraged to prepare a birth plan which specifies any special wishes and requests regarding the management of their labour. This is filed in the woman's case notes so that it is available to the staff who will be caring for her in labour.

Exercises, relaxation and breathing techniques are usually included in each class to prepare the woman for labour. Exercises to music, in water (aqua-natal) and yoga are gaining popularity in some areas now.

Postnatal period and the baby. Most classes on postnatal care include information on the physical care of the mother, including postnatal exercises, but it is also important to discuss emotional reactions to childbirth and the likelihood of an episode of postnatal blues so that parents are prepared should it occur. Most couples are anxious about the care of their baby and welcome discussion on early parenting and a demonstration of some of the skills they will need to acquire, such as bathing, changing the napkin and feeding, although this teaching will be elaborated on after delivery. Infant feeding is discussed in some detail and sometimes a breast feeding mother is invited to come and speak to the group. This is also a good opportunity to emphasize the importance of communication with the baby and highlight the baby's ability to respond. Another area for discussion is the need for new mothers to establish a network of support for the postnatal period and beyond, not only from professionals but also from family, friends and some voluntary groups who have an understanding of the great adjustments which have to be made by new mothers and the problems which may arise. Other topics for discussion include family planning, the postnatal examination and any other issues raised by the parents.

General advice

Diet. A high intake of protein is required for the growth of new tissue and can be obtained from meat, fish, eggs, milk, cheese, pulses such as dried peas, beans and lentils, and wholemeal bread, cereals and nuts.

Wholemeal bread and cereals also provide a good source of carbohydrate and roughage, whereas white bread, cakes and biscuits have limited food value and therefore intake should be reduced. Fresh fruits, salads and vegetables provide the necessary vitamins and also roughage, thereby helping to prevent constipation. Minerals such as iron, calcium, phosphorus and iodine are required and will be found in most of the protein foods described above as well as in certain fresh vegetables.

There is now evidence that vitamin deficiencies before and during the early weeks of pregnancy can cause fetal malformations such as neural tube defects (Smithels *et al.*, 1980), thus a vitamin supplementation programme may be started in the preconception period and continue during the first trimester of pregnancy in susceptible groups of women.

Exercise and rest. The well woman whose pregnancy is progressing normally should be able to continue with exercise to which she is accustomed, such as walking, cycling, swimming, aerobics, yoga and riding for as long as she feels comfortable. Many antenatal classes now include aerobics or yoga, and aqua-natal classes are proving popular. Most women need more rest in pregnancy, however, especially in the first and third trimesters, thus early nights and, where possible, a rest during the day is recommended.

Clothing. All clothes should be comfortable and without constriction. Excellent and attractive maternity clothes and patterns are available. Maternity belts are unnecessary, except for some multigravid women, and those with sacroiliac strain. Brassieres should be large enough to allow for the growth of the breasts and will be more comfortable with fairly wide shoulder straps.

General hygiene. Baths and showers should be taken as usual. Vaginal deodorants should not be used.

Dental hygiene. Free dental care is offered and should be taken advantage of as early in pregnancy as possible. A woman experiencing troublesome nausea might delay her visit until the middle trimester.

Sexual intercourse. The incidence of sexual activity varies greatly, according to the needs and preferences of individual couples. Variations in position are often helpful to reduce discomfort and supine hypotension. If the mother has a history of miscarriages, intercourse is unwise in the early months of pregnancy, especially at the time when menstruation would normally occur and around the time of previous abortions. Similarly, intercourse should be avoided following the cessation of an episode of preterm labour because it could stimulate a recurrence.

Travel. Long and very tiring journeys should, if possible, be avoided, especially late in pregnancy. After the 34th week, travel in pressurized aircraft is undesirable and, indeed, airlines may refuse to make reservations.

Smoking. Women should make every effort to cease smoking throughout pregnancy. There is evidence that it causes retardation of fetal growth and development and is associated with placental lesions, preterm labour and an increase in the perinatal mortality rate (Stimmel, 1982).

Alcohol. Evidence suggests that a low intake of alcohol in pregnancy, that is one or two units once or twice a week is not harmful, but there is conflicting evidence about a moderate alcohol intake (Alexander *et al.* 1990). Heavy drinking may lead to low-birth-weight babies, neonatal feeding and sleeping problems and/or fully developed fetal alcohol syndrome.

The advice set out above, though important, is obviously little more than a recommendation of 'moderation in all things', such as is conducive to good health in any situation. Pregnancy is a physiological state—not a disease—and most women can and should lead ordinary normal lives at this time.

Common symptoms during pregnancy and their significance

Vomiting. 'Morning sickness' (i.e. nausea, with occasional vomiting) up to the 12th week, and without ketonuria, is not serious. The woman should have a cup of tea or a biscuit before getting up, and take frequent small carbohydrate meals and, possibly, some magnesium trisilicate. For vomiting after the 14th week, or vomiting which gives rise to ketosis at any time, a doctor should be consulted.

Heartburn. Heartburn (gastro-oesophageal regurgitation) may be relieved by alkaline medicines or, if troublesome at night, by sleeping with several pillows, keeping the head high; in persistent cases, further medical advice should be sought.

Constipation. Extra fluids, fruit, vegetables and bran cereals may help. Magnesium hydroxide is a suitable aperient. Some people find senna (Senokot) necessary. Castor oil and magnesium sulphate are unsuitable, and liquid paraffin should not be taken for long periods.

Vaginal discharge. Slight, non-irritating, mucoid or whitish discharge is not abnormal. Discharge which is profuse, offensive or which causes pruritus or excoriation of the skin is abnormal and a doctor should be consulted.

Vaginal bleeding. This, at any stage of pregnancy, and however slight, is abnormal. A doctor should be informed at once.

Cramp. This may be associated with vitamin B, calcium or salt deficiency and relieved by taking wheatgerm (Bemax), extra milk or salt. Night cramps are often due to ischaemia of leg muscles and are relieved by sleeping with the foot of the bed raised about 25 cm.

Headache. This is a symptom of many conditions, some of little significance. It should never be ignored, as it may indicate severe pre-eclampsia.

Oedema. Slight ankle oedema, developing after standing and disappearing overnight, is due to increased venous pressure and is common in late pregnancy. The woman should rest with her feet higher than her pelvis and restrict her salt intake. Persistent ankle oedema or oedema of the fingers (tight rings), eyelids, face, abdominal wall and vulva occurs in severe pre-eclampsia and medical advice is necessary.

Varicose veins.
1. *Legs.* If the condition is slight and not painful, extra rest with the feet up and the avoidance of standing may help. If painful, a doctor should be consulted. He may prescribe extra rest. Well-fitting support tights give considerable relief provided they are put on before rising.
2. *Haemorrhoids.* Constipation should be avoided, and warm bathings and analgesic ointments are useful. In severe cases rest in bed is necessary.
3. *Vulva.* This is less common and, if not painful, no treatment is given. Sometimes a firm vulval pad will give comfortable support. If painful, bed rest is necessary.

Backache. Backache is generally due to an exaggerated lordosis (possibly worsened by the wearing of unsuitable shoes), and relieved by correction of posture and extra rest.

Insomnia. The possible cause should be sought and remedied. Late heavy meals should be avoided. A mild sedative, not a barbiturate, is often useful even when the insomnia is related to the activity of a lively fetus.

General malaise, feverishness, headache, nausea. This combination of symptoms generally signifies infection, and the commonest infection of pregnancy is that of the urinary tract. In any such case a doctor should be consulted.

References

Alexander J, Levy V & Roch S (1990) *Antenatal Care. A Research-based Approach.* Macmillan Education Ltd.: London.

DHSS (1970) *Domiciliary midwifery and maternity bed needs. (Peel Report).* HMSO: London.

House of Commons (1992) Health Committee Second Report, Maternity Services. Vol. 1. HMSO: London.

Kitzinger S (1987) *Freedom and Choice in Childbirth: 105.* Penguin: Harmondsworth.

Perkins ER (1980) *Education for Childbirth and Parenthood.* Croom Helm: London.

Robinson S (1985) Responsibilities of midwives and medical staff: findings from the National Survey. *Midwives Chronicle* 98 (1165): 64–71.

Smithels RW, Sheppard S, Schorah CJ, Seller MJ, Nevin NC, Harris R, Read AP & Fielding DW (1980) Possible prevention of neural tube defects by periconceptual vitamin supplementation. *Lancet* i: 339–340.

Stimmel B (ed.) (1982) *The Effects of Maternal Alcohol and Drug Abuse in the Newborn*. Haworth Press: New York.

Tew M (1990) *Safer Childbirth? A Critical History of Maternity Care*. Chapman and Hall: London.

UKCC (1991) *A Midwife's Code of Practice*. UKCC: London.

APPENDIX 4

Antenatal Tests and Investigations

There are many tests performed during pregnancy to detect already existing abnormalities or ones which occur only in pregnancy.

Blood tests

At the expectant mother's first visit to the antenatal clinic a sample of blood is taken for the following tests:

ABO group and Rhesus factor. To enable blood to be cross-matched without delay should an emergency occur.

Antibodies, especially the presence of Rhesus antibodies if the mother is Rhesus negative.

Haemoglobin value, the lower limit of normal being 11 g/dl.

Serological test for syphilis, usually:

the Venereal Disease Research Laboratory Test (VDRL)
the Treponema Pallidum Haemagglutination Test (TPHA)

If these tests are positive:

the Fluorescent Treponemal Antibody Test (FTA) is carried out to confirm the result.

Rubella screening for antibodies, because if the woman is non-immune and contracts the disease in pregnancy the virus can damage the developing fetus.

Haemoglobinopathies to detect sickle cell disease in women of African and Asian origin and thalassaemia in Mediterranean races.

HIV virus. This test may be carried out anonymously as part of the government screening programme.

Serum alpha-fetoprotein (SAFP) is estimated on maternal blood between 16 and 18 weeks gestation for the diagnosis of open neural tube defects and other abnormalities of the fetus.

A raised SAFP level is associated with:

- wrong dates;
- multiple pregnancy;
- intrauterine fetal death;
- an open neural tube defect.

Further investigations in cases of raised alpha-fetoprotein (AFP):

a repeat serum AFP test may be performed;

or scan to establish gestational age, and detect possible multiple pregnancy and fetal death. High-resolution ultrasound examination is used where available to detect open-neural tube defects.

amniocentesis, to estimate the liquor AFP as this is a more accurate test than serum AFP. It is not always carried out if there are good high-resolution ultrasound facilities.

A low AFP level is associated with:

wrong dates;

possible Down's Syndrome, therefore an amniocentesis for chromosomes studies may be performed.

Diagnosis of fetal abnormality is discussed with the parents and they may be offered:

termination of pregnancy;

genetic counselling;

counselling and support as required.

Chest X-ray

Due to the decrease in incidence of pulmonary tuberculosis and the risks to the fetus of radiation, routine chest radiography has now largely been abandoned.

Cervical cytology

A smear should be taken on first examination if one has not been done within 2 years. An Ayre's spatula is inserted against the external cervical os and rotating through 360° to scrape off cells at the squamocolumnar junction. These are then stained and examined for any malignant or premalignant cells. Because of the risk that carcinoma *in situ* will progress to become carcinoma, laser therapy or a cone biopsy is indicated after the birth unless actual malignancy is discovered, when earlier treatment may be necessary.

Ultrasonography or sonar

Ultrasound was first used in the First World War to detect enemy submarines. It is a way of discovering the internal characteristics of a solid object such as the human body, or metal, by projecting towards it a beam of very-high-frequency sound waves, inaudible to the human ear. These beams are partly reflected at each interface between tissues so that an ultrasonogram of reflected echoes can be built up.

A-scan

This is a display for measuring size and thickness accurately—especially important in cephalometry. It uses impulses from the quartz crystal in the TRANSDUCER and, after amplification, they are displayed on a cathode ray screen as vertical peaks from a horizontal line. The distances between the vertical lines are measured. The height of the narrow peak is related to the strength of the echo, so the system is named amplitude modulation—'A mode' or 'A-scan'.

B-scan or brightness modulation

This method builds up a plan or picture of the deep tissues, each of which gives an echo according to its density and its depth. It is possible to build up a valuable two-dimensional sectional view by moving the transducer at right angles to the organs below it.

GREY-SCALE DISPLAY shows more definition.

Real-time scanning

B-mode ultrasonography using an array of detectors so that scans can be made electronically at a rate of 30 frames/second and viewed as a moving image is known as real-time ultrasonography. It is of particular value when checking for fetal life, if movements or heart beat are seen on a real-time scan.

Ultrasound techniques were first developed, mainly during the 1960s, in Glasgow. Ultrasound is now used extensively as a diagnostic aid, being without the possible risks of radiography.

The woman lies on a couch, her bladder distended, as this makes for a contrast medium, and her abdomen smeared with olive oil or liquid paraffin to aid close application of the probe which is attached to the diasonagraph. The probe is moved to and fro over the abdomen, and when the sonar beam thus transmitted meets the resistance of the fetal skull or the placenta the echo is shown on an oscilloscope screen and photographed by a Polaroid camera. The whole procedure is quick and painless, and the result is known immediately.

Localization of the placenta. This is accurate and extremely useful in antepartum haemorrhage, particularly when the bleeding is slight and transient. If placenta praevia can thus be excluded, the mother may go home. The placenta should always be localized before amniocentesis.

Congenital defect. Ultrasound makes possible early diagnosis of certain fetal abnormalities, notably severe spina bifida and anencephaly. A spinal scan is done when raised ALPHA-FETOPROTEIN (AFP) levels have been obtained for further, more accurate, information before considering terminating the pregnancy.

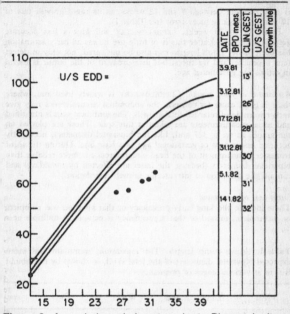

Figure 6. Amended cephalometry chart. Placental site—upper posterior.

Confirmation of pregnancy. The tiny gestation sac can be seen by 5–6 weeks as a clear area within the uterus. Its volume can be calculated by various diameters in varying planes to give a probable length of pregnancy. It is very useful to detect a missed abortion if, after a week, the size of the sac has not increased.

Duration of pregnancy. The fetus can be visualized and measured within the gestation sac by the 8th week of pregnancy. It is an oval shape and the longest diameter can be measured as the CROWN–RUMP LENGTH. It is very accurate between 8 and 12 weeks, as its rapid growth rate of 10 mm per week reduces error (*see* Table 1).

From 14 to 20 weeks, CEPHALOMETRY will give a less accurate gestational age, and after this is of little use unless an early estimation has been made. Limb lengths can also be measured, not only to detect fetal anomalies and fractures, but measurement of the femur is useful in estimating gestational age.

Assessment of fetal growth. CEPHALOMETRY is widely used and, where there is great cause for concern, the abdominal circumference may give earlier warning of retarded fetal growth. The umbilical vein is identified and serial measurements are taken at this spot. These are plotted on the graph, as on p. 327 and, like the biparietal diameters, need early accurate assessment of gestational age as a base-line. During the third trimester measurement of the head circumference is more reliable than biparietal diameters (because the latter are affected by moulding) and can aid the detection of intrauterine growth retardation.

Other uses of ultrasound

These include checking early pregnancy or that abortion was complete or incomplete, missed or that a pregnancy is ectopic or multiple or a

Table 1. Crown–rump length. The maximum, minimum and mean expected biparietal diameters of the fetal skull, as shown by ultrasound B-scan at various stages of pregnancy.

Weeks		Days		mm	Weeks		Days		mm
7	+	0	=	10	11	+	0	=	43
		2	=	12			2	=	46
		4	=	14			4	=	50
8	+	0	=	17	12	+	0	=	55
		2	=	19			2	=	59
		4	=	22			4	=	64
9	+	0	=	25	13	+	0	=	68
		2	=	27			2	=	72
		4	=	29			4	=	76
10	+	0	=	33	14	+	0	=	85
		2	=	35					
		4	=	39					

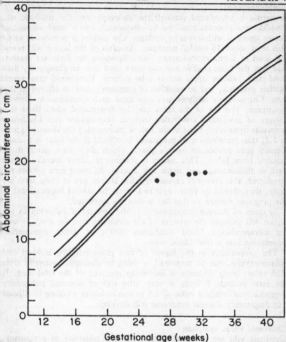

Figure 7. Fetal abdominal circumference against gestational age. Mean ± 2 SD.

hydatidiform mole. Poly and oligohydramnios can also be detected, as well as fetal ascites in severe Rhesus incompatibility. Measurement of fetal and uteroplacental blood flow is possible during an ultrasound scan, and can be useful in the diagnosis and management of intrauterine growth retardation. Fetal movements can also be observed, including sucking, swallowing, breathing and eye movements, and filling and emptying of the fetal stomach and bladder.

Amniocentesis

A needle is introduced through the abdomen into the amniotic sac, avoiding the placenta localized by ultrasound, and a small amount of liquor amnii is withdrawn by syringe. The earliest it is possible to do this is at about 16 weeks' gestation. Analysis of the liquor will reveal the level of ALPHA-FETOPROTEIN (AFP). Provided the dates are correct, and that the fetus is alive and not more than one, an abnormally high level may indicate open neural tube defects. Ultrasound may reveal further evidence, and termination of pregnancy may be offered in this case. Chromosome analysis may also show such conditions as Down's syndrome. The sex of the fetus may be determined when there is a history of sex-linked conditions such as haemophilia and Duchenne muscular dystrophy, because the risk of transmitting the disease to sons is 1:2, thus termination of pregnancy is offered if the fetus is a male. Certain gene probes are now available which allow some genes to be isolated from DNA. This makes it possible to detect specific disease such as thalassaemia and sickle cell disease. As more gene probes are developed, this area will expand rapidly. Before any of these tests are done, they should be fully explained, with the ethical implications, to the pregnant woman so that her wishes are respected.

In cases of Rhesus incompatibility, the amount of bilirubin in the liquor will indicate the severity of the condition and the need, if any, for intraperitoneal blood tranfusion (IPT), or direct intrauterine transfusion into a fetal blood vessel.

The proportions in the liquor of two phospholipids, lecithin and sphingomyelin, can be measured, a rising lecithin/sphingomyelin ratio (L/S ratio) being evidence of increasing maturity of the fetal lung. If the ratio exceeds 2 there is very little risk of neonatal pulmonary complications, while a value of 1.5 or less indicates a strong likelihood that respiratory distress syndrome will develop.

Chorionic villus sampling

Chorionic villi are obtained during the first trimester of pregnancy, usually between 8 and 10 weeks gestation by aspiration transcervically or transabdominally. The following investigations can be carried out on the sample:

DNA analysis for thalassaemia, sickle cell disease and other genetic conditions;

Diagnosis of metabolic conditions such as Tay–Sachs disease.

The main risks associated with this procedure include infection, an increased abortion rate, trauma to the fetus, placenta or uterus and Rhesus isoimmunization.

Fetoscopy

Recently the technique of entering the uterine cavity with a fetoscope has been developed to allow direct visualization of the fetus where there is a serious doubt about its normality. Both the fetus and placenta must be localized, and the gestational age known, as the best time for fetoscopy is between 15 and 20 weeks' gestation. Spina bifida, exomphalos, cleft lip and palate as well as other conditions can be diagnosed visually. Skin and tissue biopsy can detect EPIDERMOLYSIS BULLOSA, whilst fetal blood can reveal haemophilia, Tay–Sachs disease, beta-thalassaemia and SICKLE CELL DISEASE. GALACTOSAEMIA and Duchenne muscular dystrophy are also diagnosed from fetal blood. It can also be used to give a direct intrauterine transfusion for Rhesus isoimmunization. It is not without physical and psychological risk to the parents. It also gives rise to ethical issues for staff, as well as parents, to consider carefully.

Placental function tests

Although the use of biochemical tests such as assays of oestrogens in maternal blood or urine to assess fetal well-being have largely been replaced by biophysical testing, that is, ultrasound and cardiotocography in the UK, they are included here because they are still used in some parts of the world.

Measurement of the placental hormones oestriol and human placental lactogen gives some indication of placental function and thereby fetal well-being.

Oestriol is produced both by the placenta and by the fetus. The precursor is produced by the fetal adrenals and is then processed by the placenta to produce oestriol. This hormone circulates in the mother's blood and is excreted in her urine. It can thus be measured in a sample of maternal serum or in a 24 hour collection of maternal urine. It is essential that all the urine is collected, otherwise the results will be inaccurate. A series of oestriol estimations should be made and the overall levels should rise progressively throughout pregnancy. Falling or low oestriol levels are associated with fetal growth retardation which may lead to fetal death.

Human placental lactogen (HPL) is produced by the syncitiotrophoblast and is found in maternal plasma. The plasma level rises throughout pregnancy until 36 weeks when it reaches a peak and subsequently falls. Assays of HPL are carried out to determine placental function. Falling or low levels of HPL are associated with intrauterine growth retardation which, in severe cases, may lead to fetal death.

Fetal assessment

1. *Fetal movements*

A healthy fetus is active *in utero* whereas a fetus at risk of intrauterine hypoxia will be noticeably less active. Mothers in high-risk groups may be asked to count and chart fetal movements each day during the latter weeks of pregnancy. Ten movements in a 12-hour period are considered the minimum safe number. The mother will be asked to contact her midwife or doctor if she notices reduced fetal movements.

2. *Cardiotocography*

Cardiotocography is a correlation of fetal heart patterns with fetal movements or uterine contractions and is now commonly used as a method of assessing fetal well-being. In a healthy fetus the heart rate accelerates by approximately 20 beats/minute when it moves. In high-risk pregnancies serial monitoring for periods of half an hour or longer are carried out at intervals to assess the fetal condition during the antenatal period. Abnormal fetal heart problems such as decelerations or loss of beat-to-beat variation may be detected on the trace and indicate the need to expedite delivery.

Radiography

Although radiography has been largely superseded by sonar, it remains a valuable aid to diagnosis. It is used in the diagnosis of certain fetal abnormalities, and it may be employed to confirm fetal death suspected from Spalding's sign (marked overlapping of the vault bones), the ball sign (hyperflexion of the spine) or the finding of intravascular gas bubbles in the heart and great vessels.

Some authorities believe radiology to be of value in determining fetal maturity by noting the development of various ossification centres, if ultrasound is not available.

Though uncommon, cephalopelvic disproportion is still a problem; in the hands of a skilled radiographer, accurate measurement of the pelvic diameters and contours is of great value in planning the best conduct of the woman's labour. The accompanying cephalometry may be carried out by means of an ultrasound B-scan.

Chest radiography, undertaken at about the 16th week of pregnancy, is needed in the diagnosis of pulmonary tuberculosis, which, though relatively uncommon in the United Kingdom is by no means rare in immigrant women.

Radiation is not without hazard. There is some evidence to suggest that it may, in part, be responsible for the later development of leukaemia; it may also cause mutations in genes and, as a consequence, fetal malformation. This evidence, however, is slight and must be weighed carefully against the many advantages that radiological diagnosis offers.

APPENDIX 5

Social Services and Social Security, including Maternity Benefits

The midwife is often consulted about the care of babies and children deprived of a normal home environment, and she should have some knowledge of the legislation and services which exist to help and protect the mother and her child.

Social Services

The Local Authority Social Services Act of 1970 requires local authorities to establish a social services committee (department). This new department provides for:

1. The elderly.
2. The mentally and physically handicapped.
3. Children in need of care and protection.
4. Children for adoption.
5. Anyone or any family in temporary or long-term social need.

Social services departments were set up in 1971. The head in each such department is the director of social services. He or she is supported by assistants, and below that the fieldworkers are qualified and trainee social workers. In addition, he or she is responsible for the home help service, residential care, day care and meals on wheels.

The department is able to provide adaptations to the home to enable the elderly and/or handicapped to live as normal and independent a life as possible, and they can make special payments in cases of acute need. Social workers can help people obtain benefits and grants which might be due to them through the Department of Social Security.

Referral is generally through the health visitor or general practitioner, or sometimes the community midwife, although an individual may also apply direct.

Environmental Health Department

The purpose of this department is to ensure that the environment in which we all live is suitable for us to remain free from disease. To this end environmental health officers supervise commercial food preparation and working conditions. They inspect and report on premises which may be considered unfit for human habitation, and monitor the levels of noise and pollution in the atmosphere. Wherever there is an infestation of rats, mice, lice, etc., they can be called in.

Occasionally they will have to investigate the outbreak of an infectious disease.

Housing Department

Community midwives will visit many mothers and babies in local authority housing. Housing is allocated to people in order of priority, and in almost all areas the supply of houses is inadequate for the need. Under the Homeless Persons Act, 1977, the local authority has responsibility to house anyone made homeless through no fault of their own.

One-parent families

One-parent families may comprise an unsupported mother who may be unmarried, separated, divorced or widowed, or a lone father who may also be separated, divorced or widowed.

The number of single-parent families is a growing problem. The child of an unsupported parent may sometimes be 'at risk'. Poor housing, lack of emotional stimulation and social isolation contribute to this problem. The midwife should put the mother in contact with a social worker either from the local social services or from a voluntary organization (e.g. Welcare organized by the Church of England).

An unsupported mother may, if fully insured, claim the State maternity benefits; if not, she may apply for other benefits in the same way as any other person similarly placed.

Financial help includes maternity payments for those who are eligible, income support, if required, and all the additional benefits available to those receiving income support (see p. 339). Child benefit is also available and there is a special one-parent benefit. Some families also receive family credit.

The mother can continue her work if she places the child in a day nursery run by the local authority, and where her request will be given priority. If there is a crèche at her place of work, the problem is settled. Many factories, hospitals and stores have, in recent years, helped to solve their labour problems by opening and staffing a crèche. She can also leave the child with a child-minder or a foster mother, again continuing to work.

A schoolgirl may receive home tutoring in order that her studies may not be interrupted.

Affiliation

The responsibility for maintaining an illegitimate child rests with its mother. She may, however, apply, by way of summons, to a Court of Summary Jurisdiction for an affiliation order on the putative father of the child. If the court grants such an order, the father is thereby compelled to contribute a weekly sum towards the cost of the child's maintenance, continuing until the child is 16 or, if he is still receiving full-time education, 21 years old. Paternity must be admitted, or some corroborative evidence (e.g. an admission by the putative father to a third person) is necessary. Failure to comply with an affiliation order is a punishable offence though it is not always possible either to oblige the defaulter to pay or to enforce the punishment. If a mother claims income support, the Department of Social Security, through their liable relative clause, will take out their own summons.

Under the Child Support Act, 1991, one-parent families will be required to apply for maintenance. A Child Support Agency will be established in April 1993, taking over responsibility from the courts. Parents can contact the agency via a solicitor or the citizens advice bureaux. Absent parents will be required to pay maintenance which will be monitored by the Child Support Agency. Failure to pay will lead to mandatory payments, fines or imprisonment. Single parents on income support will be investigated by the agency and penalties of decreases in benefit may be levied on those who withhold information about the absent parent.

Child-minders and foster parents

These are persons undertaking for reward, the care of children other than their own offspring. They are required to notify the local authority of their undertaking, giving full details, and they must allow the local authority social services department to see their homes and the children for whom they are caring.

Adoption

As an alternative to all these possibilities, whereby she keeps her baby, the mother may place the child for adoption, thus relinquishing all claim upon the child.

Third party and private adoptions have become illegal since 1 February 1982.

A adoption order, made usually by a county court or a court of summary jurisdiction, puts the adopted child into the position of a legitimate child of the adopter or adopters. The mother now has no claim whatsoever over the child.

The Adoption Acts of 1958 and 1960 are designed to protect in every possible way the child's interests.

The Adoption Act 1958 does not allow an adoption order to be made unless the applicant:

1. is the mother or father of the infant;
2. is a relative of the infant, and has attained the age of 21 years;
3. has attained the age of 25 years.

A married couple may be granted an adoption order:

1. if either of the applicants is the mother or father of the infant;
2. if one applicant satisfies the requirements of criteria 1 or 2, above, and other has attained the age of 21 years.

Only in exceptional circumstances may a single man adopt a female child. The infant must have been continuously in the care of the applicant for at least 3 months before the order is made, not counting the first 6 weeks of life.

The applicant, at least 3 months before the date of the order, must have given written notice to the local authority in whose area he or she was then living, of his or her intention to apply for an adoption order in respect of the infant.

More recently, the Children Acts of 1975 and 1989 were introduced to put the welfare of the child first. Decisions must take into consideration the child's long-term interest. It is now mandatory for local authorities to run an adoption service. The 1975 Act also makes it easier for children to be adopted who have been in long-term care. The number of children currently being put up for adoption is small. The Abortion Act 1967, and the current trend for single parents to keep their families, have contributed to this. When an adopted person reaches the age of 18, he has the right of access to his own birth records. A counselling service is provided by the Registrar General. The social workers who are employed for this purpose have a heavy responsibility, as they can add further details to complete the family background. They also have to take into consideration the effect on the natural and the adoptive parents.

Foster parents

New rights have been granted to FOSTER PARENTS under the Children Act, 1975. Where a child has been fostered for 6 months, the natural parents must give 28 days' notice before removing the child from care. This has alleviated the 'tug of love' situation where, in the past, the child could be removed without any warning at all. It is also the intention of the Act that, after fostering a child for 3 years, a foster parent will be able to become a 'custodian'. In effect he or she will become a parent without the full adoptive parents' rights. It also gives an alternative to full adoption to grandparents who are keen to bring up their daughter's child. Many problems may result if the child is actually adopted.

With the recent streamlining and vast increase in scope of the social services departments, any unsupported mother, whatever her means, nationality or social background, should be able to approach a social worker who will give her expert advice and put her in touch with the particular authority from which she may claim monetary or other assistance.

Social Security

The Social Security Act, 1986 constituted a major revision of social security in the UK. It established three main areas from which payments can be made to meet needs, namely:

1. The Social Fund which helps people with expenses which are difficult to pay for out of regular income.
2. Income Support is a benefit to help people whose income is below a certain level.
3. Family Credit is a tax-free benefit for working families with children.

Social Fund

A maternity payment from the Social Fund can be made if expectant mothers or their partners are receiving Income Support or Family Credit. The maximum payment is £100 for each baby expected, born or adopted. To obtain this benefit the mother completes the appropriate form obtained from a social security office, antenatal clinic or health centre and sends it to the local social security office, together with a maternity certificate obtained from her midwife or doctor. She can claim at any time from 11 weeks before the week the baby is due and up to 3 months after the birth of the baby.

Statutory Maternity Pay

Statutory Maternity Pay (SMP) is only available for women who are in employment and is operated by the employer. Women eligible to receive SMP must have been in the same employment for at least 26 weeks up to and including the 15th week before the expected week of confinement (i.e. the qualifying week) and have received weekly earnings over the lower earnings limit for National Insurance. SMP can be paid up to 18 weeks, usually starting 6 weeks before the baby is due. There are two rates of SMP. Only expectant mothers who have been in employment for the specified length of time will be eligible to receive the higher rate for 6 of the 18 weeks. To claim SMP the woman must notify her employer at least 3 weeks before she intends to stop work and present her maternity certificate (MAT B1).

Maternity Allowance

Women who have recently worked, or changed jobs who cannot claim SMP may be eligible for Maternity Allowance. The woman must have paid standard rate National Insurance contributions for at least 26 weeks of the 52 week period which ends with the 15th week before the expected week of confinement. Payment is made for up to 18 weeks and starts 11 weeks before the expected date of delivery, unless the mother is still working in which case it will be deferred.

Employment rights for the expectant mother

The maternity provisions set out in the Employment Protection (Consolidation) Act 1977 were amended by the Employment Act, 1980, the Employment Act, 1982 and the Social Security Act, 1986. An employee who is expecting a baby may have the following rights, subject to various conditions:

1. not to be unreasonably refused time off work to receive antenatal care and to be paid for the time off;
2. the right to complain of unfair dismissal because of pregnancy;
3. the right to SMP;
4. the right to return to work with her employer.

Further details can be obtained from the leaflet entitled 'Employment rights for the expectant mother', published by the Department of Employment.

Other benefits available in pregnancy

Free prescriptions and free dental treatment are available for women in pregnancy and for 1 year after the birth. Families receiving Income Support can also have tokens for 7 pints of free milk per week, or 900 grams of dried baby milk, and free vitamins for mother and child. Mothers receiving Family Credit who have a child under 1 year being artificially fed can obtain powdered milk at a reduced price.

Other benefits available for low-income families

Families receiving Income Support or Family Credit can also obtain:

free NHS vouchers for glasses
free dental treatment
free prescriptions
fares paid for hospital visits, including antenatal care.

These families may also be eligible for Housing Benefit and Community Charge Benefit.

APPENDIX 6

Complications of Pregnancy

The most common complications of pregnancy are haemorrhage and pregnancy induced hypertension.

Bleeding in early pregnancy

Bleeding from the genital tract in early pregnancy, that is, before the 24th week, may be caused by implantation bleeding, abortion, ectopic pregnancy, hydatidiform mole, cervical lesions and vaginitis. After 24 weeks, bleeding from the genital tract is called antepartum haemorrhage.

Bleeding during pregnancy is always abnormal, and in any emergency the midwife's duty is to call the doctor, remain with the woman, monitor her condition, give support and carry out any emergency measures within her capabilities which may be required.

Abortion

The commonest of all the accidents of pregnancy, abortion is defined as expulsion from the uterus of the products of conception before the 24th week of pregnancy, the fetus not being born alive. A brief classification is given below.

Abortion may be spontaneous or induced. Induced abortion, or termination of pregnancy is legal, provided certain conditions are fulfilled to meet the requirements of the Abortion Act, 1967 and subsequent amendments. Up to 12 weeks, pregnancy is usually terminated by vacuum extraction or sometimes dilatation and curettage. After this time, drugs such as prostaglandins are used. Some abortions are illegally induced, either by the administration of drugs or by the introduction, through the cervix, of a foreign body. Illegal abortions are extremely dangerous, and are associated with high mortality and morbidity rates. The midwife should not give advice, information or help which could lead to an illegal abortion.

Molar pregnancy

A mole has been defined as a blighted ovum. Two types are described.

Vesicular or hydatidiform mole. This is a cystic disease of the trophoblast, the villi of which become greatly overgrown and distended with fluid. The embryo perishes soon after the pregnancy begins, but the abnormal placental tissue is overactive and the symptoms and signs of pregnancy are much exaggerated.

The dangers are haemorrhage and sepsis, and the intensely malignant condition of chorioncarcinoma may follow later. The treatment is to empty the uterus, limiting blood loss as much as possible, and to keep the woman under observation for at least 2 years subsequently in case of the development of chorioncarcinoma. The level of human chorionic gonadotrophin (HCG) in the serum is estimated until the level returns to normal.

Missed abortion. Known also as blood mole, fleshy mole and carneous mole. The pregnancy separates from the wall of the uterus and dies, but is not expelled. There is a slow oozing of blood and the gestation sac gradually becomes surrounded by layers of blood clot. Ultimately the mole may be expelled spontaneously, without difficulty or danger. Prostaglandin E_2 may be employed to encourage this, but surgical induction of abortion is avoided because it carried with it a serious risk of infection.

Ectopic pregnancy

This is a pregnancy not in its normal site, which is the body of the uterus. Theoretically it could be in the ovary, the abdominal cavity or the cervix. In fact it is almost always in the fallopian tube, usually either in the ampulla or isthmus. Occasionally the fertilized ovum embeds in the cornu of the uterus. This is termed an interstitial or angular pregnancy.

The pregnancy usually terminates within 4–10 weeks by:

1. *Tubal abortion.* The gestation sac separates from the lining of the tube and is carried to the peritoneal cavity by peristaltic action of the tube. Slight vaginal bleeding occurs as the uterine decidua is shed.

2. *Tubul rupture.* The trophoblast has penetrated the fallopian tube more deeply. This causes severe pain, intraperitoneal or intraligamentary haemorrhage and severe shock. The woman needs an immediate blood transfusion and, as quickly as possible, a laparotomy, in order that the bleeding vessels may be found and ligated.

Immediate treatment by the midwife

If the woman's condition is good, the midwife should keep her at rest and save for the doctor's inspection anything that is passed *per vaginam*. Blood-stained clothing should also be saved. The midwife should not make any vaginal examination.

If the bleeding is severe and the patient's condition deteriorating, the midwife should send an urgent message for an obstetric 'flying squad' and try to control the haemorrhage. In the commonest instance—

Table 2. Abortion.

Type	Characteristics	Treatment
Threatened abortion	Vaginal bleeding, usually slight Pain nil or very slight No dilatation of cervix	Absolute rest Possibly drugs, e.g. salbutamol
The symptoms may subside and the pregnancy continue or the condition may worsen to:		
Inevitable abortion	Bleeding, possibly severe Pain: recognizable uterine contractions Cervix dilating	Hasten process Oxytocic drugs
Two particular phases are described:		
(a) Incomplete	Some part of the products of conception—usually the placenta—is retained	Evacuation of uterus
	The dangers are haemorrhage and sepsis	Possibly blood transfusion
(b) Complete	All the products of conception are expelled spontaneously	Nil
Missed abortion	All the products of conception are retained	
Septic abortion	Infection in the uterus Pyrexia	Treat sepsis first: then evacuate uterus Blood transfusion
Habitual abortion	A term used to describe a sequence of three or more spontaneous abortions	(a) Possible hormone therapy (e.g. hydroxyprogesterone, Primolut-Depot); or (b) cervical cerclage; or

incomplete abortion with dangerous haemorrhage—she should administer intravenous ergometrine 0.5 mg or intramuscular Syntometrine, 1 ampoule, in an effort to make the uterus contract, and carry out any resuscitation treatment possible.

Following abortion or ectopic pregnancy most women are very distressed about the loss of their baby and the midwife can give them the support, information and counselling which they so often need at this time.

Antepartum haemorrhage

Antepartum haemorrhage is bleeding from the genital tract at any time from the 24th week of pregnancy until the child is born. It is a serious complication which may threaten the life of both mother and fetus. The causes are:

1. placenta praevia;
2. abruptio placentae;
3. incidental causes.

Placenta praevia

The placenta is abnormally embedded partly or wholly in the lower uterine segment, and in the last few weeks of pregnancy (when this part of the uterus stretches) the placenta, which cannot stretch, separates and haemorrhage is unavoidable. The bleeding is painless, often occurs when the mother is at rest; it always recurs, usually with increasing severity, so any suspect woman should be admitted to hospital for observation. Placenta praevia occurs in healthy women, without pre-eclampsia. The placenta occupies the lower pole of the uterus, hence a very high presenting part or an oblique lie of the fetus would suggest placenta praevia. The exact position of the placenta may be demonstrated by ultrasound scan, but in some cases diagnosis can be made only by palpation of the placenta *per vaginam*. This examination may cause very dangerous bleeding, and becomes necessary: 1. if no further serious bleeding occurs, at about the 38th week of pregnancy, when the fetus is reasonably mature; 2. if labour begins; or 3. if severe haemorrhage renders immediate active treatment essential. It is carried out only in a theatre, fully prepared for immediate caesarean section and for resuscitating a collapsed patient. The placenta may be felt just encroaching upon the lower segment (type I); the treatment is artificial rupture of the membranes. Or the placenta may be palpated at the margin of the internal os (type II). In type III placenta praevia the placenta covers the os when it is not dilated, but would not do so if it were dilated. In type IV the placenta lies centrally and would cover the os whether it were dilated or not. In all these cases a caesarean section almost always is the appropriate treatment. When the placenta is not felt or is type I anterior, then the membranes may be ruptured to induce labour.

Abruptio placentae (placental abruption)

Abruptio placentae is bleeding from partial separation of a normally situated placenta. It may be *revealed*, when all the blood escapes per vaginam, *concealed* when all the blood lost is retained in the uterus, or *revealed and concealed*, which is a mixture of both types. It may be associated with pre-eclampsia or hypertension, or it may be traumatic in origin. Trauma from a mismanaged external version is seen rather more than that resulting from a fall or blow.

The revealed type may be slight, with no pain, no apparent cause and no recurrence. No treatment is necessary, but the possibility of placenta praevia must be borne in mind. Or there may be pain and heavy bleeding, requiring examination under anaesthesia (to exclude a possible placenta praevia) and rupture of the membranes.

Concealed haemorrhage is also associated with pre-eclampsia or hypertension or, occasionally, with trauma. The patient presents a typical 'shock' picture: grey pallor, clammy skin and weak pulse, sometimes rapid but often slow. The uterus is distended, of a 'woody' consistency, and extremely tender and painful; fetal parts cannot be palpated, and the fetal heart sounds are rarely audible as the fetal mortality is high. The blood pressure may be normal, and has probably fallen from a high level. The urinary output is decreased and the urine is loaded with protein. The treatment is morphine to relieve the pain and shock, and blood transfusion. A central venous pressure (CVP) line is set up to assess the volume of blood or other substance to be transfused. The level should be kept at about $+4$ cmH$_2$O. Later, the membranes are ruptured, and a rapid labour usually follows, with quick expulsion of a stillborn fetus and placenta with considerable retroplacental blood clot. If the fetal heart sounds are heard, a quick caesarean section may save the child. Acute renal failure, due to lower nephron nephrosis or cortical necrosis of the kidneys, and blood coagulation disorders may occur as complications.

Many women experience slight antepartum haemorrhage, with no other symptoms, which does not recur. Its cause is unexplained, but since it may be serious it cannot be ignored. Biophysical tests to assess fetal well-being should be done serially to detect any deterioration.

Incidental haemorrhage

Incidental haemorrhage is extraplacental, arising from cervical polyps or erosion, acute vaginitis and, occasionally, carcinoma of cervix. It is uncommon, easily recognized on inspection of the cervix and vagina with a speculum, and rarely causes dangerous haemorrhage. The treatment is that of the cause.

Treatment

The midwife's responsibility if called to any woman who has vaginal bleeding in late pregnancy is the same:

1. To call a doctor and, in serious haemorrhage, an obstetric 'flying squad'.
2. To keep the mother as quiet as possible. Even in severe bleeding it is better not to carry out any active treatment, such as the application of vaginal packs, because this may aggravate rather than arrest the haemorrhage.
3. Give analgesia such as pethidine 100 mg intramuscularly if the woman is in severe pain.
4. Never to make a vaginal examination, as torrential haemorrhage can occur.
5. To keep a record of the patient's pulse rate and blood pressure and of the fetal heart rate, and to save all blood that is lost.
6. Take blood for X-matching.
7. Give support to the woman and her partner.

Pregnancy-induced hypertension (PIH)

This includes three conditions:

1. Gestational hypertension, which may occur in women who are normotensive in early pregnancy but who subsequently develop hypertension without proteinuria.
2. Pre-eclampsia, which may occur in women who are normotensive in early pregnancy but who subsequently develop hypertension *with* proteinuria.
3. Eclampsia is a life-threatening condition characterized by fits, which may follow pre-eclampsia if it is not adequately controlled.

PIH complicates 5–20 per cent (British Birth Survey) of all pregnancies but the cause, despite much research, remains unknown. It is seen more frequently in primigravidae, in multiple pregnancy, and associated with essential hypertension or diabetes mellitus. It is seen commonly in the last 8 weeks of pregnancy, uncommonly between the 24th and 27th week and rarely in early pregnancy. PIH is diagnosed on physical signs and not on symptoms, so all women need to be screened regularly and carefully.

Signs
Signs of PIH are:

1. A rise of 10–15 mmHg diastolic above the baseline blood pressure, but a blood pressure of over 140/85 always gives cause for concern. However, permanently raised blood pressure does not cause pre-eclampsia in the absence of renal complications.
2. Oedema is often a feature of normotensive as well as hypertensive pregnancies and, indeed, is associated with large babies unless proteinuria develops (MacGillivray, 1985). Severe oedema affecting feet, legs, hands, face and abdominal wall may be a sign of pregnancy-induced hypertension, however, and excessive weight gain (exceeding 0.5 kg per week in the latter half of pregnancy) may be due to occult oedema.
3. Proteinuria—the third sign—is the most serious, signifying that renal function is impaired and that the fetoplacental unit's function may be in danger. Protein from contaminants or from urinary tract infection must be excluded by obtaining a midstream urine specimen

The woman with gestational PIH may be monitored at home under the supervision of the community midwife. Assessment of both maternal and fetal well-being is essential. Any deterioration, including the detection of proteinuria, indicates the need for immediate hospitalization, even though at this stage the woman usually feels well. Anti-hypertensive drugs may be prescribed to try and control the blood pressure. If her condition deteriorates, the signs become worse and she may experience unpleasant symptoms. Severe frontal headache may result from cerebral oedema; retinal oedema may cause various visual disturbances; vomiting and epigastric pain suggest liver haemorrhage and may herald eclamptic fits. Oliguria is a further dangerous sign.

The dangers are eclampsia, abruptio placentae, renal and cardiac failure and cerebral haemorrhage. The placenta may become infarcted, and this placental insufficiency limits the oxygen and food available to the fetus, so that intrauterine growth is retarded. The fetus could die in extreme cases from anoxia, or be SMALL FOR GESTATIONAL AGE.

Management
Rest may lower the blood pressure, lessen the oedema and clear up the proteinuria by improving the renal and placental circulations.

Observation, which is important, includes:

1. A twice-daily, 4-hourly, or more frequent blood pressure recording
2. A fluid intake and output measurement, with daily checks for proteinuria.
3. Daily examination of the abdomen to monitor fetal growth, amount

of amniotic fluid and to auscultate the fetal heart, the latter usually twice daily, or 4-hourly.
4. Oedema is noted and daily weighing may be undertaken.
5. Assessment of renal function includes serial estimations of plasma electrolytes, blood urea and creatinine and uric acid.
6. Assessment of liver function includes serial measurements of liver enzymes and liver function tests.

Monitoring the fetal condition may also be carried out:

1. A kick chart can be completed by the mother.
2. Cardiotocography is used regularly.
3. Estimation of fetal growth by ULTRASOUND by cephalometry, abdominal girth and length of femur (see Appendix 4).

The records should be set out in graph form, so that the obstetrician can see the mother's progress at a glance.

There may be great improvement, but close observation must continue. The condition may remain static, when, in mild cases, labour is induced shortly before term. If proteinuria is present or tests show that fetal well-being is not being maintained, earlier induction or caesarian section is advisable.

Worsening may occur, shown by increasing proteinuria and diminishing urinary output; in such a case, immediate induction of labour or caesarean section is necessary. In severe early pre-eclampsia with rapid worsening or fetal distress, caesarian section is often necessary.

Delivery is usually followed by quick recovery.

Eclampsia

This is a serious condition in which there are fits identical to 'grand mal' seizures. It is rare, the fits occurring sometimes in pregnancy but more often towards the end of labour or shortly afterwards. The fits consist of a tonic phase of violent muscular spasm, with rigidity, apnoea and deepening cyanosis. A clonic phase, when jerky, violent and uncontrollable movements, occur. Then a return to breathing with a risk of inhaling mucus or blood from the mouth or pharynx. These two stages, tonic and clonic, last about 2 minutes. A period of coma lasting a short time ensues.

Dangers

Repeated fits are very dangerous and may lead to cardiac failure, while a markedly hypertensive person may suffer a cerebral haemorrhage. Grossly oedematous patients may develop pulmonary oedema or renal failure. Pneumonia may result from inhalation of debris. Hepatic failure may occur. The commonest causes of death are cerebral haemorrhage and oedema. In antenatal eclampsia, the fetus, already hypoxic from placental insufficiency, is especially at risk during the mother's apnoeic phase.

Prevention

By prompt recognition and treatment of pre-eclampsia, most cases (except the very rare fulminating cases of eclampsia) should be prevented.

Treatment

Call medical aid, and then gently but swiftly:

1. Lie the patient on her side and maintain a clear airway.
2. Give oxygen once the airways are cleared and breathing restarts.
3. Protect the patient from injuring herself.
4. Insert an airway as soon as the jaw muscles relax. It is useless to try to insert a mouth gag before this because the teeth are clenched tightly, although traditionally this was recommended.
5. Give drugs ordered by the doctor as soon as possible, to control any further fits. Various drugs are used—some to reduce the blood pressure (such as hydrallazine hydrochloride, Apresoline), others to prevent further fits (such as phenytoin, Epanutin). A number of other regimens are in use, such as:
    (a) CHLORMETHIAZOLE (Heminevrin);
    (b) Lytic cocktail, consisting of promethazine, chlorpromazine and pethidine;
    (c) Diazepam (Valium).

These are usually given intravenously in a solution such as 5% dextrose.

6. Diuretic treatment is indicated when the urinary output is less than 20 ml/hour.
7. Antibiotics may be prescribed to prevent pulmonary infection.

General management follows two main principles:

1. The prevention of further fits by keeping the patient as quiet as possible and by administering drugs as the condition demands.
2. The prevention of deterioration in the patient's general condition—achieved by close observation and well organized nursing care. This includes maintaining a clear airway, giving oxygen when needed, giving attention, when the patient is heavily sedated, to the mouth and pressure points, changing position, blanket bathing. All these, together with the necessary observation of temperature, pulse, blood pressure, respiration and intake and output are carried out with a minimum of disturbance. Intravenous rather than oral fluids will be

given and a second infusion is usually set up for the administration of drugs. A central venous pressure line should be established for accurate measurement of fluid volume. The indwelling catheter is released hourly and urinary output measured and recorded. All specimens are tested, especially for protein. The fetal condition is monitored carefully for signs of hypoxia. (*See* Appendix 16.)

In the rare antepartum eclampsia, labour—which must be watched for—is usually quick and easy. As soon as the fits and blood pressure are under control in antepartum eclampsia, arrangements are made for delivery.

If the fetus is alive a caesarian section may be performed, or labour is induced by artificial rupture of the membranes and an oxytocic infusion. Effective analgesia is achieved by epidural anaesthesia. An elective forceps delivery is usually performed and the mother is then heavily sedated to reduce the risk of postpartum fits. A paediatrician should be present at delivery to resuscitate the baby. After delivery, most mothers make a fairly rapid and generally complete recovery. While a fit may occur up to 48 hours postnatally, eclampsia rarely recurs, though a subsequent pregnancy may occasionally be complicated by pre-eclampsia.

Essential hypertension

The diagnosis is made if, in early pregnancy, the blood pressure (after checking) is 140/90 mmHg or more. During pregnancy the hypertension may improve, remain static or worsen. Anti-hypertensive drugs may be given, though these are used cautiously because they can decrease the renal and placental blood flow.

The dangers are increasing hypertension, abruptio placentae, superimposed pre-eclampsia and occasionally, subarachnoid haemorrhage, cardiac failure or renal failure. The fetus is exposed to the risk of placental insufficiency and may be small for gestational age or even stillborn.

Renal disease

Chronic renal disease is a rare but serious problem in pregnancy. There may be a background of nephritis in childhood, but this is not always so. Proteinuria in early pregnancy is suspicious, the diagnosis then being made on renal function tests.

These women need close observation, often with long periods in hospital. The risks are miscarriage, pre-eclampsia, abruptio placentae and further renal impairment. The fetus, malnourished and small, may die *in utero*.

In contrast, it must be stated that some nephritic patients seem able to go through their pregnancies without deterioration and are delivered of healthy mature infants.

Women with renal transplants which have good function, and who are stable, have a good chance of a successful pregnancy—in marked contrast to those undergoing dialysis.

Anaemia

Anaemia, in both mild and more severe forms, is commonly seen in childbearing women. It is debilitating in pregnancy, dangerous in the third stage of labour and apt to worsen with successive pregnancies.

Iron deficiency anaemia is the most common type. It is probably related initially to poor nutrition and is aggravated in early pregnancy by the changes in the blood, with a greater increase in plasma than in red cells; later, the increasing demands of the fetus further deplete the mother's reserves. In all pregnancies, the haemoglobin value should be estimated at 'booking' and on three or four occasions after that, particularly in the third trimester. Readings of less than 11 g/dl should be noted, and further investigation (e.g. a blood film) should be done. It is no longer routine practice to give iron to all women in pregnancy (Hytten, 1976), but only to those who have iron-deficiency anaemia, as indicated by a low serum ferritin value. Some women taking oral iron have digestive upsets, but so many preparations are available that a suitable one can usually be found. Severely anaemic women may need intravenous iron, which raises the haemoglobin by 1 g per week; rarely, blood transfusion is necessary to prevent the risk of a woman going into labour in a dangerously anaemic state.

Sometimes a woman whose anaemia fails to respond to the administration of iron is found, on investigation, to have megaloblastic anaemia of pregnancy which is due to folic acid deficiency. It should be specially looked for in epileptic women since they are likely to be taking, over long periods, the anticonvulsant drug phenytoin (Epanutin) which is a folic acid antagonist and so may produce this unfortunate side effect. The condition is corrected by the administration of folic acid with the iron.

Haemoglobinopathies

Sickle cell disease (Haemoglobin (Hb) S or C) and thalassaemia (Hb A2 + HbF) are two haemoglobinopathies which may complicate pregnancy. Abnormal HbS and/or HbC may be found in people who originate from Central and West Africa and parts of Asia. In sickle cell disease, the erythrocytes are sickle shaped and easily haemolysed, thus severe anaemia is common. Folic acid but not iron is given routinely in pregnancy and blood transfusions may be required for severe anaemia. Acute episodes known as crises may occur which can endanger the life of the mother and her unborn child.

Thalassaemia is most common in people of Mediterranean origin.

Again the abnormal red cells cause severe anaemia and folic acid is given because the bone marrow is very active in replacing the short-lived red cells.

Heart disease

The most frequent heart lesion seen in pregnancy was mitral stenosis, usually related to rheumatic fever or chorea in childhood, but not always easily accounted for. Congenital heart disease (CHD) now forms the majority of cases in the United Kingdom. The obstetrician, when he or she examines the mother's heart, may suspect an abnormality; he or she will then refer the mother to a specialist physican and she will continue her pregnancy under their joint care. Cardiac disease may worsen in pregnancy, so careful monitoring is essential. The woman may remain well-compensated throughout pregnancy, needing only extra rest at home, or she may need bed rest in hospital, possibly for a few weeks. A few women go into cardiac failure during pregnancy and require prolonged rest, oxygen, digoxin and diuretics. Mitral valvotomy is carried out during pregnancy in suitable cases.

Women with cardiac disease usually have normal and often short and easy labours. They should be supported by a wedge or pillows so that their breathing is not embarrassed. They benefit from epidural anaesthesia unless anticoagulated, whilst forceps delivery spares them the exertion of the second stage. Caesarian section is indicated only when there is a further complication, such as fetal distress. In the third stage, strong uterine contractions squeeze about 1 litre of extra blood into the general circulation. This increase in blood volume may so embarrass the heart as to initiate cardiac failure. The administration of an OXYTOCIC drug may accentuate this. The midwife therefore should consult the doctor present at delivery about the administration of oxytocic drugs. These women must be carefully protected from infection because the risk of subacute bacterial endocarditis is always serious and may be fatal. Any hazard—from dental extraction to labour itself—is to be negotiated with full antibiotic cover. Induction of labour is therefore not usually attempted.

Finally, women with symptomatic cardiac lesions should, during pregnancy, see a social worker, who may make arrangements for domestic help during pregnancy, and upon return home after delivery; in appropriate cases, rehousing, in a flat with a lift or a house with fewer stairs, may be arranged.

Diabetes mellitus

The British Diabetic Association has adopted the World Health Organisation (WHO) classification of Diabetics Mellitus (Editorial, 1983) which is as follows:

1. *Type I*. Insulin-dependent diabetes (formerly called clinical diabetes). The glucose tolerance test (GTT) is abnormal and women have the signs and symptoms of the disease and require treatment.

2. *Type II*. Non-insulin-dependent diabetes (formerly known as chemical diabetes), where there are no signs and symptoms but the GTT is abnormal.

3. *Impaired glucose tolerance*. (IGT) (formerly known as latent diabetes or, in pregnancy, gestational diabetes). The GTT is abnormal during pregnancy but reverts to normal after delivery. These women tend to develop overt clinical diabetes later in life.

4. *Other*. This group would include potential diabetics who have a normal GTT but have a higher incidence of diabetes than normal women. They may have a history of:
   (a) a previous baby weighing 4.5 kg or more;
   (b) an unexplained perinatal death;
   (c) mother, father or siblings with diabetes;

   and on clinical examination:

   (d) glycosuria on two or more occasions;
   (e) polyhydramnios;
   (f) obesity.

Pre-pregnancy
Diabetic women should seek advice before they become pregnant.

Management during pregnancy
Any woman with diabetes mellitus as described above requires careful investigation and supervision, as she may shift from one category to another due to pregnancy. There are risks to both mother and fetus.

Maternal complications:
1. The diabetes becomes unstable and ketoacidosis can develop with all the associated risks.
2. Infections, especially vaginal and urinary, are common.
3. Pregnancy-induced hypertension.
4. Polyhydramnios.

Fetal/neonatal complications:
1. Intrauterine death.
2. Congenital abnormalities (the causes of which are not known).
3. Excessive size of the fetus, if the mother's diabetes is poorly controlled.
4. Birth trauma is more likely, especially shoulder dystocia leading to ERB'S PARALYSIS.
5. Fetal hypoxia.
6. Respiratory distress syndrome (RDS) (*see* Appendix 17).
7. Hypoglycaemia (*see* Appendix 17).

A midwife should encourage any woman with diabetes to attend a specialized consultant clinic where a physician can carry out joint management with the obstetrician, as the mortality and morbidity are directly related to the standard of care given. A well-controlled woman with diabetes should deliver a normal-sized baby. To achieve this, the blood glucose level should be kept within normal limits (i.e. 3–6 mmol/l). In recent years the perinatal mortality rate has improved greatly due to good diabetic control.

Care in pregnancy
Diabetic women with no obstetric complications are usually managed at home with regular, self-monitoring of the blood glucose levels under the supervision of the community midwife. The woman is also taught to test her urine daily to detect ketone bodies. Measurement of glycosylated haemoglobin (HbA1) helps to assess diabetic control. Only if diabetic control is poor or obstetric complications arise is hospital admission necessary. Insulin requirements increase during pregnancy and are adjusted according to the blood glucose levels. Better diabetic control is generally achieved if a combination of short and intermediate-acting insulins are given twice daily (Gillmer, 1983). Oral hypoglycaemic drugs are not recommended because they may cause severe hypoglycaemia in the baby after birth due to their slow metabolism in the infants immature liver. Close monitoring of mother and fetus is required throughout pregnancy to detect any obstetric complications which may arise.

Care in labour
If the diabetes is well controlled and there are no other complications, the woman may be delivered at term; otherwise labour will be induced earlier, or a caesarean section performed. The L/S RATIO is estimated if delivered before term because, if less than 2.0, there is a high risk that the baby will develop respiratory distress syndrome. In labour an intravenous infusion of dextrose and soluble insulin are administered,

as prescribed by the physician. Blood glucose levels are monitored hourly and maintained between 4.4 and 5.5 mmol/l. Continuous monitoring of the fetal heart and regular assessment of maternal condition and progress are necessary to detect complications. If labour proceeds normally the woman will be delivered vaginally. Otherwise a caesarean section is performed. A paediatrician should be present at delivery because there is a danger of asphyxia and hypoglycaemia.

Postnatal care

The mother's insulin requirements fall sharply after delivery, so frequent blood glucose estimations are necessary to detect hypoglycaemia. Insulin dosage is reduced. Extra carbohydrate is required while the mother is breast feeding and insulin requirements may need further adjustment.

Urinary tract infection

This is a common complication of pregnancy, particularly between the 20th and 28th weeks. The infecting organism, usually *Escherichia coli* but sometimes *Proteus vulgaris*, enters the urinary tract via the blood stream, the descending colon or through the urethra, and the static urine in the dilated ureter favours multiplication of the bacteria. The woman becomes feverish, with loin pain, often nausea or vomiting and in some cases, increased frequency of micturition with dysuria. In acute cases, she is hyperpyrexial, with rigors and severe pain. Chronic infection may present as general malaise, backache or vomiting. In acute case the pain is often spasmodic and the diagnosis is confused with preterm labour. It is further complicated because the pyrexia may precipitate labour.

The diagnosis is established when, on microscopy, pus cells and bacteria are seen in the urine, a count of 100 000 organisms/ml or more being significant. The mother is given an antibiotic to which the bacteria are sensitive, copious fluids, and analgesics varying according to the severity of the pain, from codeine tablets to, occasionally, morphine. She is likely to make quite a quick recovery, but is often left with a residual bacteriuria. Thus the infection readily recurs, and prolonged follow-up has shown that some women develop chronic pyelonephritis and, ultimately, renal failure. Thus all women, at the first clinic visit should be routinely screened for asymptomatic bacteriura.

Pulmonary tuberculosis

A few years ago this condition was fairly uncommon in the United Kingdom. However, in areas with a large immigrant population, poor housing and overcrowding it has again become a problem.

Whether a woman is already receiving treatment for tuberculosis or whether it is first discovered following a chest X-ray in the antenatal period, the management is along the same lines. The woman receives care from a chest physician together with an obstetrician, usually on an out-patient basis, unless she has positive sputum when hospital admission and isolation are usually necessary. Then she is attended by staff who are Mantoux-positive. Treatment is often with streptomycin and isoniazid with either para-aminosalicyclic acid or ethambutol. Rifampicin should not be used in the first trimester.

Labour should be made as easy as possible, preferably with epidural analgesia and, probably, forceps delivery at full dilatation and intravenous ergometrine as the baby's anterior shoulder is born, to limit blood loss.

In the few mothers who have positive sputum, lactation is suppressed and, a few days after delivery, the mother returns to the chest hospital for as long as necessary. The baby, who is extremely vulnerable to the infection, is segregated from the mother with open tuberculosis until she is Mantoux-positive. Having had a BACILLE CALMETTE-GUÉRIN (BCG) vaccination as soon as possible after delivery, the baby is discharged to a healthy relative or foster parent, his name being entered on the paediatric 'at risk' register.

Multiple pregnancy

In the UK the incidence of twins is about 1 in 80. Higher order births, although less common, now occur more frequently due to treatment for infertility with drugs that stimulate ovulation, or *in vitro* or *in vivo* fertilization.

Twins may be one of two types:

Monozygotic or uniovular twins develop from one ovum and one spermatozoon which divide. They are both the same sex and there is only one placenta and one chorion but two amniotic sacs. Developmental abnormalities are more common in monozygotic twins.

Dizygotic or binovular twins are more common and arise from the fertilization of two ova with two spermatozoa, thus they may be of different sexes. They have two placentae, often fused together, two amnions and two chorions.

Diagnosis

The midwife should suspect a multiple pregnancy if the uterus is large for dates, two heads or three poles are palpable, or a small head is found in a large uterus. Polyhydramnios is often present and renders palpation difficult. Most women now have an ultrasound scan between 16 and 18 weeks, and a multiple pregnancy is usually diagnosed then.

Pregnancy

The minor disorders of pregnancy, especially pressure symptoms, are exacerbated and more serious complications such as pregnancy-induced hypertension, anaemia, polyhydramnios and preterm labour are more likely to occur. The mother therefore needs careful monitoring at more frequent intervals in pregnancy, as well as support and advice about the alleviation of minor disorders, and preparation for childbirth and parenthood.

Labour

Preterm labour and malpresentations are common complications, thus the woman is delivered in a consultant obstetric unit with neonatal intensive care facilities. The first and second stage of labour are conducted normally until after the delivery of the first twin. The umbilical cord is then clamped securely before being divided, because the second twin may share the same placenta. The first baby and cord are labelled twin I. Next it is essential to palpate the uterus to determine the lie and presentation of the second twin, and to auscultate the fetal heart. If the lie is not longitudinal it is corrected and the presentation confirmed on vaginal examination. The membranes are then ruptured and a careful examination made to detect cord prolapse. Normally uterine contractions recommence soon after the delivery of the first twin and the second baby is delivered within a few minutes. If uterine activity is delayed, or poor, an intravenous infusion of Syntocinon will be necessary. An intravenous injection of ergometrine 0.5 mg is usually given with the delivery of the second baby because of the high risk of postpartum haemorrhage. As soon as the uterus contracts, controlled cord traction is applied to both cords together. When the placenta is examined the number of amnions, chorions and placentae is noted.

Postnatal care

This is often a very tiring and sometimes anxious time for the mother, especially if one or both babies are in the neonatal unit. She may need much support from her midwife and help, as she learns to care for her babies and develop confidence. Voluntary groups such as The Twins and Multiple Births Association may have a local group where support and practical help is available once the mother is discharged. The midwife should be aware of such groups in her area so that she can give mothers information and telephone numbers.

References

British Diabetic Association (1983) *Classification of Diabetes Mellitus.*
Gillmer M (1983) Diabetes in pregnancy. *Medicine International* 1(35): 1639–1640.

Hytten FE (1976) Metabolic adaptations of pregnancy. In Turnbull AC & Woodford EP (eds) *Prevention of Handicap Through Antenatal Care.* Elsevier/North-Holland. Amsterdam. pp. 35–39.

MacGillivray I (1985) Pre-eclampsia. *Midwifery* 1: 12–18.

APPENDIX 7

Normal Labour

Labour which begins spontaneously usually starts at or about term. It is regarded as normal if the fetus presents by the vertex and the process is completed within 12–18 hours, depending on the woman's parity, without active assistance and without injury to mother or child. Labour is divided into three stages: a first stage of dilatation of the cervix, a second stage of expulsion of the fetus and a third stage of expulsion of the placenta and membranes.

All primigravidae and many multigravidae are likely to benefit from some form of preparation for labour (*see* Appendix 3), and a well-prepared woman approaches her labour in a calm, confident and hopeful state of mind especially if she knows the midwife who is likely to care for her in labour. The expectant mother, in collaboration with her partner and midwife, will be able to carry out the particular type of exercise, breathing and relaxation she has practised during pregnancy, and adopt the position of her choice. Her special wishes with regard to her care in labour will be documented in her birth plan.

Onset of labour
The first symptom may be that the woman is aware of uterine contractions amounting to discomfort felt intermittently in the lumbar region, which may be noted by placing a hand on the abdomen. There may be a 'show', which consists of blood-stained mucus which comes from the cervix through the vagina. Sometimes the membranes may rupture at the onset of labour and liquor amnii escapes. Once regular contractions have begun, or the membranes have ruptured, or if the expectant mother is worried or in doubt about what is happening, she should contact her midwife or the hospital for advice. In most cases, if a 'show' only has occurred, she may safely wait until more positive signs of labour are evident.

Initial examination
The midwife greets the expectant mother and her partner warmly at the beginning of labour and tries to put them at ease, since they may have mixed feelings of excitement and fear at this time. The birth plan is discussed with the mother and her partner and clear, simple explanations are given about all examinations and procedures carried out.

The woman's general condition is observed and she is asked how she feels, her temperature, pulse rate, and blood pressure are ascertained, her urine is tested for protein, ketones and glucose, and her abdomen is examined. If she is calm and cheerful and physically well, the uterus is of normal size for 40 weeks, the fetus is presenting by the vertex with the head engaged, the occiput anterior or lateral, and the fetal heart sounds are strong and regular, a normal labour may be anticipated. An experienced person can gauge the progress of labour sufficiently accurately by observation of the patient, but in most cases it is wise to make a vaginal examination, mainly to ascertain the dilatation of the cervix and the descent of the head. It is no longer routine practice to give women an enema or suppositories at the beginning of labour; evacuation of the bowel is only required if the rectum is full and the woman unable to open her bowels (Romney & Gordon, 1981). Most women appreciate a warm bath and some may wish to remain in the bath if they find it eases the discomfort of labour and helps them to relax.

First stage

Most women prefer not to be alone in labour, and if she so wishes, an expectant mother should be able to have her partner or mother, or a close friend with her during labour, while the midwife should be at hand.

Ambulation is encouraged and the woman chooses the position she finds most comfortable during contractions, and practices her breathing techniques and relaxation. Support and encouragement are given and the couple are kept fully informed of progress and involved in decisions relating to the management of their labour. Leisure pursuits such as listening to music or playing cards or games may help the time pass, especially in early labour.

In very early labour the woman may have a small, light meal such as toast or breakfast cereal or soup but, as labour progresses, food is generally withheld and only oral fluids are given because, if complications arise an anaesthetic may become necessary. To reduce the risk of acid-aspiration syndrome (Mendelson's syndrome) an antacid such as magnesium trisilicate 15 ml 2-hourly is given, or some doctors prescribe sodium citrate 30 ml of a 3 mol/l solution.

High standards of hygiene are necessary to prevent infection of the genital tract and the midwife must use sterile equipment and aseptic technique to prevent the introduction of infection during examinations *per vaginam* and at delivery.

Observations

Maternal

1. *Temperature*: 4-hourly.
2. *Pulse rate*: 2-hourly, increasing in frequency until taken every 15 minutes in the active phase of labour.
3. *Blood pressure*: 2-hourly unless an epidural is in process (*see* Appendix 8).
4. *Urinalysis*: this should be carried out every time the bladder is emptied, which should be approximately 2-hourly. Ketones and protein are important to find. If, however, the blood pressure is normal, proteinuria can be caused by liquor amnii if the membranes have been ruptured.
5. *Liquor colour*: a dark green meconium stain may indicate fetal hypoxia (*see* Appendix 16). Bleeding, as opposed to a 'show', is also abnormal during labour.
6. *Reaction to labour*: the need for pain relief, explanation and company should be carefully considered.
7. *Contractions*: length, strength and frequency should be recorded at increasingly frequent intervals either manually or, more accurately by, either an intrauterine catheter or a strain gauge transducer applied to the abdomen.
8. *Progress of labour*: this is assessed by:
   (a) uterine contractions;
   (b) descent of the fetal head which can be assessed by abdominal examination (determined by fifths which remain palpable above the pelvic brim) (*see* Figure 8) and by vaginal examination;
   (c) effacement and dilatation of the cervix.

Dilatation of the cervix should occur in two phases: slow at first (latent phase) and then much more rapidly (active phase). The normal rate can be seen from the cervicogram (*see* Figure 9).

The progress of labour depends on the rate and efficiency of the contractions, which should be recorded together with all other observations on a partogram (*see* Figure 10). This provides a graphical record of the whole labour so that when normal progress does not occur, action, such as augmentation, can be taken if there is no reason for the delay except poor contractions.

Fetal

1. *Heart sounds* as heard with the fetal (Pinard) stethoscope (normal rate is 120–160 beats/minute). They should be counted for 15 seconds and multiplied by four. Listening between contractions will give a baseline but recordings must also be taken during and after a contraction

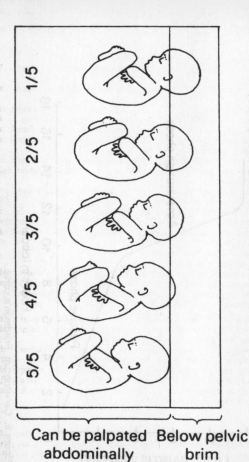

| 1/5 | 2/5 | 3/5 | 4/5 | 5/5 |

Can be palpated abdominally   Below pelvic brim

Figure 8. Diagram illustrating descent of the fetal head into the pelvis.

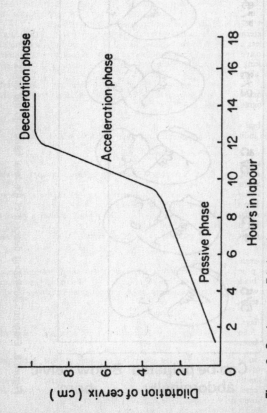

Figure 9. Cervicogram: Friedman's curve.

to detect any deceleration. Should any occur, particularly after a contraction, or there is persistent tachycardia or bradycardia, continuous monitoring should be used as soon as possible.

2. *Continuous fetal ECG.* The most accurate method uses an electrode attached to the fetal scalp or buttock. The types of electrodes can be seen in Figure 11. The disadvantage of these electrodes is that they must be applied after the membranes have been ruptured.

External monitoring is done by using either an ultrasound TRANSDUCER or, less commonly, a microphone placed on the mother's abdomen.

To avoid a woman's being confined to bed when continuous monitoring is taking place, some units use TELEMETRY (*see* Appendix 16) for normal and abnormal tracings).

3. *Fetal blood sampling.* This may be carried out if intrauterine hypoxia is suspected. A high pH indicates any acidosis resulting from hypoxia (*see* Appendix 16 for details).

Vaginal examination

The indications for vaginal examination in labour are as follows:

● to diagnose the onset of labour;
● to assess progress in labour;
● to rupture the membranes and in some cases, to apply a scalp electrode;
● to diagnose a prolapsed cord following rupture of the membranes when there is an ill-fitting presenting part;
● to diagnose the presentation, if in doubt (this is always necessary after the birth of the first twin);
● to determine the cause of delay in any stage of labour.

Preparation

The procedure is explained to the mother and she is asked to empty her bladder before the midwife makes an abdominal examination followed by a vaginal examination. A vaginal examination in labour is an aseptic procedure.

Findings

The following findings can be determined from a vaginal examination in labour:

● Condition of the external genitalia, including oedema, varicosities, vulval warts, vaginal discharge and the presence of scars.
● Condition of the vagina which is normally warm and moist. Occasionally in a mulliparous woman, a cystocele may be found and, more rarely a rectocele; a full rectum will be noted.

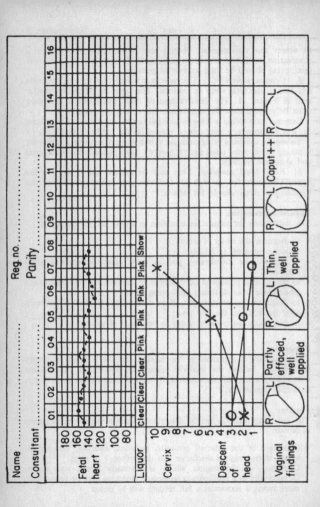

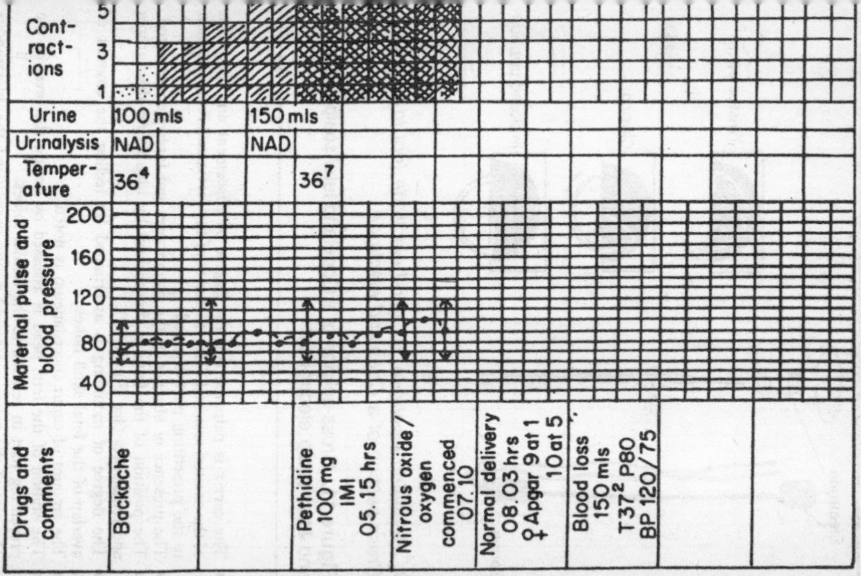

Contractions	5 3 1		
Urine	100 mls	150 mls	
Urinalysis	NAD	NAD	
Temperature	36^4	36^7	
Maternal pulse and blood pressure	200 160 120 80 40		

Drugs and comments

Backache

Pethidine 100 mg IMI 05.15 hrs

Nitrous oxide/oxygen commenced 07.10

Normal delivery 08.03 hrs ♀ Apgar 9 at 1 10 at 5

Blood loss 150 mls $T37^2$ P80 BP 120/75

Figure 10. Continued.

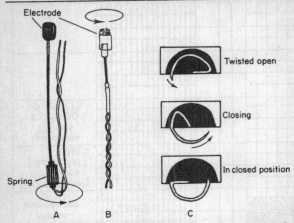

A. *Copeland electrode;* B. *spiral electrode (not to scale);* C. *Cross-section of a Copeland electrode.*

Figure 11. Cross-section of a Copeland fetal scalp electrode and fetal scalp electrodes.

- The cervix is palpated and the degree of effacement and dilatation of the os uteri assessed. The thickness of the cervix and its application to the presenting part is noted.
- The presence or absence of the membranes and forewaters is noted.
- The position of the fetus is determined by identifying the sutures and fontanelles (see Figure 12).
- The degree of moulding is ascertained by feeling the amount of overlap of the fetal skull bones.
- The amount of caput succedaneum is noted.
- The station of the fetal head is assessed by noting the level of the presenting part in relation to the ischial spines.
- The size of the pelvis is assessed noting particularly the interspinous and intertuberous diameters and the size of the subpubic angle which should be about 90°.

On completion of the examination the midwife makes the mother comfortable and explains the findings to her. Finally she records her findings in the notes.

With a well-flexed vertex presentation, the membranes often rupture at or near full dilatation of the cervix, if they have not already been artificially ruptured for internal fetal monitoring, and during the next few contractions the midwife should watch for signs that the mother is in the second stage of labour. Should the anus gape, the perineum bulge and the head be seen at the vulva, the midwife should prepare for the delivery.

Second stage

The second stage of labour starts at the time of full dilatation of the cervix which is normally confirmed by vaginal examination and is completed with the complete expulsion of the baby. Like the first stage it is divided into two phases, the latent and the active phases. During the latent phase when the fetal head is not visible the woman has little or no desire to bear down with contractions and should not be exhorted to do so. Once the active phase is reached and the head is exerting pressure on the perineum the desire to bear down with contractions becomes irresistible.

The length of the second stage varies from a few minutes in multigravidae to an hour or more in primigravidae. Providing the presenting part is progressively descending and the maternal and fetal condition remain satisfactory, the woman should be able to deliver spontaneously within a reasonable length of time, thus rigid time limits are unnecessary. If progress is slow the adoption of an upright or squatting position often aids progress.

During this stage the woman should adopt the position which she finds most comfortable, which is often a well-supported semi-sitting position with the aid of a foam wedge. However, she may prefer to lie on her side, squat, kneel or adopt an all-fours posture, or use a birthing chair, stool or Gardosi cushion, should they be available. Some delivery beds can be divided to allow the woman to adopt a more comfortable sitting position.

The midwife stays with the mother and her partner throughout the second stage, supporting and encouraging them, keeping them informed of progress and involving them in all decisions related to their care. Physical care includes:

● ensuring that the bladder is empty because a full bladder can delay progress and be damaged by the pressure of the fetal head.
● observing high standards of hygiene and an aseptic technique during delivery.

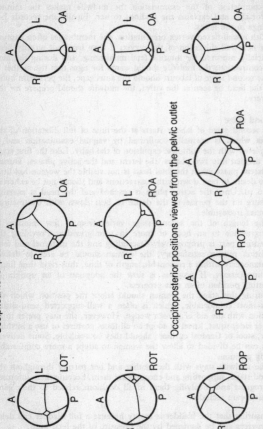

Figure 12. Identifying the position of the fetus on vaginal examination by identifying the position

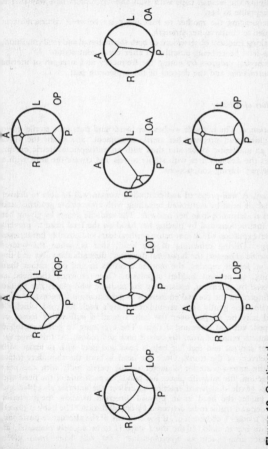

Figure 12. Continued.

- helping the woman cope with pain and discomfort in a way that is acceptable to her.
- encouraging the mother to rest and relax between contractions in order to conserve her strength.
- making frequent observations of both the maternal and fetal condition, the fetal heart being auscultated after every contraction.
- observing progress by noting the frequency and strength of uterine contractions and the descent of the presenting part.

Conduct of delivery

Preparation. The midwife washes her hands and puts on a sterile gown and gloves and prepares her sterile equipment. She swabs the vulva with an antiseptic lotion and then with an antiseptic obstetric cream, drapes the delivery area with sterile towels and covers the anus with a sterile pad during contractions.

Delivery. A well-prepared and controlled woman will be able to deliver her baby's head by controlled breathing with appropriate guidance and minimal assistance from her midwife. The midwife assists by giving her clear instructions and by placing her hand on the fetal head to prevent sudden expulsion which may cause perineal tears and possibly intracranial damage. During crowning of the head, that is, when the widest transverse diameter, the biparietal diameter, distends the vulva and the head no longer recedes, the mother breathes in and out, rather than pushing, to prevent sudden expulsion. Once crowned the head is delivered by extension, assisted by the midwife who places her thumb and fingers on the parietal eminences to aid extension if necessary. The midwife then gently feels around the baby's neck for cord which, if found may be slipped over the baby's head if sufficiently loose, or clamped, cut and unwound if tight. The eyes may be gently swabbed and mucus removed from the baby's nose and mouth. At this stage the mother can see and feel her baby's head and may wish to assist with the delivery of the trunk. Once the head is born the shoulders rotate into the antero-posterior diameter of the pelvis and, with the next contraction, the midwife places her hands on each side of the head and applies gentle downward traction to deliver the anterior shoulder and then guides the head in an upward direction to allow the posterior shoulder and trunk to be delivered by lateral flexion. The baby is placed on the mother's abdomen or, if she is in one of the alternative positions, given to her to hold. If the third stage is to be actively managed, an oxytocic drug such as Syntometrine 1 ml will have been given intramuscularly by an assistant with the birth of the anterior shoulder. This causes the uterus to contract strongly in 2.5 minutes.

The time of delivery is noted and the baby gently dried and covered warmly to prevent chilling. Skin to skin contact with the mother not only aids bonding, but also helps to keep the baby warm. The cord will be clamped and cut soon after delivery or, if there is no contraindication, it may be left until it has stopped pulsating. If the mother wishes to breast feed the baby may be put to the breast at this stage.

Third stage

The third stage of labour starts as soon as the baby is born and is completed with the expulsion of the placenta and membranes. With active management it rarely lasts more than 5 or 10 minutes whereas passive or physiological management may take up to an hour. The aim is to deliver the placenta and membranes complete, and prevent postpartum haemorrhage.

Active management

An oxytocic drug such as Syntometrine 1 ml is given with the crowning of the head or the birth of the anterior shoulder and takes effect in 2.5 minutes. The midwife covers the mother's abdomen with a sterile towel and places a hand gently on the uterine fundus to note its consistency. A sterile receiver is placed against the vulva to collect blood loss and receive the placenta. When the uterus contracts, the midwife places the ulnar border of her left hand in the suprapubic region and gently pushes the contracted uterus upwards, while with her right hand she gains a firm hold on the cord and exerts gentle steady traction. This traction is first downwards (towards the bed) to ease the placenta from the lower uterine segment and then forwards (towards the ceiling) to withdraw it from the vagina. The membranes, which tear easily, are eased out slowly and carefully. It is now common to apply cord traction with the first contraction about 2½ minutes after the administration of Syntometrine with the birth of the baby's anterior shoulder, without waiting for signs of separation and descent of the placenta and membranes.

Passive or physiological management

The placenta separates from the uterine wall physiologically without the use of an oxytocic drug to expedite the process. The following signs of separation and descent are awaited before attempts are made to deliver the placenta and membranes: the uterus rises, feels small, hard and mobile, the cord lengthens and there is a small gush of blood from the vagina.

Maternal effort

When the uterus is well contracted, the mother is asked to push down as for the delivery to expel the placenta and membranes.

Fundal pressure

The midwife pushes the contracted uterus, with her left hand, towards the pelvis. This acts as a piston and pushes the placenta out of the vagina. The drawbacks to this method are that it can be very uncomfortable for the mother and it imposes a strain on the uterine ligaments as they are also displaced.

Aftercare

Following delivery of the placenta and membranes it is important to palpate the uterus to check that it remains well contracted. The vulva is then gently cleansed and the perineum and vagina inspected for lacerations before being covered with a sterile pad. The placenta and membranes are examined to ensure that they are complete. If incomplete the doctor is notified because retained products of conception may lead to haemorrhage and infection. Perineal repair, if required, may be carried out by the midwife provided she has been taught and pronounced proficient in the procedure. The mother's temperature, pulse and blood pressure are then recorded and both she and her partner are offered a drink and left together to get acquainted with their baby. If the baby was not put to the breast earlier, the midwife will help the mother who wishes to breast feed put her baby to the breast now. A mother who wishes to artificially feed is encouraged to offer her baby a bottle feed.

After a short rest the mother is encouraged to pass urine and then has an assisted shower or wash and changes into a fresh nightdress. The midwife examines the baby beside the parents, clamps and shortens the cord, weighs, measures, labels, washes and dresses the baby. The mother should not be left for at least an hour following delivery, and the midwife must then be satisfied that the uterus is well contracted, the pulse slow and strong, the blood pressure within normal limits and, preferably, the bladder empty. She must satisfy herself also that the baby's colour and respiration are normal and that there is no bleeding from the umbilical cord. All the records are fully completed and then, if in hospital, mother and baby are transferred together to a postnatal ward.

Reference

Romney ML & Gordon H (1981) Is your enema really necessary? *British Medical Journal* 282: 1269–1271.

APPENDIX 8

Anaesthesia and Analgesia

Anaesthesia means 'absence of sensation' and anaesthetic drugs are used to abolish painful sensations. General anaesthetics produce unconsciousness; local anaesthetics abolish sensation in a particular region.

Analgesia means absence of or relief from pain without loss of consciousness. Many drugs (e.g. nitrous oxide and chloroform) will produce analgesia or, if given in higher concentrations, anaesthesia. The chief use of analgesic drugs in midwifery is to relieve the pain of labour in a way that leaves the woman conscious and able to cooperate.

General anaesthetics

These are avoided where practicable, to prevent deaths from MENDELSON'S SYNDROME. One midwife, or nurse, must assist the anaesthetist during induction and apply cricoid pressure (Sellick manoeuvre). Once the endotracheal tube is passed and the cuff inflated, the danger of aspirating acid gastric juice has gone.

Local analgesics

Various synthetic preparations of cocaine are used, of which the most popular is lignocaine hydrochloride (Xylocaine). It is used as a local infiltration before episiotomy, usually 10 ml of a 0.5% solution (for episiotomy) or 5 ml of a 10% solution, as an epidural or paracervical block, or as a pudendal nerve block for forceps delivery or ventouse extraction. Bupivacaine (Marcain) is a long-acting local anaesthetic used in epidural analgesia.

Pain relief in labour

There is now greater emphasis on natural methods of pain relief in labour and the use of complementary therapies.

Antenatal education and psychological support can empower the woman to achieve a well-controlled delivery which is both pleasurable and fulfilling.

Psychophysical preparation includes learning controlled, conscious breathing and relaxation techniques.

Ambulation and a variety of positions can be adopted to enhance the woman's comfort. The upright position has physiological advantages in that the pressure of the fetal head on the cervix is increased and this stimulates uterine action, thereby resulting in a shorter labour, less need for analgesia and a reduction in fetal heart abnormalities (Flynn, 1978). Some women like to be in a warm bath which can ease painful contractions and promote relaxation.

Complementary medicine for pain relief

Complementary medicine, also known as alternative therapies, includes such therapies as hypnosis, massage, acupuncture and reflexology. There is now increasing interest and use of such methods for pain relief in labour.

Hypnosis (often self-induced) is a trance-like state induced in response to certain stimuli. Whilst in the hypnotic state the woman is responsive to suggestion, for instance, that the contractions are not painful.

Massage, sometimes with the use of highly concentrated oils (aromatherapy), is used to relieve pain and promote relaxation in labour.

Acupuncture is a therapeutic method of using needles on acupuncture points in the body. Lines of energy within the body are known as meridians. These pass from the organs of the body to the extremities, that is, the fingers and toes. The auricle of the ear has a complete set of acupuncture points which correspond approximately with the anatomy of the body. The auricle is particularly suitable for acupuncture when women are ambulant in early labour. Later the foot or lower leg may be used. Acupuncture in labour is used to encourage relaxation and aid pain control.

Reflexology is massage of the reflex areas found in the feet which are linked by meridians to the various organs of the body. It works on the same principles as acupressure.

Transcutaneous Electrical Nerve Stimulation (TENS)

TENS is the application of pulsed electrical current through surface electrodes placed on the skin and is now widely used for the relief of pain in labour in the UK. The electrodes are usually placed parallel to and each side of the spine, the first pair reaching from the 10th thoracic to the first lumbar vertebra and the second pair from the second to the fourth sacral vertebra. It works through the gate control theory, closing the 'gate' to pain and also increases the release of cerebrospinal endorphins (Melzack and Wall, 1965). The mother should be taught to use the apparatus during the antenatal period and control its use herself in labour.

Narcotics

Pethidine is the narcotic drug most widely used in labour in the UK. It is usually given intramuscularly in doses of 50–150 mg, or can be administered intravenously in doses of 25 mg on demand from the mother via a Cardiff palliator. Pethidine causes depression of the fetal respiratory centre and therefore can delay the onset of respiration at birth if given to the mother within about 2 hours of delivery. Longer term effects on the baby include being less alert, quicker to cry when disturbed, more difficult to console, and sucking is less frequent and effective (Redshaw and Rosenblatt, 1982).

Meptazinol is a more recent analgesic drug with partial opiate antagonistic properties. The usual dose is 100 mg administered intramuscularly.

Pentazocine hydrochloride (fortral) is a mild analgesic, used sometimes in the first stage of labour. The dose is 50 mg orally.

Tranquillizers such as promazine 25–50 mg or promethazine 25–50 mg intramuscularly are sometimes given with narcotic drugs.

Epidural analgesia
See the dictionary entry for definition and a diagram.

Dangers
1. Sudden hypotension leading to fetal hypoxia.
2. Spinal tap is rare but causes total spinal blockade.
3. Toxic reactions are not common but can occur if the drug is given intravenously in error.
4. Neurological sequelae from injury or haematoma formation.
5. Descent and rotation of the presenting part are not encouraged so the instrumental delivery rate is higher.
6. Dural tap.
7. Infection.

Prevention
1. Intravenous infusion should be commenced *prior* to the insertion and the woman must be nursed on her side to prevent postural hypotension increasing the hypotension. The bed must be able to be tipped head down.
2. Facilities for resuscitation must be in the room.
3. A test dose must be given first and at each 'top-up' a check made that the catheter has *not* entered a vein.
4. The mother should be fully monitored.

Indications for use
1. Prolonged labour, especially when the occiput is posterior.
2. Breech labour and delivery. It removes the urge to push before the cervix is fully dilatated.

3. Rotation or other forceps delivery.
4. Hypertension and pre-eclampsia as the blood pressure is lowered.
5. Client demand where a full service is available.
6. Multiple and preterm delivery.
7. Operative deliveries such as caesarean section.
8. Cardiac and respiratory disease.

'Topping up'

After the anaesthetist has given the test *and* first *full* dose of analgesia, a midwife may give the subsequent injections in certain circumstances. The UKCC permits 'topping up' provided that: 1. the ultimate responsibility lies with the doctor; 2. written instructions are given; 3. the midwife has been instructed in the technique; 4. in all cases the dose given by the midwife must be checked by one other person; and 5. instructions given by the doctor contain details such as posture of the woman at the time of injection, observations required and measures to be taken in the event of any side effects.

Management

The woman must not be nursed flat on her back but other positions may be adopted. Immediately after the 'top-up' she remains on one side for 5 minutes and is then turned onto the other side to allow the analgesia to be bilateral. Late in labour or for suturing the patient may be asked to sit up for 10 minutes.

Observations

Blood pressure is taken every 5 minutes for 30 minutes and every 15 minutes at other times between 'top ups'.

Inhalational analgesics

Entonox

The UKCC has approved for use by midwives the Entonox apparatus whereby the mother inhales a mixture of 50% nitrous oxide and 50% oxygen. The nitrous oxide and oxygen are premixed in a single cylinder to which is attached a simple reducing and demand valve with corrugated tubing and face mask or mouthpiece. It is non-cumulative, therefore, can be used for long periods if required. Care must be taken to avoid storing the cylinder at temperatures of less than 8°C because then the two gases may separate and, after initially inhaling pure oxygen, the mother would receive pure nitrous oxide.

Trichlorethylene (Trilene)

Trichlorethylene is no longer approved for use by midwives in the UK, but is still used in some other countries. It can be administered via the Tecota Mark 6 or Emotril machines in concentrations of 0.35% or 0.5% mixed with air. It is cumulative in effect and therefore should not be used for prolonged periods.

Other drugs that a midwife may administer

Midwives, though not permitted to give general anaesthetics, may give certain tranquillizers, analgesics and local anaesthetics which assist greatly in relieving pain at various points in labour.

References

Flynn AM, Kelly J, Hollins G & Linch PF (1978) Ambulation in labour. *British Medical Journal*, Aug 20, 591–593.

Melzack R & Wall PD (1965) Pain mechanisms: a new theory. *Science* 150, 971–979.

Redshaw M & Rosenblatt DB (1982) The influence of analgesia in labour on the baby. *Midwife, Health Visitor & Community Nurse* 18 (4): 126–132.

APPENDIX 9

Complications of Labour (First and Second Stages)

Delay in the first stage of labour

The midwife informs the doctor if progress in labour is slow. The diagnosis of delay is simplified now with the use of partograms. Average rates of cervical dilatation show two phases: latent and active (*see* the cervicogram, p. 362). The latent phase lasts until the cervix is fully effaced and is 2–3 cm dilated; in the active phase the rate in a primigravida is 1 cm dilatation per hour, whilst in a multigravida it is approximately 1.5 cm.

Diagnosis of delay in labour

With the use of a partogram it can be seen at a glance if the rate of cervical dilatation, assessed on 2- to 4-hourly vaginal examinations, is lagging behind the predicted line. If the lag is 2 hours or more, action should be taken to augment the contractions.

Augmentation of labour

1. Rupture of the membranes, if not already ruptured.

2. Oxytocin (Syntocinon) infusion. Before this is started, full internal monitoring should be commenced, as there is always a danger that hyperstimulation can occur which may cause sudden fetal hypoxia (*see* Appendix 16).

Various methods to deliver the oxytocin are available. In one, a peristaltic pump such as the Ivac or Tekmar is used to deliver the drug, the rate of which is controlled by the midwife until satisfactory contractions of 1 minute's duration occur every 2–3 minutes. Automatic infusion systems (e.g. Cardiff system) are also used.

These are programmed to increase the dose until satisfactory contractions occur.

3. Posture. Contractions are better when the mother is as upright as possible. This position militates against the standard oxytocin infusion and full monitoring, both of which keep the mother lying in bed. There is growing concern amongst the public about their overzealous use for this reason. They also render the labour under the control of the attendants, instead of the woman's own body.

TELEMETRY is a means of monitoring the fetal condition by 'remote control', thus enabling the woman to be mobile and vertical.

In the absence of a partogram and active management, the first stage of labour must be considered as having lasted too long: 1. if there are signs of fetal or maternal distress or exhaustion; and 2. if 18 hours have elapsed, without augmentation, since the onset of labour and the cervix is not fully dilated. This is especially important if the membranes have been ruptured since the onset of labour. A doctor should be called and the domiciliary patient should be admitted to hospital. In fetal distress immediate delivery is necessary, thus caesarean section would be performed. If the uterine contractions are weak and infrequent, augmentation by one of the means discussed can be commenced. If the contractions are very strong and painful but ineffective, cephalopelvic disproportion should be reconsidered and suitable analgesia administered.

Delay in second stage of labour

The usual duration of this stage is 30–105 minutes in a primigravida, and 10–30 minutes in multigravida but, provided maternal and fetal condition are good, rigid time limits are no longer considered necessary (Skelton, 1984; Morrin, 1985). The midwife should send for a doctor immediately if signs of fetal or maternal distress appear, if the contractions of the uterus are too weak to expel the baby, or if any malpresentation is present.

Induction of labour

Labour should only be induced when the life or health of the mother or fetus is endangered by the continuation of pregnancy.

Indications

1. Intrauterine growth retardation diagnosed by clinical examination and confirmed by ultrasound estimation of fetal growth.
2. Other evidence of diminished fetal well-being such as reduced fetal movements and abnormal cardiotocographs.
3. Rhesus isoimmunization.
4. Medical disorders such as diabetes, hypertension and renal disease when there is increased risk for mother and fetus.
5. Prolonged pregnancy, i.e. 42 weeks when there is risk of placental dysfunction.
6. Pregnancy-induced hypertension because of the increased risk of placental dysfunction and also maternal complications.
7. Severe abruptio placentae because rupturing the membranes reduces the intrauterine pressure and expedites delivery.
8. Breech delivery, between 38 and 40 weeks to facilitate easier delivery of the head.
9. Previous large baby, to reduce the risk of a difficult delivery of a large baby.

10. Unstable lie after the lie has been corrected. This reduces the risks of cord prolapse following spontaneous rupture of the membranes and obstructed labour.

11. Intrauterine death to reduce the risk of disseminated intravascular coagulation.

Preparation

The state of the cervix must be assessed by the 'Bishop's score' as seen below in Table 3.

Table 3. 'Bishop's score'.

Criteria	Score			
	0	1	2	3
Cervix				
Dilation (cm)	Closed	1–2	3–4	5+
Length (cm)	3	2	1	0
Consistency	Firm	Medium	Soft	
Position	Posterior	Central	Anterior	
Head				
Station (in cm)				
above ischial spines	−3	−2	−1	0

Score 5 or below: in a primigravida this is *unfavourable*. *Action*. Ripeness of the cervix is encouraged by the insertion of prostaglandin E₂ (Prostin E) in the form of a vaginal pessary on the evening prior to induction.

Score 6 or more: indicates a favourable cervix for induction.

Methods of induction

Prostaglandin

A prostaglandin E₂ (Prostin E) pessary is inserted into the posterior vaginal fornix. The woman is asked to lie on her side for 30 minutes to prevent supine hypotension and loss of the pessary. After this she may be mobile. As labour is established, the normal observations must be made (*see* Appendix 7).

Amniotomy

Position. For this procedure the woman is in either the lithotomy or the dorsal position. The Amnihook or Kocher's forceps (*see* Figure 13) are directed through the cervical canal to rupture the forewaters.

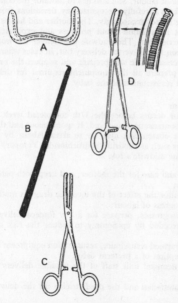

A. *Sim's speculum*; B. *Amnihook*; C. *straight Kocher forceps*; D. *curved Kocher forceps*.

Figure 13. Instruments for artificial rupture of the membranes.

Intravenous oxytocin
(*See* Appendix 9, Augmentation of labour.)

Midwife's role
Although the doctor will be responsible for the woman when labour is induced the midwife has a vital role to play in establishing a good rapport with her, and supporting and caring for her throughout what may be a difficult labour. She also has to monitor the condition of both mother and fetus carefully, recognize any deviations from the normal and notify the doctor accordingly. The mother and her partner will also want frequent information about progress and explanations about all procedures carried out. The midwife will deliver the woman if labour results in a spontaneous vertex delivery but, in cases where an operative delivery is necessary, she will prepare and support the mother and her partner, and prepare all the equipment required for delivery and for reception and resuscitation of the baby.

Preterm labour
Preterm labour occurs before the 37th completed week of pregnancy and may be spontaneous or induced. If spontaneous and the membranes are intact, the obstetrician may try to arrest labour by administering tocolytic drugs such as ritodrine hydrochloride (Yutopar) or salbutamol (Ventolin). The midwife's role is:

- to support and care for the mother, and keep both parents informed of progress;
- closely monitor the effect of the tocolytic drug on mother and fetus, and the progress of labour;
- if labour progresses, prepare for a low forceps delivery (Wrigley's forceps) preceded by episiotomy to reduce the risk of intracranial injury;
- prepare a warmed resuscitaire, resuscitation equipment and incubator for the reception of a preterm baby;
- notify the neonatal unit staff of the possible delivery of a preterm baby;
- call the obstetrician and the paediatrician for the delivery.

Malpositions (occipitoposterior positions)
Occipitoposterior positions, also known as malpositions, are cephalic presentations with the occiput directed towards the right or left sacroiliac joint. The positions are therefore right and left occipitoposterior (ROP and LOP). Occipitoposterior positions are the commonest of all the causes of mechanical difficulty in labour.

Cause. No definite cause is known, but it is favoured by abnormal shape of the maternal pelvis. Both android and anthropoid pelves predispose to this position. Frequently the fetus is in an attitude of deficient flexion of the head and spine, and this gives rise to numerous difficulties. It is most troublesome in primigravidae whose good muscles keep the baby's spine in the military attitude and whose contractions may not be efficient enough to cause flexion and descent of the head.

Incidence. It is found in 10 per cent of all pregnancies.

Diagnosis. On inspection, the *abdomen* often appears flattened below the umbilicus. Palpation reveals a high, deflexed head; limbs are felt over a large area of the abdomen, on both sides of the middle line; the back may be felt, with difficulty, in one flank, or it may not be palpable. The fetal heart sounds are heard in the flank and in the middle.

By means of a *vaginal examination* the degree of flexion of the head may be assessed during labour. The head, often high, is palpated with the bregma lying anteriorly or centrally. The posterior fontanelle is usually out of reach.

Dangers. To the mother, prolonged and painful labour (with all its attendant risks), delay in the second stage, difficult and traumatic delivery, and infection. To the child, hypoxia following early rupture of membranes and prolonged labour, and intracranial haemorrhage from abnormal, upward moulding.

Pregnancy. With the head deflexed, the occipitofrontal diameter of 11.5 cm presents instead of the suboccipitobregmatic diameter of 9.5 cm, and the head does not engage easily. This is the commonest of all causes of failure of the head to engage. The midwife should consult the doctor, in order that cephalopelvic disproportion may be excluded.

Labour. In two-thirds of the cases in which the occiput is posterior after the head is engaged, the head flexes, the occiput, meeting the resistance of the pelvic floor makes a long forwards rotation (three-eighths of a circle) and no difficulty is experienced, the child being born in the occipitoanterior position.

In one-third of the cases, flexion remains deficient. The head does not fit the lower uterine segment accurately and liquor is forced into the bag of forewaters, which ruptures early. The ovoid presenting part is a poor dilator, the cervix is not well applied and the stimulus to good contractions is absent. Thus the first stage is long and tedious, with severe backache. The cord may occasionally prolapse and be compressed, causing fetal distress.

In the *second stage*, the mechanism of internal rotation is affected by the following.

1. *Deep transverse arrest.* An attempt at long rotation fails, the head being arrested with its long diameter between the ischial spines, which may be unduly prominent. This condition requires Kielland's forceps rotation and delivery or manual rotation followed by forceps delivery.

2. *Persistent occipitoposterior position.* The sinciput, lying lower than the occiput, is rotated forwards, through one-eighth of a circle to the symphysis pubis, and the occiput turns to the hollow of the sacrum. The head therefore remains deflexed with a wider presenting diameter, the occipitofrontal which measures 11.5 cm. Delay in the second stage commonly occurs and the midwife can help to accelerate progress by encouraging the woman to adopt an upright position such as squatting. With good contractions, the head advances, the root of the nose engages under the pubic arch; the head is then born in a face-to-pubes position. This causes extreme stretching of the pelvic floor and perineal tissues, often with deep lacerations. With poor contractions, no advance occurs. Forceps delivery, usually after rotation of the head through a half circle, is sometimes necessary.

The midwife can help by massaging the woman's back, helping her to find a comfortable position, attending to her needs for adequate hydration, regular micturition, prevention of infection, information about progress and psychological support. Close observation of the fetal and maternal condition and progress in labour is also essential.

The midwife may need to call a doctor for prolongation of the first stage, fetal distress, maternal distress or delay in the second stage, or to resuscitate an asphyxiated baby. Occipitoposterior labours are better conducted in a consultant unit with medical help at hand. It is then possible to offer the mother an epidural analgesia and, in cases of delay, labour may be augmented and carefully monitored.

Malpresentations

Breech presentation

The buttocks lie lowermost in the uterus. Four types are described: the *frank* or *extended breech*, where the thighs are flexed, but the legs extended alongside the trunk, with the feet near the head; the *full* or *flexed breech*, the child sitting tailor-wise, buttocks and feet over the pelvis; and *footling* and *knee presentations*, with foot or knee, respectively, below the buttocks. The frank breech is the commonest type in a primigravida.

Cause. Up to 34 weeks' gestation, a fetus frequently presents by the breech. Extended legs, and also a septate uterus, can prevent the fetus from 'kicking his way round'. In twin pregnancies, frequently one fetus presents by the breech. There may be a serious underlying cause, such as contracted pelvis or placenta praevia.

Incidence. About 2.5 per cent of all deliveries. It is common in earlier pregnancy, but the frequency diminishes as some breeches are turned and many turn spontaneously.

Diagnosis. On *abdominal palpation*, the presenting part is softer and less round and regular than the fetal head, which is felt—hard, round, and ballotable—in the fundus uteri. Often this is an easy diagnosis, but sometimes, especially when the legs are extended and the breech deep in the pelvis, it is very difficult, and confirmation (in pregnancy by sonar and in labour by vaginal examination) is necessary.

On *vaginal examination* the buttocks feel firm, but softer than the head; the anal orific, natal cleft, sacrum, genitalia, and possibly the feet, may be palpable.

Dangers. To the mother there is very little risk.

To the child there is a considerable risk of intracranial haemorrhage from a tear of the tentorium cerebelli, which is submitted to severe strain by the necessarily rapid passage of the after-coming head through the pelvis. The presenting diameter—the occipi frontal—which enters the pelvic brim is larger than if full flexion has occurred, so is vulnerable to rapid abnormal moulding. A lesser but still serious risk is that of hypoxia from compression of the cord, delay in the birth of the head and premature inspiration and inhalation of liquor or meconium. Without expert care there are additional hazards of fractures, dislocations and trauma to abdominal viscera.

Pregnancy. The midwife should refer to a doctor any woman with a breech presentation noted after the 32nd week. To avoid breech labour, the doctor may perform an external cephalic version. This manoeuvre must be gentle, since forceful version—with its risks of rupture of membranes, preterm labour, separation of the placenta and antepartum haemorrhage—is even more dangerous than breech delivery. Because of the risks, and the tendency for the fetus to return to its original presentation, there has been a decline in this practice.

Labour. The woman should be in hospital and, since a head fitting is not possible, antenatal X-ray pelvimetry is carried out. Even with a minor degree of contracted pelvis, caesarean section is preferable to breech delivery. A doctor is normally responsible for the woman in labour with a breech presentation and he or she conducts the delivery. In an emergency when there is no doctor present the midwife takes responsibility and therefore must have sound knowledge of the management of a breech delivery.

The *first stage* differs little from the normal. When the membranes rupture, a vaginal examination is necessary to exclude—or diagnose—prolapse of the cord, which is a particular hazard in the flexed and footling types of breech. The mother must be discouraged from 'pushing', which, in a frank breech, might be initiated by the small presenting part slipping through the incompletely dilated cervix; otherwise the arms and head may become extended, with consequent delay. Nowadays it is common practice to offer an epidural anaesthesia to women in labour with a breech presentation because it solves the problem of premature pushing and is suitable for operative delivery.

The *second stage* is conducted with the mother in the lithotomy position. In a primigravida, an episiotomy should be performed as the anterior buttock is born. This minimizes compression later on the baby's head. The feet are guided over the perineum, a loop of cord is pulled down to prevent traction on the umbilicus, and cord tone and time are noted; if the arms are flexed, the shoulders are born with the next contraction. Extended arms are delivered by the *Lövset manoeuvre*. For this, the baby's whole body is gently held and the trunk is rotated through a half circle, back upwards, bringing the posterior shoulder to the front of the pelvis, whence it is easily released. The trunk is then similarly rotated in the reverse direction, bringing back the shoulder which was originally anterior, to be freed in the same way.

The child is now allowed to hang by his own weight for about 1 minute (*Burns–Marshall manoeuvre*) to aid flexion and descent of the head. When the hair line appears at the vulva, the head is at the outlet, ready for delivery. This is effected by raising the trunk (holding the child by the ankles and exerting slight traction) and carrying it through a wide arc up and over the mother's abdomen. The perineum is retracted, exposing the child's mouth and nose, permitting the airway to be cleared and oxygen to be given, while the birth of the head is completed very slowly, usually with the aid of obstetric forceps to the after-coming head.

If the head is extended and fails to descend, delivery may be effected by the *Mauriceau–Smellie–Veit manoeuvre* of the jaw flexion and shoulder traction. This method allows far better control over the delivery of the head than does the Burns–Marshall in cases where forceps delivery is not possible.

The *third stage* is usually short, the placenta having separated during the slow birth of the head.

A paediatrician should be present at delivery to resuscitate the baby since birth asphyxia is a common complication.

Face presentation
This is a cephalic presentation, with complete extension of the head and spine.

Cause. Sometimes in an occipitoposterior labour the deficient flexion increases as the biparietal diameter (BPD) gets caught on the sacrocotyloid diameter until the head is extended. An android pelvis may favour this. Fetal abnormalities such as anencephaly also cause face presentation.

Incidence. Approximately 1 labour in 500.

Diagnosis. Abdominal examination is inconclusive, and the diagnosis is usually made in labour, when vaginal examination reveals the mouth and alveolar margins, and the orbital ridges.

Dangers. For the mother, though labour is often easy, it can present serious difficulty and, in mentoposterior positions, may become obstructed.
To the child, there is some risk of trauma to the facial tissues.

Labour. The midwife, if she suspects a face presentation should consult a doctor. In a mentoanterior position, labour may be easy, the chin rotating forwards through 45° (an eighth of a circle) to escape under the pubic arch and the head being born by flexion; episiotomy is essential to prevent undue trauma to the pelvic floor as the sub-mentovertical diameter passes through the vaginal orifice. With the chin posterior, long rotation is not easy and there is a risk of persistent mentoposterior position with complete obstruction. To avoid this, the doctor would attempt manually to rotate the head to bring the chin forwards, and complete the delivery with forceps. In a primigravida, delivery by caesarean section would be preferable.
The infant's face is so markedly bruised and oedematous that the mother should be told of its state and reassured that it will quickly improve, as she sees the baby.

Brow presentation
The head presents partially extended, with the mentovertical diameter of 13.5 cm attempting to enter the 13.0 cm transverse diameter of the pelvic brim.

Cause. The causes are those of face presentation.

Incidence. It is rare: hardly ever seen in pregnancy, and occurring once in about 1000–1500 labours.

Diagnosis. Abdominal examination reveals that the presenting head is very high; it feels unusually large. Vaginally, the presenting part is often too high to palpate. If not, the diagnostic features are the bregma and the orbital ridges.

Dangers. It is always dangerous, since, with fetus and pelvis of normal size, labour *must* become obstructed. Only with a very small fetus and an ample pelvis can delivery occur.

A midwife suspecting this condition should send an urgent message for a doctor, and the mother, if at home, should immediately be transferred to hospital.

The best treatment, especially for a primigravida, is caesarean section. In areas where this is not feasible it may be possible by vaginal manipulation to flex the head so that the vertex presents, or to extend it further, into a face presentation, and then apply forceps. Failing this, and without hospital facilities, delivery may be affected by internal podalic version and breech extraction.

Transverse lie and shoulder presentation

A transverse or oblique lie in pregnancy will, if not corrected, become a shoulder presentation in labour. This in turn may lead to prolapse of the cord and/or the fetal arm, and it will cause obstructed labour.

Cause of transverse lie. Most commonly this is lax abdominal and uterine muscle, in a multigravida. It sometimes occurs in twin pregnancy, placenta praevia or a contracted pelvis.

Diagnosis. This is generally easy. On abdominal inspection, the uterus is typically broad and asymmetrical, with the fundus low for the period of amenorrhoea. On palpation, the head is usually felt in the flank or in the iliac fossa.

Management. The midwife should consult a doctor about any unstable or transverse lie persisting after the 30th week of pregnancy.

The lie is corrected by external cephalic version every time it is seen during antenatal examination. If the lie is not stable by the 37th week, the mother is admitted to hospital for observation. The lie can then be corrected at any time and particularly at the onset of labour. Sometimes the lie is corrected and the membranes are ruptured, to stabilize the fetus and to induce labour (stabilizing induction). This prevents the development of shoulder presentation.

If a serious cause, such as placenta praevia, is found, delivery is effected by caesarean section.

Shoulder presentation. On abdominal examination the uterus appears broad and the fundal height is less than expected for the period of gestation. On vaginal examination, if the presenting part is not too high, the fetal ribs (which are quite distinctive) are palpated; an arm may have prolapsed into the vagina.

If this emergency occurs in domiciliary practice, a midwife should summon an obstetric 'flying squad'. The mother should be transferred to hospital for an emergency caesarean section or, in parts of the world where this is unsafe or not possible, an internal podalic version and breech extraction would be carried out on a live fetus, and possibly a destructive operation on a dead fetus. These latter procedures may cause uterine rupture thus are highly dangerous for the mother.

Obstructed labour

Obstructed labour is a rare condition in which there is an insuperable barrier to the passage of the child, so that, in spite of good uterine contractions, there is no advance of the presenting part. This may be because the mother's pelvis is grossly contracted, because the available space is encroached upon by a large tumour, or because of a shoulder or brow presentation, a persistent mentoposterior position or a fetal abnormality such as hydrocephalus.

With adequate care in pregnancy and early labour this condition is largely preventable. Thus it is rare in the United Kingdom, but it is bound to be seen from time to time in any country where good midwifery services are not available.

In the advanced state the mother is in great distress, and looks anxious and ill. Her pulse rate is much increased and her temperature probably raised. Her urine is scanty and loaded with ketones. Her tongue is coated, sores appear on her lips, vomiting may occur and there is persistent severe abdominal pain.

The uterus appears 'moulded' around the fetus; on palpation it is continuously hard (tonic reaction) and fetal parts cannot be felt. This extreme retraction causes fetal death from anoxia and therefore the fetal heart sounds cannot be heard; Bandl's reaction ring may be observed as a ridge running obliquely across the abdomen and marks the junction between the grossly thickened upper segment, and the dangerously thinned and overstretched lower segment of the uterus.

Vaginal examination may reveal, hot, dry, oedematous vaginal walls, a high presenting part with considerable caput formation, and with a thick 'curtain' of cervix hanging around and below it.

At this stage a multigravid patient is in imminent danger of death from exhaustion or from rupture of the uterus. More favourably, the primigravid uterus may cease to contract (secondary uterine inertia), allowing a little time in which to consider treatment.

Long before this the woman's pulse rate would have increased steadily and ketonuria would be present. Whatever the cause of this, a midwife should call a doctor when it is first noted. This cannot be emphasized too strongly.

In a neglected case first seen in the advanced state, the midwife should send urgently for medical aid and administer an injection of pethidine 100–150 mg to relieve severe pain. Blood is taken for crossmatching and an intravenous infusion is started to treat dehydration and shock. In hospital the treatment is immediate caesarean section to deliver the fetus whether alive or dead. Only if this is not possible are manipulative or destructive procedures carried out because such treatments carry a very high risk of rupturing the thinned, overstretched lower uterine segment.

Presentation and prolapse of the umbilical cord

Presentation of the cord means that it lies below the presenting part of the fetus when the membranes are intact. Once the membranes rupture the cord is described as prolapsed. This is an extremely dangerous condition as the cord will be compressed between the presenting part and maternal pelvis, especially during contractions, thereby impeding the oxygen supply to the fetus.

Diagnosis. This is made by noting fetal distress when auscultating the fetal heart and making a vaginal examination following rupture of the membranes to detect the presence of cord. In some cases it is visible at the vulva.

Management. This depends on whether the fetus is alive and on the stage of labour. In the first stage the mother is placed in the exaggerated Sim's position with the foot of the bed raised to try and relieve pressure on the cord. The midwife may introduce two fingers into the vagina and push the presenting part away from the cord, especially during contractions. If the cord is outside the vagina it is gently replaced, if possible, or covered warmly to prevent spasm. The fetal heart is monitored closely, the mother given oxygen to inhale and prepared for emergency caesarean section. In the second stage, delivery is expedited, if imminent, by encouraging the mother to push and by making an episiotomy; otherwise an emergency forceps delivery is performed or, if the presenting part is high, a caesarean section may be necessary.

References

Morrin N (1985) The second stage. *Nursing Mirror* **161**(3): S7–S11.
Skelton SWK (1984) The second stage of labour—Do we clock watch? *Midwives' Chronicle* July: 212–213.

APPENDIX 10

Episiotomy, Perineal Repair and Operative Deliveries

Episiotomy
See the dictionary entry for the definition and details.

Perineal repair
Midwives who have received instruction, have been supervised in the technique of repair of the perineum, and pronounced proficient may now undertake this procedure for the repair of first and second degree tears and episiotomies.

Principles
1. The repair should be carried out as soon after delivery as possible.
2. A good light is essential to identify the apex of the episiotomy.
3. Adequate analgesia, using 15–20 ml of 1 per cent lignocaine if an epidural is not topped up.
4. Lithotomy is the best position.
5. A tampon is inserted into the vault of the vagina to prevent blood obscuring the area being sutured.

Procedure (*see* Figures 14 *and* 15)
The perineum is closed in three layers.

1. The vagina is sutured, commencing just above the apex of the incision. Interrupted sutures are most commonly used.
2. Deep and superficial muscle layers are next sutured. Some authorities suggest starting in the centre of the incision to give good approximation. The suturing of this layer should restore the efficient functioning of the pelvic floor.
3. Perineal skin is finally sutured.
4. Remove the tampon.
5. A gloved finger should then be passed into the rectum to ensure that no sutures encroach into it.

Forceps delivery
Forceps delivery is a method of extracting the fetal head using obstetric forceps and is one of the commonest obstetric operations carried out in the United Kingdom. The main indications are:

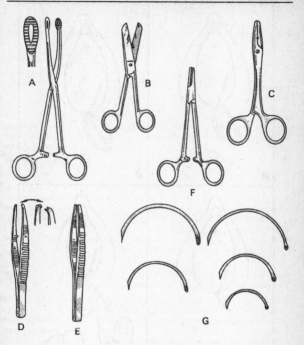

A. *Sponge-holding forceps*; B. *blunt-ended scissors*; C. *needle holder*; D. *toothed dissecting forceps*; E. *non-toothed dissecting forceps*; F. *small Spencer Wells artery forceps*; G. *needles*: left, *round-bodied Nos. 8 and 12*; right, *cutting, Nos. 6, 8 and 12. A traumatic needle 40 mm on Dexon suture now commonly used.*

Figure 14. Instruments for perineal repair.

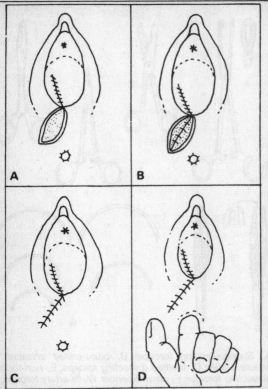

A. *Vagina sutured with continuous catgut*; B. *muscle layer sutured with interrupted catgut*; C. *perineal skin sutured with interrupted catgut or silk*; D. *rectal examination to exclude rectal involvement*.

Figure 15. PERINEAL REPAIR (COMMONLY USED METHOD).

1. Delay in the second stage of labour which could be caused by poor uterine contractions, deep transverse arrest or persistent occipitoposterior position.
2. Fetal or maternal distress.
3. To avoid undue exertion in conditions such as severe hypertension or cardiac disease.
4. To reduce the risk of intracranial injury in the birth of a preterm baby, or the after-coming head of a breech.

Conditions necessary for a forceps delivery:
1. Os uteri fully dilated.
2. Ruptured membranes.
3. No cephalopelvic disproportion.
4. Normal uterine action.
5. Fetal head engaged and position identified.
6. Bladder empty.

Role of the midwife
1. The midwife can be a great source of support and comfort to the mother and her partner in what is a frightening method of delivery for them. During the delivery the midwife should be close to the mother where she can have eye to eye contact, hold her hand and keep her informed of progress. This close contact together with clear, ongoing explanations, encouragement and praise can transform a frightening situation into a more positive experience for the mother and her partner.
2. Preparation of equipment for delivery which will include:

> delivery pack;
> obstetric forceps;
> episiotomy scissors;
> equipment for perineal repair;
> analgesia;
> resuscitation equipment for the baby;
> oxytocic drug.

3. Monitor the fetal and maternal condition.
4. The midwife, together with an assistant, will carefully place the woman in the lithotomy position for the delivery.
5. Call a paediatrician to receive and resuscitate the baby, if required.
6. Assist with the administration of inhalational analgesia to the mother, if required.
7. Assist the doctor, as necessary.

Anaesthesia

A pudendal nerve block or epidural analgesia is usually adequate. General anaesthesia is rarely used because of the danger of MENDELSON'S SYNDROME. Inhalational analgesia (Entonox) may also be used if the mother wishes.

Types of obstetric forceps (see Figure 16)

Wrigley's forceps are small, light and have a short shank. They are used to 'lift out' a head which is on the perineum and, sometimes, to apply to the after-coming head of a breech. Kielland's forceps have no pelvic curve and a sliding lock and can be applied to a head in any position in the pelvis (e.g. in the transverse diameter). The forceps are then used to rotate the head until it is directly occipitoanterior, when it can be extracted. Axis-traction forceps were designed to permit traction in the axis of the birth canal. There are several varieties, the Neville–Barnes, Haig Ferguson and Milne Murray types being popular. The blades have a pelvic curve which fits into the curve of the sacrum (thus the fetal head must be occipitoanterior), and the forceps have an extra handle, originally designed for the correct application of traction, but now rarely used.

The mother is placed in the lithotomy position and the obstetrician introduces, first, the left blade and, second, the right blade; only thus will the forceps lock accurately. Traction is exerted gently, and, coinciding with uterine contractions, the fetal head is brought down to the perineum, an episiotomy is performed and the head is brought down to the point of 'crowning', when the forceps blades are removed and the delivery is completed.

In the UK, forceps delivery is normally carried out by a doctor but, in some parts of the world, midwives carry out this procedure.

Ventouse extraction

The Malmström vacuum extractor (*see* Figure 17) or ventouse is a simple suction apparatus sometimes used as an alternative to the obstetric forceps. It can also be employed towards the end of the first stage, to hasten dilatation of the cervix.

The apparatus consists of a metal or plastic cup, narrower at the rim, to which are attached a chain and handle, for traction, and a pump. The cup is made in three sizes, the smaller two for application in the first stage. The cup is applied closely to the fetal head and the pump is used to create a vacuum of 0.8 kg/cm^2. This is done gradually, over about 10 minutes. The fetal scalp is drawn into the cup in the form of an artificially induced caput. Traction is then exerted, coinciding with uterine contractions, and the head gradually descends through the pelvic cavity and outlet and is born. The vacuum is then released and the

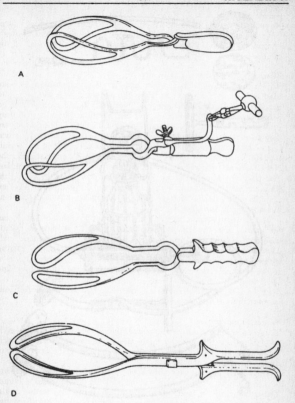

A. *Wrigley's*; B. *axis-traction*; C. *Anderson's*; D. *Kielland's*.

Figure 16. OBSTETRIC FORCEPS.

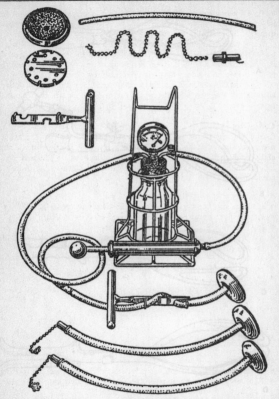

Figure 17. Malmström vacuum extractor, showing the vacuum pump and three sizes of cup; chain and handle, and components of the extraction pump.

infant is seen to have a large oedematous bruised swelling, known, from its appearance, as a 'chignon' on the scalp. The swelling subsides quickly, the discoloration more slowly.

Ventouse extraction can be carried out under pudendal block analgesia or epidural anaesthesia. Since it takes longer than forceps delivery, it is not used where rapid delivery is necessary (e.g. in fetal distress). Nor is it suitable in malpresentations or in preterm labour.

The midwife's role is similar to that described for forceps delivery, although in some parts of the world the midwife herself carries out this procedure.

Caesarean section

Caesarean section is an operation whereby the fetus, placenta and membranes are delivered from the uterus through incisions made in the abdominal and uterine walls, after the 28th week of pregnancy. The incidence in the UK is now about 11% of all births. The indications are:

- cephalopelvic disproportion;
- placenta praevia if grade 3 or 4 and sometimes grade 2;
- abruptio placentae (moderate or severe if fetus is alive);
- fetal distress in the first stage of labour;
- malpresentations such as brow, posterior face, shoulder and often breech presentations;
- failure to progress in labour;
- severe pregnancy-induced hypertension;
- eclampsia;
- intrauterine growth retardation;
- poor obstetric history;
- diabetes (in some cases).

Midwife's role

Preparation of the mother:
- Support and explanation are given to the mother and her partner.
- Skin preparation: pubic shaving may be required and, if an elective LSCS, the mother has a shower or bath.
- Bowel preparation: the night before an elective lower segment caesarean section (LSCS) it is usual to give two glycerin suppositories.
- Clothing and removal of jewellery: the mother is dressed in a back-fastening operation gown and all other clothing and jewellery are removed, apart from the wedding ring which should be taped in position.

- Dentures and contact lenses must be removed.
- An antacid preparation such as sodium citrate or mist magnesium trisilicate to render the gastric juices alkaline is given as prescribed to reduce the risk of Mendelson's syndrome.
- Premedication as prescribed by the anaesthetist is given.
- A urinary catheter is passed, the bladder emptied and the catheter spigotted and left *in situ*.
- Blood is taken for cross-matching and haemoglobin estimation.
- Consent for operation should be obtained by the doctor.

Preparation of equipment:
- Intravenous infusion.
- Cross-matched blood available.
- Anaesthetic trolley and/or equipment for epidural anaesthesia.
- General laparotomy set.
- Obstetric forceps (usually small Wrigley's forceps).
- Ergometrine 0.5 mg drawn up in syringe and further supply of oxytocic drugs.
- Resuscitation equipment for the baby.
- Incubator plugged into heat.

The partner may accompany the mother to the theatre and stay with her if she is having an epidural anaesthesia. A midwife should be free of other duties to stay with the couple to give support, comfort and information. Another midwife should be available to receive the baby and assist the paediatrician if resuscitative measures are required.

Immediately before the operation the spigot is removed from the indwelling urinary catheter and it is left to drain freely.

Operative procedure
The skin is cleansed and after the abdomen is suitably draped, a vertical midline incision is made extending from the umbilicus to the symphysis pubis, or a transverse (Pfannenstiel) incision just above the symphysis pubis, the rectus muscles are separated and the peritoneum is opened. The front of the lower segment of the uterus appears in the wound and is recognized by the loosely attached peritoneum covering it. This is divided by a curved incision, concave upwards, about 10 cm in length, and the lower edge of the peritoneum and the bladder are displaced downwards by a gauze swab. The myometrium of the lower segment is then similarly incised. The membranes which bulge in the wound are ruptured and the fetus is then extracted. If the presentation is by the vertex delivery of the head through the incision, it is aided by the application of fundal pressure. The cord is clamped and cut, and the baby is placed quickly in a warmed cot or on a Resuscitaire or, provided

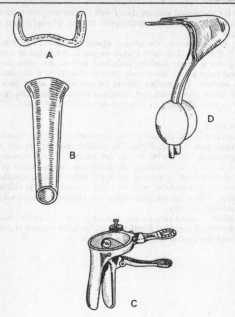

A. *Sim's*; B. *Fergusson's*; C. *Cusco's*; D. *Auvard's*.

Figure 18. VARIOUS SPECULA.

its condition is good, given directly to the mother. The placenta and membranes are then extracted from the uterus and inspected to see if they are complete. The uterus is massaged to encourage retraction, and 0.5 mg of ergometrine may be given intravenously. The uterine wall is then closed, first by a row of interrupted catgut sutures and then by a continuous catgut stitch. The peritoneum covering the lower segment is closed by a second continuous catgut suture and, after the swabs are counted and found to be correct, the peritoneum and anterior rectus sheath of the abdominal wall are closed with continuous catgut, the skin edges being approximated by interrupted sutures, Michel's clips or a subcuticular stitch.

During the puerperium the mother should be allowed up from the first day if she is fit. The baby should be put to the breast as soon as possible if she is breast feeding. Help and support are given so that mother and baby get to know each other as quickly as if the delivery has been normal. The mother should be encouraged at all times to undertake active movements and breathing exercises, and not remain immobile in bed. She may go home on about the 4th–6th day.

Symphysiotomy

Symphysiotomy is the incision of the fibrocartilage of the symphysis pubis through part of its thickness. The bladder must be emptied prior to this procedure, otherwise it may be injured. Symphysiotomy is performed in labour and enlarges the transverse measurements of the pelvis. It is carried out in areas of the world where caesarean section is not possible, or is associated with very high mortality, or is culturally unacceptable. Following symphysiotomy the vacuum extractor may be used to facilitate delivery.

After delivery, broad strapping is applied around the pelvis and the legs may be bound together. A self-retaining catheter remains *in situ* for 4–5 days and the mother is nursed on her side.

APPENDIX 11

Complications of the Third Stage and Obstetric Shock

Postpartum haemorrhage (PPH)

Definition: Excessive bleeding from the genital tract at any time from the birth of the child up to the end of the puerperium (usually 6 weeks).

Primary postpartum haemorrhage: This occurs within the first 24 hours following the delivery of the baby.

Secondary postpartum haemorrhage: This occurs after the first 24 hours and up to 6 weeks after the birth of the baby.

The amount of blood loss which constitutes a primary postpartum haemorrhage is usually considered to be 500 ml or more, but a lesser amount which adversely affects the mothers condition is also recognized as a PPH.

Cause of primary PPH
This is mainly the failure of the uterus to contract and retract and therefore bleeding occurs from the placental site. Cases when this most commonly occurs include:

- multiparous women;
- multiple births;
- polyhydramnios;
- prolonged and difficult labour;
- general anaesthesia;
- following antepartum haemorrhage;
- previous postpartum haemorrhage;
- anaemic and debilitated women who are less likely to withstand blood loss;
- women with fibroids;
- retained products of conception;
- mismanagement of the third stage, including a full bladder.

Some of these factors can be avoided by good antenatal care and careful conduct of labour, but others are unavoidable. In any case where a postpartum haemorrhage might be anticipated, delivery in a consultant unit is planned.

Whatever the circumstances of postpartum haemorrhage, the midwife should call a doctor as quickly as possible. In severe haemorrhage occurring in the patient's home she should herself call an obstetric 'flying squad', where this service is available.

Management

The aim is to arrest haemorrhage as soon as possible, the objectives being: 1. to help the uterus to contract firmly; and then 2. deliver the placenta if still *in situ*.

Method

1. Call a skilled obstetrician, or the 'flying squad' if there is one in the community.
2. Repeat or give an initial dose of an oxytocic drug. Intravenous ergometrine 0.5 mg acts in 40 seconds but if the midwife is inexperienced, rather than waste time, it is better to give intramuscular Syntometrine 1 ml containing 5 units oxytocin and 0.5 mg ergometrine. This will be effective in 2½ minutes.
3. Lightly massage the fundus of the uterus to encourage further contraction of the uterus and expel clots if the placenta and membranes are delivered.
4. Catheterize the bladder.
5. When the uterus is well contracted, attempt controlled cord traction (CCT).
6. Prepare equipment ready for the doctor to erect an infusion of oxytocin (Syntocinon), and to remove the placenta manually if it is still undelivered. Take blood for cross-matching before the veins collapse.
7. In the rare case when no doctor is available and the uterus is uncontracted despite the placenta being delivered, bimanual compression of the uterus will be life-saving.

Manual removal. A midwife working in a region with no medical assistance or hospital available will have to manage the entire case unaided. In these circumstances she should, as early as possible (and before the patient's condition deteriorates), carry out a manual removal of placenta, which is performed as follows:

1. Spread antiseptic cream quickly over the gloved right hand.
2. Introduce the hand in the vagina and follow up the umbilical cord to the uterus and placenta, supporting the uterus through the abdominal wall with the left hand.

3. Find the separated part of the placenta, peel off the remainder and withdraw it from the uterus.
4. If bleeding continues, immediately apply bimanual compression.

In an emergency, this procedure may have to be carried out without anaesthesia, but it should stop the bleeding. The risk of inducing shock by performing a manual removal is greater when no anaesthetic is given.

Traumatic haemorrhage
This uncommon form may be recognized by the time of occurrence and by its continuance in spite of good uterine contraction. The bleeding starts as the baby is delivered. It may be from the cervix, vaginal walls or perineal body. It is treated by applying direct pressure to the bleeding point with pad, artery forceps or sponge-holding forceps, or by digital pressure until lacerations can be sutured.

Secondary haemorrhage
This occurs in association with retention of placental tissue and/or sepsis. If the uterus is palpable abdominally (often it is subinvoluted) massage may be of value. Intravenous ergometrine 0.5 mg may be given, but it is of doubtful value. Retained products are detected by ultasound. If they are present, an evacuation of retained products (ERPC) is carried out under anaesthesia.

Coagulation disorders
These occur in some cases of severe abruptio placentae, intrauterine death, endotoxic shock and, rarely, amniotic fluid embolism. All labile clotting factors are reduced; fibrinogen is low and there is THROMBOCYTOPENIA. Profuse bleeding occurs and it will be noted that the blood fails to clot. Medical aid must be summoned urgently and immediate action is taken to maintain the blood volume. Investigations include cross-matching, full blood count, prothrombin time and clotting time, platelet counts and fibrinogen and fibrinogen degradation products (FDP). Fresh blood is obtained and transfused as soon as possible. Until it is available fresh frozen plasma, platelet concentrates and packed red cells will be transfused.

Acute inversion of the uterus
This is a rare, but serious complication of the third stage when the uterus becomes partly or wholly turned inside out.

Causes:
1. Mismanagement of the third stage, by exerting pressure on the

fundus and/or traction on the cord when the uterus is relaxed. It is particularly likely to occur when the placenta is situated in the uterine fundus.
2. Spontaneous occurrence associated with uterine atony and a sudden increase in the intra-abdominal pressure such as occurs with coughing, sneezing or a straining effort.

Diagnosis:
1. Sudden, profound shock accompanied by severe abdominal pain.
2. Bleeding if the placenta is partially or wholly separated.
3. Palpation of a concave-shaped fundus in the abdomen or no uterus felt at all if the inversion is complete.
4. Palpation of the uterus in the cervix or vagina.
5. Uterus visible at the vulva.

Management: Urgent medical assistance is called. Meanwhile the midwife raises the foot of the bed to relieve tension and alleviate shock and attempts to replace the placenta by applying pressure to the lower segment near the cervix and working upwards to the fundus. If replacement of a totally inverted uterus is not possible it should be gently placed inside the vagina to reduce traction on the fallopian tubes and ovaries.

Severe shock is treated by an intravenous infusion and blood is cross-matched. A narcotic drug such as morphine 15 mg is given to relieve pain. Once shock is treated the mother is given a general anaesthetic and the uterus is replaced manually or by the hydrostatic method. In the latter method several litres of warm sterile fluid such as saline are run into the posterior vaginal fornix through a douche nozzle and the operator's forearm is placed over the vaginal outlet to effect a seal. The fluid pressure in the vagina pushes the uterine fundus up until it resumes a normal position. An intravenous injection of ergometrine 0.25 to 0.5 mg is then given to cause the uterus to contract and control bleeding.

If all attempts to replace the uterus fail, a hysterectomy will be necessary.

Shock
Shock is collapse due to circulatory failure. There are two varieties of shock which can occur during pregnancy, or, more commonly, after delivery: haemorrhagic (hypovolaemic) and non-haemorrhagic.

Main causes
1. Haemorrhage, ante or post partum, is the commonest cause.
2. Uterine causes include inversion or rupture.
3. Acid aspiration syndrome.
4. Pulmonary embolism.
5. Amniotic fluid embolism.
6. Hypotension caused by regional anaesthesia or as a result of drug reaction.
7. Endotoxic shock caused by septicaemia.

Clinical signs
The blood pressure falls and the pulse rate rises—although these do not always occur immediately and may not be particularly noticeable, especially when the woman has had pre-eclampsia, until the condition becomes serious. The CENTRAL VENOUS PRESSURE (CVP) is a more reliable guide. The skin may be cold and clammy as well as white, and air hunger occurs when the condition is severe.

Management
Urgent resuscitative measures are necessary before the condition becomes irreversible. The principles underlying the treatment, whatever the cause of the shock are:

1. Maintainance of an airway.
2. Administration of intravenous fluids to increase the blood volume. Until cross-matched blood is available, plasma substitutes can be given. Physiological saline is of use as a temporary measure only. The volume of fluid needed can only be estimated by the use of a CVP line; otherwise insufficient or excess fluids may be given.
3. Raising the foot of the bed (except in late pregnancy, when this embarrasses the respiration). The woman should be nursed on her side to prevent the uterus pressing on to the vena cava, which would increase the shock.
4. A sedative may be ordered. The woman should be kept as quiet and undisturbed as possible.
5. Administration of oxygen, especially if dyspnoea is present.
6. Avoidance of overheating the patient. The cold pale skin is evidence that the body's defence mechanism is at work. The superficial arterioles and capillaries have contracted in order to direct the blood to essential parts of the body—i.e. the heart, brain and kidneys.

Non-haemorrhagic shock

Endotoxic shock. This occurs when there is a serious infection by Gram-negative organisms, especially *Escherichia coli* and *Clostridium welchii*. There is a widespread dilatation of arterioles so that the venous return is diminished and shock occurs. The signs are similar to hypovolaemic shock but sometimes rigors occur too. The infection must be treated urgently with the appropriate antibiotics.

Transfusion fluids

Fresh blood. This is particularly useful in cases of active sepsis or haemolytic disease because the cells will not have undergone change.

Stored blood. This is stored at 4°C and may be kept for up to 3 weeks. A slight reaction is likely at the end of this period. It is particularly useful for all emergency cases of haemorrhage (e.g. antepartum or postpartum haemorrhage).

Packed cells. A proportion of the plasma is removed by pipette and this means that haemolysis of the cells takes place much more readily. Fresh blood must be used and transfused into the patient within 24 hours. It is given when it is desired to increase the number of cells without overloading the circulation with fluid, as sometimes in exchange and intraperitoneal transfusion.

Plasma. Dried plasma is supplied in one bottle and in a companion bottle is distilled water for reconstituting the plasma. The blood that becomes out of date at the blood bank makes a good source of supply. It is stored at room temperature and is useful in the treatment of shock and to increase the plasma proteins.

Infusion fluids

An infusion is the introduction of fluid into the circulation by any route other than the mouth. The most common route is the intravenous one. The fluids are all used to combat dehydration and maintain the body's electrolyte and water balance.

Physiological saline. This is an infusion fluid given intravenously which is only of temporary value in shock and haemorrhage, as it is quickly lost into the tissues.

Dextrose saline. This is used in varying strengths, sometimes with the addition of other substances, to correct a state of ketoacidosis.

Ringer's solution. This is an isotonic solution containing salts of sodium, potassium and calcium. It is not used as often as saline solution or Hartmann's.

Hartmann's solution. This is Ringer's solution with lactic acid added.

Dextran saline intravenous (Intradex, Dextraven). This is a plasma substitute in which the dextran molecules remain in the circulation a long time and so exert osmotic pressure. It is useful in the treatment of shock where there is no blood loss. A sample of blood should be obtained before the infusion, since afterwards there is rouleaux formation of the red blood cells which interferes with cross-matching.

Exchange transfusion

An exchange or replacement transfusion may be carried out when a Rhesus-positive infant born to a Rhesus-negative mother is seriously affected by this blood incompatibility (*see* Appendix 17).

A syringe with a three-way tap may be used. Alternatively, the donor blood may be set up to drip through a tube introduced into the umbilical vein while a second tube introduced into one umbilical artery carries the blood which is to be discarded, set to drip at the same rate.

APPENDIX 12

Postnatal Care and Family Planning

Postnatal care

The puerperium

The puerperium starts with the completion of labour and lasts until the reproductive organs have returned to their pre-gravid state, usually a period of 6–8 weeks. During this time certain physiological changes take place:

1. Involution of the uterus and other soft parts of the genital tract.
2. Secretion of breast milk.
3. Physiological changes in all other systems of the body which are affected by pregnancy.

Postnatal care

Postnatal period means a period of not less than 10 or not more than 28 days after the end of labour, during which the continued attendance of a midwife on the mother and baby is requisite (UKCC, 1991).

Most mothers are now transferred home from hospital between 6 hours and 3 days after delivery, thus the majority of postnatal care takes place in the community. The midwife's role in postnatal care is to:

- monitor the mother's psychological and emotional condition, and give support;
- monitor the mother and baby's physical condition, and give midwifery care and appropriate advice;
- educate the mother with regards to her own health and in the care of her baby, thereby building up her confidence and competence;
- assist with the establishment of feeding.

Psychological and emotional care

The midwife has a major role in giving psychological support during the postnatal period. Many women become very anxious about the care of their baby and minor problems are magnified, especially when the mother is overtired and/or the baby is fretful or has a problem such as jaundice. About 60% of women develop the 'blues' sometime between the third and tenth day. They become overwhelmed by feelings of tearfulness, inadequacy and often a feeling of panic. A caring, understanding and competent midwife can help the mother through this difficult period and most recover within 24 hours or so.

Physical care

Most healthy women following a normal delivery are ambulant within an hour or two of the birth for toilet and washing purposes. They are encouraged to empty their bladder soon after delivery and should have a bowel action within 2 or 3 days, with the help of an aperient such as Senokot, if required. High standards of hygiene to prevent infection are essential, thus the mother is encouraged to use a bidet after using the toilet, change her pads frequently and have a shower or bath once or twice a day. Adequate rest and sleep are required and a good nourishing diet is encouraged.

Daily observations and recordings

1. Psychological and emotional condition, including reaction to the baby and ability to cope.
2. General well-being, such as whether well-rested, eating well and socializing normally.
3. Temperature and pulse rate to detect signs of infection.
4. Blood pressure only if there is a special indication such as hypertension or haemorrhage.
5. Urinary output, and any problems such as frequency and dysuria.
6. Bowel action.
7. Breasts, including the condition of the nipples and areola, amount and flow of milk, signs of infection or blocked ducts.
8. Involution of the uterus which should progress daily until no longer palpable by about the tenth postnatal day. Autolysis (self-digestion) and ischaemia are the processes which bring about involution. The uterus may be displaced by a full bladder or a full rectum. Actual subinvolution may result from uterine infection and/or from retention of placental tissue.
9. Lochia, noting the amount, colour, consistency and odour. It is normally bright red and fairly profuse for 2 or 3 days, red-brown and diminishing for 3 days, and then scanty becoming brown and then almost colourless, during the next 3 or 4 days. Slight losses of bright red blood occur intermittently during the first 3 weeks, generally coinciding with breast feeding or increased exercise. Profuse lochia after the third day, or offensive lochia at any time, is abnormal and may signify infection.
10. Perineum, if sutured, to observe oedema, bruising, healing and signs of infection.

11. Legs for signs of oedema, inflammation and/or pain which could be associated with superficial or deep vein thrombosis.

Haemoglobin. This is normally checked within a few days of delivery to diagnose anaemia and iron supplements are prescribed, if necessary.

Postnatal exercises

Postnatal exercises include deep breathing and leg exercises if the woman is in bed, and exercises for the pelvic floor, abdominal muscles and improved posture. Pelvic floor exercises are particularly important as many women suffer from stress incontinence, hence these exercises should be carried out several times daily for at least 6–8 weeks after delivery.

'Bonding'—mother/baby relationship

When a baby is born, the mother does not automatically 'take to' or love the new arrival. Love at first sight is very rare. The formation of a permanent attachment, or 'bonding', is preceded by acquaintance.

1. Acquaintance. A mother becomes familiar with her baby by feeling, looking, examining and hearing him/her. The baby also uses its senses by looking, hearing, feeling and smelling its mother, thus soon recognizing her. As they stimulate each other and respond, the relationship becomes firmer.
2. Attachment occurs after they have become acquainted, when both recognize each other and expect certain behaviour as one responds to the other.
3. 'Bonding'. A permanent relationship then develops, and, even if the baby is separated from the mother, it will not be damaged. The development of this relationship is a fluid one and can be adversely affected. If either participant does not respond in the expected way, the attachment can diminish, as in the case of a baby who is handicapped. This may lead to rejection by the mother and/or father. A baby who is in the intensive care unit amongst an imposing array of equipment, does not immediately appeal to the mother. Instead she may be frightened and feel guilty. Even when encouraged, getting to known the baby by feeling and examining is difficult. The baby is also unable to respond, so attachment is often delayed. This may be one of the factors leading to NON-ACCIDENTAL INJURY when the baby goes home (*see* Appendix 17).

Health education and parentcraft teaching

The mother is advised about the care of her own health and about the care of her baby. As well as teaching the mother the basic principles of physical care such as good hygiene, prevention of infection and feeding, the midwife also encourages the mother to get to know her baby, to talk to him and to give him love and a sense of security. The midwife helps the mother make her own decisions about the care of her baby by talking through the various options with her. This strategy not only helps to increase the mother's confidence, but also reduces the problem of conflicting advice.

In some cases postnatal support groups have been established where mothers can meet together for company and discuss any problems. A network of support for some months after the birth of a baby is a great help to mothers.

Infant feeding
See Appendix 14.

Discharge and postnatal examination

When transferred home from hospital, the community midwife takes over the care of the mother and baby. Medical care is provided by the general practitioner. The midwife discharges the mother and baby to the care of the health visitor between the 10th and 28th postnatal day. Before discharging the mother, family planning is discussed and the mother is reminded that although she will not menstruate for about 5 weeks or more, she will, however, ovulate before this, and could become pregnant if she has unprotected intercourse. Anxieties about perineal pain and discomfort and about the resumption of intercourse are common. An opportunity to discuss these and any other problems should be provided before discharge. At her postnatal clinic visit, usually 6 weeks after delivery, the mother is asked how she feels, and is given an opportunity to report any symptoms. Tiredness associated with her increased domestic duties, and with anaemia, is common and the haemoglobin should be estimated, iron being prescribed if necessary. Backache, usually due to faulty posture, is another common complaint. Whether or not she is still breast-feeding, the breasts are examined and any necessary advice is given. The muscle tone of the abdominal wall is noted. If it is lax, exercises may still be of value.

A detailed pelvic examination is carried out and a repeat smear may be obtained for cervical cytology. The vulva, vaginal walls and cervix are inspected. Lacerations should be healed, bleeding should have ceased and the cervix should be closed and healthy. Cervical erosion is common, but does not usually require treatment. The uterus is palpated bimanually, its size and position being noted. The mother is asked to strain or cough, in order to observe descent of the vaginal walls of uterus. For a very slight degree of prolapse, treatment may not be necessary; exercises may be recommended, but in later life sometimes operative repair may be necessary.

Adequate time should be allowed for discussion of problems at the postnatal examination because to women this was regarded as the most important part of the visit, yet it was often unsatisfactory (Bowers, 1984).

If everything has proved satisfactory, the mother is finally discharged.

Family planning

Family planning has far-reaching effects on social and epidemiological factors, as there is now a range of relatively reliable artificial methods of birth control available which will allow couples to control their own fertility. Family size and spacing can now be controlled.

Since 1974, the family planning service has been the responsibility of the National Health Service and has been provided free. The service is increasingly being provided by general practitioners, but there are also family planning clinics in some hospitals and the community provided by health authorities, and a limited domiciliary service for a few selected clients who fail to attend clinics. The Family Planning Association also provides clinics in some parts of the country, but charges are made for the service.

Barrier methods of contraception

The cap. The woman may use an occlusive cap, covering the cervix, combined with a chemical contraceptive which has a spermicidal action. The diaphragm is the type most commonly recommended. This is a thin rubber dome attached to a metal ring, which fits across the vaginal vault, extending from the posterior fornix to the retropubic groove. It is available in a variety of sizes and, if accurately fitted, should prevent semen from reaching the cervix. For additional safety, the woman should apply a spermicidal paste to the cap prior to insertion. It should be left in place for at least 6 hours after intercourse. She has the cap fitted, is carefully instructed in its insertion and removal, returns in a week or two to confirm that the fit is correct and that she is able to manage the device and, subsequently, attends about every year for further checks. Postnatally it may need checking at 1 week and 3 months before annual visits are arranged, to ensure a good fit as the muscle tone improves.

If the woman has a cystocele, a vault cap, which clings by suction to the vaginal vault, may be more satisfactory; for a woman with a long cervix, a cervical cap, which fits closely over the vaginal part of the cervix, may be preferable.

Condom. These are sheaths to cover the erect penis. They are made of plain latex and are prelubricated, and can be either round or teat-ended. The latter is designed to collect the ejaculate.

They should be applied before any genital contact occurs, and removed very carefully after intercourse to ensure that no sperm can escape. When used with a spermicide, they are reasonably safe and do not have any side effects.

They are sometimes called rubbers or french letters, and are disposable. Non-allergic condoms can be obtained for those allergic to rubber compounds. The use of condoms is strongly recommended to provide protection from sexually transmitted diseases, and especially to reduce the spread of AIDS.

Chemical contraceptives also may be used; these are spermicidal chemicals prepared in the form of jelly, paste, cream pessary or aerosol foam. They are generally prescribed for use with a mechanical barrier. Sometimes, where maximum efficiency is not essential, the aerosol foam may be used alone.

Systemic methods of contraception

Oral contraceptives. Known as 'the pill'. These are preparations of hormones.

Combined pill. This is a preparation of oestrogen and progesterone. The former prevents ovulation by suppressing the production of follicle-stimulating hormone (FSH) by the anterior pituitary gland. The progesterone causes the cervical mucus to remain dense and impenetrable to sperm. This pill, if taken as instructed by the manufacturer, is completely effective. This pill is not taken daily; there is a 6 or 7 day break in the cycle when 'menstruation' occurs. This menstruation is due to oestrogen withdrawal and is scantier than a normal period. The 'pill' does, however, have a number of side effects, hypertension and thromboembolic disease being two of the most serious. Nausea, weight gain, depression and CHLOASMA also may occur.

The 'pill' is contraindicated in the presence of a history of hypertension, thromboembolic disease, epilepsy, diabetes, heavy smoking and severe migraine. Lactation will be reduced by the oestrogen content of the pill. It should also be avoided for 6 weeks before major surgery.

Progesterone-only pill (POP). The cervical mucus becomes thick, tenacious and impenetrable to sperm. The endometrium atrophies, and motility of the fallopian tube slows down.

In newly delivered mothers, lactation is not suppressed with progesterone only. It is vital to advise that the pill is taken at the same time each day; otherwise, pregnancy can occur because ovulation is not suppressed. This pill is taken daily.

Failure of the 'pill' can be due not only to forgetting a pill, but also if there is any illness, such as gastroenteritis, affecting absorption.

Injectable progestogen. The action of a high-level progestogen, such as Depot-Provera given every 3 months, is to suppress ovulation as with the combined pill. It is not widely used in Britain except in the short term. It is useful in the puerperium, when rubella vaccination is given, or when a vasectomy is planned.

Other methods

Intrauterine contraceptive devices. For many years it has been realized that pregnancy is unlikely to occur if the uterus contains a foreign body. The metal rings in use 50 years ago were fairly effective as contraceptives, but they appeared sometimes to aggravate pelvic inflammatory conditions and to cause uterine bleeding. Modern devices, made from plastics, while not infallible, are reasonably effective. Various shapes are used; e.g. the Safe-T-Coil, Lippe's Loop, Copper 7, Copper T, Multi-load 250 and Novagard.

With a special introducer, the doctor inserts the device, which passes without difficulty through the cervix into the uterine cavity. The woman may experience a little bleeding or some pelvic discomfort, though many have no adverse symptoms. The discomfort is felt at the time of insertion and continues for 1–2 hours. Occasionally the contraceptive device is expelled; this is most likely to occur during the first period after insertion. However, the threads should be checked monthly after periods for maximum efficiency. All copper devices require to be changed 3-yearly.

The great advantage of the intrauterine device is that, once it has settled into place in the uterus, it can be forgotten except when the woman attends for re-examination—at 6 weeks, 6 months and, thereafter, yearly. Thus it may well be the method of choice for women unable to give good and intelligent cooperation, and in those in whom continued supervision might prove difficult. It is of undoubted value in contraceptive campaigns in developing countries. Complications associated with the use of intrauterine contraceptive devices include: the risk of perforated uterus, pelvic inflammatory disease, abnormal uterine bleeding, pelvic pain, vaginal discharge and ectopic gestation.

The rhythm method or 'safe period'. This method is, apart from total abstinence, the only one permitted to Roman Catholics. Intercourse is avoided during the fertile phase of the menstrual cycle at the time of ovulation, and restricted to the 'safe', or infertile, phase. Calculation, which is not easy, is based on the assumption that spermatozoa can survive for 48 hours and the ovum, after ovulation, remains viable for 24 hours. Ovulation is thought to take place between 12 and 16 days before the onset of a menstrual period but cycles are frequently not absolutely regular.

Temperature method. The time of ovulation may be found if the woman records her basal temperature every morning before getting up. The pattern is characteristic: lower during the follicular phase and higher in the luteal phase. It is thus advised that intercourse should not take place until the higher temperature has been maintained for 3 days. This temperature-taking is tedious for the woman and is immediately valueless if she should develop the mildest pyrexial disorder.

Billings' method. This method of assessing changes in cervical mucus at ovulation is gaining popularity in Britain. It is commonly used in Australia. With ovulation, the mucus can be pulled into thin threads, whereas it is thick and firm at other times and impenetrable to sperm.

Coitus interruptus. This method requires withdrawal before semen can be deposited in the vagina. It may prove satisfactory to couples who do not wish to use any appliance. The failure rate is fairly high, and this in itself may be a cause of anxiety.

Sterilization

Female sterilization. This is a surgical procedure in which the fallopian tubes are completely and permanently occluded. This is not lightly undertaken, and careful counselling should be given. Now that divorce and remarriage are more common, women are seeking reanastomosis of their tubes—which is not always successful. If the current marriage is not stable, other means of contraception should be carefully considered. Some serious medical diseases or persistent contraceptive failures resulting in high parity are less controversial reasons for sterilization.

There are two basic methods.

Laparoscopy. This is a minor operation and the fallopian tubes can have a Yoon ring, Filshie clip or Hulka/Clemens clip applied to occlude them. Diathermy is less commonly used, as reversal cannot be peformed.

Laparatomy. Pomeroy's techique. This involves partial salpingectomy with the ends of tubes buried in the uterus.

Male sterilization by vasectomy. In this simple operation under local analgesia, the vasa deferentia are divided so that sperm cannot be transported to the seminal vesicles. However, this does not immediately become effective, as some sperm are already in the ducts. Sperm counts are done at intervals, usually 6 weeks and 3 months or until free of sperm. Alternative methods of contraception will need to be used until a sperm-free specimen is obtained.

References

Bowers J (1984) The six week postnatal examination. Parts I and II. *Research & The Midwife Conference Proceedings*. pp. 28–50. London.

UKCC (1991) *Midwives Rules*, UKCC: London.

APPENDIX 13

The Normal Baby

From the eighth week after conception the human embryo is called the *fetus*. At five weeks it measures 2 cm long and has a head with eyes and ears, limb buds and a tail. The heart and circulation are already developing. By the eighth week the length is 3 cm, the hands and feet may be recognized and the tail has almost disappeared. By the 12th week the fetus is about 9 cm long, the sex is distinguishable and ossification centres are present. At the 20th week the fetus is 20–21 cm long and the length now increases at a fairly constant rate of 2.5 cm in 2 weeks. Lanugo is present on the skin. By the 24th week vernix caseosa covers the skin and there is hair on the scalp.

At the 24th week the fetus is said to be *viable*, but usually, if born at this time, will only survive by having intensive care to aid its immature systems, particularly the respiratory system. Twenty-five years ago most babies born between 24–28 weeks died, but now a baby weighing less than 1000 g, of 24 or more weeks' gestation, has a good chance of survival if skilled intensive care is available.

Care of the normal baby

A normal baby is one born at or near term with no congenital malformations and no birth trauma.

Care at birth

Profound physiological changes occur at birth and the baby has to adapt to a dry, light, noisy environment, from its warm, quiet, dark familiar one. Dr Leboyer has laid emphasis on reducing the sudden shock (see Dictionary).

Changes and management

Initiation of respiration. The fetal circulation ceases as soon as efficient respiration occurs, and as the pulmonary circulation opens up fully the FORAMEN OVALE closes. This should occur within a very few minutes of birth. A failure or delay means inadequate oxygenation of the vital centres, so an assessment of the baby's respiratory function should be carried out routinely. This is commonly done by the Apgar score.

The *Apgar score* is take routinely at 1 and 5 minutes, and again later if necessary; 0, 1 or 2 points are given for each item listed in the table.

A score of 8 or more at 1 minute is satisfactory. At 5 minutes it is usually 10 (*see* Appendix 16 for the management of the babies with low Apgar scores).

Normal management. As the baby is born, mucus may gently be removed from the nose and mouth using swabs, if necessary. Mechanical suction can be used in cases of excessive mucus, but care must be taken not to damage the larynx and the vocal cords. If the baby is laid face down either on the mother's abdomen or on the delivery bed, the mucus and liquor may drain away by gravity.

Cessation of placental circulation. The cord is normally clamped and cut as soon as the baby is born, unless it is left until pulsations have ceased. It is usually clamped using a sterilized plastic device such as a Hollister clamp. The purpose is to prevent bleeding and, as the cord shrinks, the clamp closes tighter. However, varous thick ligatures can be used, but must be checked that bleeding does not occur when shrinkage occurs. The stump should be inspected to check on the number of arteries. If only one is present, instead of two, renal abnormalities should be looked for. The stump is prone to infection, so it should be kept as clean and dry as possible.

Thermoregulation. The neonate's system is not well developed and

Table 4. Apgar scores

Sign	Score		
	0	1	2
Colour	Blue to pale	Body pink, limbs blue	Pink
Respiratory effort	Absent	Irregular gasps	Strong cry
Heart rate	Absent	Less than 100/minute	Over 100/minute
Muscle tone	Limp	Some flexion of limbs	Strong active movements
Reflex irritability	Nil	Grimace or sneeze	Cry

hypothermia can ensue very soon after delivery if the baby is allowed to lose heat, which is particularly likely if the liquor is allowed to evaporate. The baby should be dried as soon as possible with a warm towel and wrapped warmly to be given to its mother. Alternatively, the baby may be laid on the mother's bare abdomen or breasts where her body will transmit warmth to the baby. In this case, unless the delivery room is very warm 21°C (70°F), a blanket over both or an overhead heater will be needed.

Mother/baby relationship. After delivery, mother and baby need to get acquainted completely by feel, sight, smell and hearing. The sooner they develop a satisfactory relationship which becomes a deep attachment, the better. Then if separation does occur, the relationship will not be permanently damaged, so reducing the incidence of NON-ACCIDENTAL INJURY (NAI). Skin-to-skin contact, early breast-feeding, and general encouragement should be given to the parents to get to know their baby. The baby should remain by the mother's side until they can both be transferred together from the delivery room.

Full examination. This should be carried out as soon as possible to detect any abnormalities that need urgent or later attention. The mother will appreciate seeing this done and can be reassured that all is well in the majority of cases. The baby is also weighed and measured; the normal weight range is 3–4 kg, the length 50–52 cm and the head circumference between 32 and 35 cm. The skin should be smooth and pink and the baby should be quite plump.

Prevention of infection. In utero the fetus is in a sterile environment. After delivery, immunity takes time to develop as various organisms are encountered. Should there be a sudden exposure to many pathogens, a baby may become easily infected before its immunity has built up. It is essential to pay meticulous attention to hand-washing before attending to a baby, particularly when the face and cord are being dealt with. These areas should be the first to be cleansed whether the baby is 'topped and tailed' or bathed.

Bathing was traditional, but is not essential. It removes blood and meconium effectively, but it involves unnecessary exposure and chilling is probable. The vernix, moreover, is probably better not removed, as it may protect the skin from infection. The bath, whenever it is carried out, includes washing the face with water and wool swabs from a separate bowl, washing the hair with soap and water, washing the child's body, immersing him or her in the water to rinse off the soap, and drying by a patting or 'blotting' procedure. The drying cannot be hurried as rubbing will injure the skin and care is necessary to be sure the creases and crevices are absolutely dry. Powder may be used, but is not a necessity. In the first few days, zinc and castor oil cream or petroleum jelly should be applied to the buttocks to protect the skin and facilitate the removal of meconium. The eyes, ears, nostrils and mouth are inspected, but do not require cleansing.

Subsequent care

Daily observations.

The umbilical cord. The umbilical cord is inspected daily. It undergoes a process of dry gangrene, and separates after 6 or 7 days, leaving a small scar which soon heals. It should be left entirely alone as studies have shown that there is no increase in infection and the application of spirit and powder to the cord delays separation (Lawrence, 1982; Magowan *et al.*, 1980; Barr, 1984).

The skin. The colour is observed for pallor, cyanosis or jaundice, and creases for soreness. Minor infections are fairly common, and spots should be recognized and treated promptly. In hospital the baby should be isolated to prevent cross-infection.

The orifices. The nostrils, mouth and ears are inspected daily, but not treated unless infection occurs. In particular, the mouth is inspected for white plaques of candida infection (thrush), and the buttocks for redness.

The eyes. These are observed and not treated unless infection occurs. Ophthalmia neonatorum is any purulent discharge occurring within 21 days of birth, which must be notified.

Stools. Meconium, a greenish-black substance, is passed for 2–3 days, and the stool then changes through a greenish-brown to the typical mustard yellow by the fourth day or so. The stool is passed frequently during the first 2–3 weeks, the frequency gradually diminishing to one motion daily, or less. It is not uncommon for a breast-fed baby a month old to pass only one stool in 2–3 days. Provided the stool is normal and the child well, this is unimportant. The midwife should appreciate that this is a matter about which anxious parents will consult her frequently.

Urine. This is usually passed either at birth or within a few hours. Failure to pass urine should raise the suspicion, at birth, of some obstruction or, later on, of dehydration.

Vomiting. Commonly a little mucus, possibly blood-stained, is vomited soon after birth. This is usually of no significance. POSSETTING is also a normal event, and not to be confused with vomiting which persists, and is abnormal. Persistent vomiting should be reported, as there are many causes, some serious.

Weight. A weight loss of up to 10 per cent of the birth weight is normal in the first few days of life. It should be regained by 10–14 days. Subsequently, the baby should gain approximately 200 g per week.

Temperature. It is probably wise to take the neonate's temperature soon after delivery, and if he or she has any sign of infection. This will usually be manifested by fretfulness, lack of appetite and, possibly, greyish pallor. Conversely, if colour, appetite and muscle tone are good, the baby probably is well. Temperature readings may reveal unsuspected hypothermia. The temperature may be taken rectally or in the axilla.

Neonatal abilities.

A normal newborn baby possesses a number of simple reflexes at birth, which are enough to set him/her off to learn appropriate behaviour for the future. These are particularly easy to see in the alert period immediately after delivery.

Grasp reflex. A baby will clench his hand or foot if any pressure is applied.

Rooting reflex. A touch on the cheek or side of the mouth stimulates the baby to turn to the side touched seeking for food.

Sucking reflex. A baby will usually suck very well if put to the breast as soon as delivered. Not only will this be satisfying to the baby, but will engender the mother's maternal feelings and help her to become attached to the baby.

Moro reflex. This often occurs spontaneously as the baby is delivered and is usually stimulated by the doctor during the routine examination of the baby soon after birth. The reflex will be absent or barely present in preterm babies, and in cases of severe brain damage and depression by drugs.

Walking reflex. A baby held upright with one foot on a hard surface will step out with the other foot and make alternate stepping movements.

General behaviour.

Sleep. This occupies a large part of the day at first, but is very variable in individual babies.

Alert periods. As well as waking when hungry or uncomfortable, a baby will lie quietly in the cot. During these alert periods the baby explores the environment, and when held to look over one's shoulder, stays alert and looks round.

Vision. The human face is particularly interesting and the baby will recognize the mother by the end of a week. Opportunity should be given for mother to hold her baby 'en-face'—i.e. with the baby's face about 9 inches away from the mother's face. They then look into one another's eyes. Mothers find this contact exciting and it stimulates more and more contact between them.

Hearing. A baby responds to noise and particularly to the human

Table 5. The normal baby after birth.

Age (months)	Average weight (g)	Progress
1	3600	Regards face, responds to a bell. Lifts head
2	4500	Smiles responsively
3	5500	Holds up head. Smiles spontaneously. Puts hands together
4	6400	Sits supported. Laughs and gurgles. Grasps object firmly. Rolls over
5	6800	Uses eyes and hands with some coordination. Pull to sit without head lag
6	7300	Sits resting forward on hands. Two teeth. Attempts to feed self rusk
7	7700	Tries to drink from cup. Plays peek-a-boo
8	8100	Sits unsupported. Says repetitive words; e.g. dada, baba
9	8500	Crawls. Understands a few words, including 'No'. Thumb, finger grasp
10	9000	Understands more words. Hauls self to standing position. Mimics sound. Plays pat-a-cake
11	9400	Stands supported. Better understanding of words
12	9700	Says a few words. Walks with support. Six to eight teeth. Tries to feed self. Fine pincer-grasp. Stands momentarily

voice. Habituation soon occurs, so that the baby responds only to sounds which have some significance to him. Constant rhythmical sounds will lull the baby to sleep.

Smell. The baby is very soon able to recognize its mother. One way that has been shown is by her breast milk.

It used to be thought that babies were passive objects, but it is now recognized that they can initiate responses from parents and others to meet their needs. In fact, babies have very individual behaviour patterns, and rigid baby care is quite inappropriate. Their appetites and other needs can vary in the same way as adults.

References

Barr RJ (1984) The umbilical cord: to treat or not to treat? *Midwives' Chronicle* July, 224–226.

Lawrence CR (1982) Effect of two different methods of umbilical cord care on its separation time. *Midwives' Chronicle* June, 204–205.

Magowan M, Andrews A & Pinder B (1980) The effect of an antibiotic spray on the umbilical cord separation times. *Nursing Times* October 16, 1841.

APPENDIX 14

Baby Feeding

Breast feeding

Breast feeding is so clearly the natural way to feed a baby that it should hardly need advocating. However, women often need help and advice from the midwife.

Advantages to the baby

1. The constituents of breast milk vary to meet the needs of the baby both during a feed and during the day, from day to day and from week to week. The protein is mostly lactalbumin which is more easily digested than caseinogen, the protein predominantly found in cow's milk. Fat too is more easily digested and absorbed by the baby because it contains more polyunsaturated fatty acids and also lipase, a fat-digesting enzyme. The fat content of breast milk is very variable both during a feed and throughout the day, there being a marked increase in fat in the 'hind' milk, that is the last milk of the feed. Most of the carbohydrate in human milk is lactose which helps to promote the growth of lactobacilli in the intestine and leads to increased acidity of stools. The mineral content of breast milk is lower than cows' milk, thus the immature kidneys of the newborn cope more easily with the solute load presented to them. The vitamin content of breast milk depends largely on the mother's intake of these substances.

2. Breast feeding is also a way of promoting interaction and thereby attachment between mother and child. The breast-fed infant has close skin-to-skin and eye-to-eye contact with its mother during feeds and more readily initiates interaction to which the mother responds and two-way communications develop.

3. Asthma, eczema or hay fever are less likely to be severe. The onset of any allergies will be delayed provided breast-feeding is complete. This is particularly important if there is any family history of these conditions. Even one cows' milk feed will stimulate sensitization, so only clear fluid complements should be given in this case.

4. Breast milk is easily available and ready for consumption, so there is no delay or frustration.

5. The breast-fed baby is less likely to develop a severe infection; this is especially true for gastroenteritis and respiratory conditions. The immunoglobulin, IgA, found in high concentrations in COLOSTRUM and breast milk, lines the baby's gut. This together with lactoferrin,

aids the colonization of the gut with non-pathogenic lactobacilli, thereby increasing acidity. Lactose also facilitates this process. Growth of pathogenic ESCHERICHIA COLI is thus inhibited. Another anti-infective agent found in breast milk is the enzyme lysozyme, a protein with a non-specific anti-bacterial effect. Breast milk also contains large numbers of white cells and an anti-viral substance, both of which help combat infection. In some developing countries where bottle-feeding has been advocated, epidemics of gastroenteritis have caused widespread mortality and morbidity. Facilities for sterilization and education of the mothers did not accompany the commercial drive to sell artificial milk. These are not needed for breast-feeding.

6. Biochemical disturbances are less likely. Where unmodified cows' milk is used as an alternative, hypocalcaemia can occur due to the high phosphate level. Also, the high sodium content can lead to HYPERNATRAEMIA, as the baby's kidneys are not very efficient. Mistakes in preparation can occur in any society, whereas breast milk is always appropriate for the individual baby's needs.

7. Cot death is much less common in breast-fed babies.

8. Obesity is less likely to occur.

Advantages to the mother

1. Satisfaction. Successful breast-feeding brings a great sense of calm, emotional pleasure and satisfaction. This is enhanced by the knowledge that it is also beneficial to the baby.

2. It is more restful and labour saving, because the mother also has a rest as she feeds her baby, although no one else can help with feeding. No feed preparation is needed, however, and there are no utensils to be cleaned, or sterilization liquid to prepare.

3. Involution of uterus is promoted by the release of oxytocin which occurs during breast feeding.

4. Figure. This is more likely to return to normal as fat stores are used up and the uterus involutes. The breasts themselves, however, must be well supported, as there is an increase in size and weight.

5. Carcinoma of the breast is less common in women who have breast fed.

Management of breast feeding

Antenatal. Studies have shown that the majority of women decide on breast feeding before or very early in pregnancy (Beske & Garvis, 1982). There is no evidence to support the various forms of antenatal breast preparation which have traditionally been taught from early pregnancy, thus discussion about the mother's chosen method of feeding can be delayed until later in pregnancy. Advice about wearing a well-fitting brassiere, ordinary cleanliness of the breasts and good education which increases the mother's confidence in her ability to breast feed is all that is required during the antenatal period.

Physiology of lactation. An understanding of the physiology of lactation helps the mother and midwife in the management of successful breast feeding. The level of prolactin, the lactating hormone from the anterior pituitary gland, rises throughout pregnancy but milk production is inhibited by the high level of oestrogen and progesterone produced by the placenta. Two to four days after delivery when the level of these placental hormones has fallen, prolactin initiates the production of milk. At the time the baby is put to the breast, or even earlier, oxytocin is released from the posterior pituitary gland and causes the myoepithelial cells around the milk-producing cells, the alveoli, to contract, thereby expelling the milk through the ducts to the ampullae which lie just behind the nipple. This is known as the let-down reflex. Correct attachment of the baby to the breast and unrestricted sucking enables the milk to be removed effectively and maintains lactation.

Postnatal management. There is considerable evidence that mothers who breast feed soon after delivery feed for longer (Salariya *et al.*, 1978; Thomson *et al.*, 1979). The baby is particularly responsive during the first hour or two after birth, so the midwife should help the mother make this first feed a successful experience, thereby promoting her confidence and positive response to her baby. It is the midwife's responsibility to help the mother achieve a successful first feed within half an hour after delivery if possible, or certainly within 2 hours.

The single, most important factor which promotes effective breast feeding is the correct attachment of the baby to the breast. This is achieved by holding the baby facing the mother's breast and brushing his lips with the nipple to stimulate the rooting reflex which results in the baby opening his mouth. Then, supporting the breast underneath if necessary, the mother moves her baby on to the breast, ensuring that both the nipple and most of the areola are placed inside the baby's wide open mouth. Indications that the baby is correctly attached are:

- The baby's mouth will be wide open and the lower lip will be curled back and further away from the base of the nipple than the top lip.
- The baby will have the nipple, much of the areola and underlying breast tissue in his mouth.
- The jaw action soon becomes rhythmical and steady and this action extends back to the ears; there is no sucking inwards of the cheeks.

Pauses are uncommon early in the feed once the milk has been let-down but increase later (RCM, 1991). The length of time the baby suckles at the breast should be unrestricted, as the rate of milk transfer to babies is very variable and also the hind milk has a higher calorific value (Howie et al., 1981). Once satisfied, the baby will release the nipple spontaneously. The second breast is offered but the baby may refuse it if he is already satisfied. Unrestricted suckling time does not result in nipple damage if the baby is correctly attached to the breast. The frequency of feeds should also be baby-led, that is, the baby is fed on demand.

Some babies will feed every hour or two from about the third day, but after a time the interval between feeds increases. Complementary feeds should not be given to healthy breast-fed babies. Colostrum is rich in all the nutrients required by the baby during the first 2 or 3 days and then, when the milk comes in, the supply is regulated by demand. The baby will feed less at the breast if he is topped up with artificial feeds and thus the mother's milk supply will diminish.

Problems. Once the mother has learned to recognize when her baby is correctly attached to the breast and allows unrestricted feeding on demand, breast feeding should be successful and the problems of nipple damage and milk engorgement should not occur. Vascular engorgement during the first few days after delivery is physiological and may cause some discomfort. If nipple damage does occur, it is invariably due to incorrect attachment of the baby to the breast and repositioning the baby is the best method of managing this problem. The use of a nipple shield is not recommended as it has been shown that the baby receives less milk (Woolridge et al., 1980). If milk engorgement occurs, the midwife should supervise a feed to check that the baby is correctly attached to the breast and that the mother is allowing unrestricted feeding on demand. It may be necessary to express a little milk before the feed to aid attachment and afterwards to relieve discomfort.

Mastitis may be non-infective or infective. Non-infective mastitis is often the result of engorgement, thus antibiotics are not required. Infective mastitis is usually treated with antibiotics and the mother continues to breast feed. She expresses and discards excess milk after feeds until the condition resolves.

Artificial feeding

Although breast feeding is the recommended method of feeding, not all mothers wish to breast feed, some fail in their attempt to do so and in a small number there is a contraindication, as listed in Table 5.

Table 5. Contraindications to breast feeding.

Maternal	Baby
Certain drugs	Metabolic disorders
e.g. cytotoxics, antithyroid	e.g. galactosaemia, lactose
Some infections	intolerance,
e.g. tuberculosis, HIV	phenylketonia
positive	Certain congenital malformations
Possibly breast injury or surgery	make breast feeding difficult
	if not impossible
	e.g. cleft lip and palate,
	Pierre Robins syndrome

Types of artificial milk

Dried cows' milk. This milk, which has been modified to resemble human milk as far as possible, is most commonly used for infant feeding. The protein in cows' milk is mainly caseinogen whereas in human milk there is more lactalbumin. Much of the casein is therefore removed and it is replaced by whey-milk protein which contains more lactalbumin. Some of the indigestible milk fat from cows' milk is removed and replaced by vegetable fat. Lactose is added to increase the energy value. Finally, cows' milk is demineralized to reduce the high mineral content, thereby reducing the solute load presented to the kidneys. Vitamins and iron are added to the milk. When the baby is a few weeks old, a milk formula containing a higher ratio of casein is recommended.

Evaporated milk. This is of a smooth consistency and easy to mix, but is not recommended because it is not modified. It is evaporated to one-third of its original volume, so it is reconstituted by mixing one part of the milk with two parts of water and adding sugar. For a 120 ml feed, 40 ml of evaporated milk is mixed with 80 ml of water and 4 g of sugar is added.

Fresh cows' milk This is not recommended for babies under 6 months of age, except in an emergency. Then it should be boiled, diluted with boiled water and have sugar added. The following formula would be suitable in an emergency for a baby weighing 3.5 kg:

90 ml boiled milk (240 kJ, 60 Cal).

30 ml boiled water.

4 g (1 teaspoon) sugar (60 kJ, 15 Cal).

Energy (calorific) requirement

The term, healthy baby requires approximately 440 kJ (110 Cal) per kg body weight per day, and 150–165 ml fluid per kg body weight per day. Thirty millilitres of cows' milk contains about 80 kJ (20 Cal), thus a baby weighing 3.5 kg will require approximately 1540 kJ (385 Cal) in 24 hours, i.e. about 575 ml of milk. In practice, babies vary greatly in the amount of milk they take and this should not be a cause for concern if the baby is thriving.

Preparation for feeds

All mothers who are artificially feeding should be shown how to make up feeds and instructed in the cleansing and the sterilization of the feeding equipment. The instructions on the packet of milk must be followed closely.

Dried milks are supplied with their own scoops, made to very exact measurements. To reconstitute the feed it is necessary to mix it in the proportion of one scoop of food to 30 ml of cooled boiled water. The scoop must be filled—not packed—and then levelled flat with a knife. This should be stressed when the preparation of feeds is being demonstrated to mothers. It is now realized that the danger of giving overconcentrated feeds, where the sodium level is already higher than that of breast milk, causes the kidney to concentrate the urine to preserve the water balance of the body. Should there by an excessive water loss, as in diarrhoea or vomiting, hypernatraemic dehydration occurs, with a risk of permanent neurological trauma. This is now reduced with the use of modified milks.

A long-term effect of overconcentration is that of obesity, with all its attendant risks.

Sterilization of equipment

Bottles and teats are rinsed in cold, running water and then washed thoroughly with a bottle brush in warm soapy water. The teat is cleaned inside and out with salt. After rinsing in clean water the equipment is either boiled for 5 minutes or more commonly immersed in a sterilizing solution such as 1 in 80 sodium hypochlorite which sterilizes in 1½ hours.

Management of artificial feeding

The mother is encouraged to cuddle her baby closely when bottle feeding so that, like the breast fed baby, he or she feels secure and loved. Feeds should be room temperature or above, up to 30°C, and the mother is taught to test the temperature by sprinkling a little milk on her forearm. The bottle is held like a pen so that the neck is filled with milk rather than air. Feeding should be baby-led, that is, the baby is fed when he/she is hungry and takes the amount of milk he/she requires at each feed. This may vary during the course of the day but should not cause anxiety if the baby is healthy and gaining weight.

References

Beske EJ & Garvis MS (1982) Important factors in breastfeeding. *Maternal and Child Nursing* 7: 174–179.

Howie PW, Houston MJ, Cook A, Smart L, McArdle F, McNeilly AS (1981) How long should a breast feed last? *Early Human Development* 5: 71–77.

Royal College of Midwives (1991) *Successful Breastfeeding.* p. 18. Churchill Livingstone: London.

Salariyia EM, Easton PM & Carter JI (1978) Duration of feeding after early initiation and frequent feeding. *Lancet* ii: 1141–1143.

Thomson ME, Hartstock TG & Larson C (1979) The importance of immediate postnatal contact: its effects on breastfeeding. *Canadian Family Physician* 25: 1374–1378.

Woolridge MW, Braum D & Drewett RF (1980) Effect of a traditional and of a new nipple shield on sucking patterns and milk flow. *Early Human Development* 4(4): 357–364.

APPENDIX 15

Immunization Schedule

Immunization cannot be commenced until a baby is 3 months old, as the production of the specific antibodies will not occur effectively until this age. Infectious diseases which can be avoided by immunization are listed below.

Smallpox
World-wide vaccination has been so successful that the disease has virtually been eradicated, so it is no longer given as a routine.

Whooping cough (pertussis)
In about 1974 anxiety grew about the danger associated with immunization. A nationwide inquiry since then has revealed that there is a risk of 1 in 110 000 children developing serious neurological damage. These rare cases were given so much prominence in the media that many parents have not had their children immunized. An epidemic of whooping cough has resulted. The illness may last as long as 8 weeks, and most children recover without apparent long-term ill-effects, but fatalities occur in babies under 6 months of age. Health authorities are being exhorted by the Department of Health to run local campaigns to improve the uptake of immunization. It is given as a triple antigen with diphtheria and tetanus toxoids.

Triple antigen
This contains dead organisms of whooping cough (*Bordetella pertussis*) together with the toxoids of diphtheria and tetanus. The dose is 0.5 ml on three occasions.

Contraindications. The triple vaccine should not be given if there is a family history of epilepsy, disease of the central nervous system, fits or other abnormality of the baby's own central nervous system. Any severe reaction from the first injection such as dyspnoea, fits or encephalopathy, indicates that the programme should continue with *only* diphtheria and tetanus toxoids.

Storage. The triple vaccine should not be frozen, but refrigerated between 2° and 10°C.

Rubella

In 1970 the Joint Committee on Vaccination and Immunisation (JCVI) recommended the routine use of rubella vaccine for girls between 11 and 14 years of age. The uptake of rubella vaccination was only about 80%, and, in an effort to improve this, from 1 September 1981, the younger age of 10 became Department of Health policy.

Poliomyelitis

This is given as a syrup on a lump of sugar, usually at the same time as the triple antigen initially, but needs a booster dose on leaving school (as does tetanus).

Table 6. Typical scheme of immunization.

Age	Avoidable disease
4–6 months 1st	Diphtheria, tetanus, pertussis and poliomyelitis
6–8 months 2nd	As above
10–14 months 3rd	As above
1–2 years	Measles, mumps and rubella
5 years (school entry)	Diphtheria, tetanus and polio boosters
10–13 years	Tuberculosis BCG (if immunity tests are negative)
10–14 (girls only)	Rubella (German measles)
15–19 (school-leaving age)	Tetanus, poliomyelitis

APPENDIX 16
Fetal Hypoxia and Neonatal Asphyxia

Fetal hypoxia

Diminution of oxygen to the fetus (fetal hypoxia) may arise through interference with the passage of oxygen at any time from its inspiration by the mother to its reaching the fetal tissues and, in particular, the vital centres. Very often an acute episode of fetal distress is preceded by a period of chronic intrauterine hypoxia before the onset of labour. One of the aims of antenatal care is to select high-risk cases early in pregnancy in order that the fetal condition can be carefully monitored to detect such problems. The causes of intrauterine hypoxia are:

1. *In the mother*: failure of respiration, as in eclamptic fits or epilepsy; less commonly, inadequate circulation, as in cardiac failure or profound anaemia, hypertension and hypotension, both of which result in a reduced blood supply to the placenta; diabetes mellitus and maternal infections.
2. *In the uterus*: hypertonicity; or excessive retraction in obstructed labour.
3. *At the placental site*: partial separation of the placenta, as in abruptio placentae and placenta praevia.
4. *In the placenta*: placental insufficiency, as in postmaturity and pre-eclampsia.
5. *In the umbilical cord*: prolapse, pressure during delivery, tight coiling, traction or true knot.
6. *In the fetus*: circulatory failure resulting from intracranial birth trauma, severe Rhesus incompatibility causing gross anaemia; certain congenital abnormalities; intrauterine infection; the risk is also increased in multiple pregnancy, malpresentations and malpositions.

Fetal hypoxia is manifested clinically as 'fetal distress'.

Fetal distress

Danger. Hypoxia can lead to irreversible brain damage. This either presents in the form of cerebral palsy or, if anoxia ensues, stillbirth will result. It is therefore vital to detect any sign of hypoxia as soon as possible to prevent these conditions.

Detection

Auscultation. The midwife records the fetal heart intermittently with a fetal (Pinard) stethoscope. Suspicious alterations in the fetal heart include:

1. Sometimes fetal tachycardia, above 160 per minute, especially if followed by fetal bradycardia.
2. Fetal bradycardia, which persists particularly when it occurs between contractions (*see* Appendix 7).
3. Irregularity.

Observation. The passage of meconium or meconium-stained liquor *per vaginam*, especially when the head is presenting. This sign is not too reliable, but cannot be ignored.

Movement. Tumultuous movements of the fetus. These may be noted by the mother, and indicate that the fetus could be in a terminal condition.

It should be emphasized that none of these signs is entirely reliable. After disquieting variations in the fetal heart sounds and the passage of fresh meconium, the child may yet be born in excellent condition. Conversely, with apparently no warning the infant is occasionally born severely asphyxiated.

A more accurate assessment of the fetal condition can be made by the use of more complex apparatus than the simple Pinard stethoscope or the Doptone machine.

Continuous electrocardiogram. The best signal is obtained from an electrode on the fetal scalp, but an ultrasound transducer on the maternal abdomen can be used as an alternative. The interval between paired heart beats is measured by the monitor and converted into beats per minute to be recorded on the chart (*see* Figure 19).

Normal recordings.
1. Heart rate between 120 and 160 beats per minute.
2. No significant variation between contractions.
3. Base-line irregularity or variability of at least 5 beats per minute.
4. Accelerations of more than 15 beats per minute which occur with contractions are usually also considered normal.

Suspicious recordings. The midwife should report the following to the obstetrician:
1. Base-line tachycardia. This may be associated with maternal pyrexia or ketosis. If base-line irregularity is lost or decelerations occur, FETAL BLOOD SAMPLING (FBS) should be done to assess the degree of hypoxia.
2. Base-line bradycardia. This is not usually ominous alone but with the above complications.

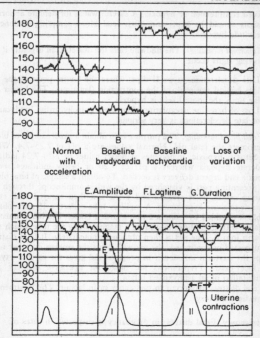

I. *Early deceleration (type 1 dip)*; II. *late deceleration (type II dip)*

Figure 19. Fetal heart recordings.

3. Loss of baseline irregularity. Unless this is associated with maternal drug administration (e.g. pethidine), it should be considered a serious sign of hypoxia.

4. Early decelerations (type I dips) which are variable in shape and alter more than 15 beats per minute, may indicate head compression,

cord compression or hypoxia. A careful watch for definite abnormal signs should be kept, and often fetal blood sampling is done to exclude hypoxia.

Abnormal recordings. The midwife calls the obstetrician urgently if the following signs occur:

1. Late decelerations (type II dips) where the lowest point of the dip lags behind the peak of the contraction (lag time). The longer the lag time, the more likely is hypoxia.
2. Loss of base-line irregularity when there is tachycardia, bradycardia or late decelerations is very serious.

Fetal blood sampling. The purpose is to obtain a small sample of blood to estimate the fetal pH. Normal values are a pH of 7.25–7.4. When the fetus is hypoxic, it becomes acidotic; values of 7.20–7.24 indicate moderate hypoxia whereas a pH of 7.20 or below indicates severe hypoxia and urgent delivery is needed. To obtain a sample of fetal blood the presenting part is visualized by the widest amnioscope through the dilating cervix. It is cleaned and dried and then sprayed with ethyl chloride to cause hyperaemia. A capillary tube collects a 15 mm column of blood obtained by using a 2 mm guarded blade. The blood must be agitated with iron filings moved by a magnet along the tube which mix heparin into it. The pH is then estimated immediately. If fetal distress is suspected or confirmed, the midwife turns the woman onto her side, stops the oxytocin infusion if in progress and gives the mother oxygen by face mask. Preparations are made for operative delivery and resuscitation of an asphyxiated infant.

Fetal distress may occur in pregnancy or in labour. The treatment is immediate delivery.

In pregnancy. Fetal distress in pregnancy is suspected in cases of:

- diminished fetal movements;
- intrauterine growth retardation, which may be detected on abdominal examination and by ultrasound measurements of the fetal head and abdominal girth;
- poor maternal weight gain;
- reduced amniotic fluid;
- abnormal cardiotocography which includes a trace which is non-reactive to fetal movements, has loss of beat-to-beat variation and type II decelerations.

These are serious signs of fetal distress and immediate caesarean section would be necessary.

Cardiotocography in labour. For the early detection of fetal hypoxia, women at risk should have the fetal heart sounds monitored continuously throughout labour. Such mothers are those with known placental insufficiency, whatever the cause—e.g. severe pre-eclampsia, renal disease, diabetes, post-maturity and many others.

For hitherto normal and healthy women, in the first stage of labour regular recordings of the fetal heart sounds are made at increasingly frequent intervals, 2-hourly or hourly, then, every 10 or 15 minutes, as labour advances. In some units the fetal heart is monitored continuously for about 30 minutes when the woman is admitted in labour and then, if the trace is normal it is discontinued, although it may be repeated later for short periods. Other units monitor every woman. This is a controversial issue, as there are hazards in applying scalp clips and using intrauterine catheters. The necessity for keeping a woman in bed, unless telemetry is used, is also undesirable. Labour is more rapid, less painful and fetal distress less likely when the mother is upright.

In the second stage the fetal heart sounds are recorded after every contraction as fetal hypoxia is more common at this time and should be recognized early and reported to the doctor immediately. The treatment is almost always forceps delivery, though at the end of the second stage an episiotomy may be sufficient to hasten delivery and if appropriate, the midwife can help the woman adopt a more upright position which usually increases expulsive efforts and descent of the fetus. In addition to preparing for delivery, the midwife checks and prepares the neonatal resuscitation equipment and calls a paediatrician to resuscitate the baby at birth.

Neonatal asphyxia

Asphyxia neonatorum is failure of the child to breathe after birth. In order that respiration may be established, the lungs must be normally developed, the respiratory centre functioning normally and the air passages clear. It is rare for the lungs to be malformed, but it is not uncommon for the airway to be blocked or the respiratory centre to be depressed. In preterm babies there is often difficulty in establishing satisfactory breathing at birth because of the immaturity of the lungs, respiratory centre and respiratory muscles.

Depression of the medulla has three main causes:

1. Drugs given to mother (i.e. pethidine, papaveretum (Omnopon) or morphine). Naloxone (Narcan) 0.01 mg/kg administered intramuscularly to the baby at birth will reverse the depression.
2. Hypoxia. This is the commonest reason for depression, the many causes are those of fetal distress already listed in this appendix.
3. Intracranial damage occurring during birth where excessive or

abnormal MOULDING is allowed to occur. A breech delivery is particularly vulnerable and also a preterm baby.

Management of asphyxia neonatorum

Asphyxia neonatorum should be anticipated if there are any signs of fetal hypoxia in labour and the midwife will check and prepare the resuscitation equipment ready for use and alert the paediatrician. After delivery the midwife will:

1. Note the time.
2. Aspirate mucus from the nasopharynx and oropharynx.
3. Cut the cord.
4. Dry the baby with a warm towel, then wrap warmly.
5. Transfer the baby to a pre-heated resuscitaire and position under a radiant heater in the supine position with the head slightly lower and extended.
6. Assess the Apgar score at 1 minute (see Appendix 13).
   (a) Apgar score 8–10: no further treatment necessary unless the score has dropped when it is reassessed at 5 minutes.
   (b) Apgar score 5–8 (mild asphyxia):
      (i) Call a paediatrician.
      (ii) Give oxygen by intermittent positive pressure ventilation (IPPV) with equipment such as an Ambu, Cardiff or Penlon bag and face mask. If this is not available, mouth-to-mouth respiration should be applied.
      (iii) Stimulate by gently flicking the soles of the feet.
      (iv) Check if any maternal drug was given and give naloxone (Narcan) if appropriate; dose, 0.01 mg/kg body weight.
   (c) Apgar score 4 or below (severe asphyxia): this baby has circulatory collapse and is therefore shocked. A paediatrician should be summoned urgently if not already present. Attempts to stimulate the baby should not be made because the shock will deepen. Act swiftly, as oxygen is urgently needed by the medulla; otherwise, it may be permanently damaged.

Action:

1. Clear airways gently.
2. Give oxygen by IPPV as described above, or careful endotracheal intubation if trained to do so. The pressure of oxygen should never exceed 30/cmH$_2$O pressure. The endotracheal tube should be attached to a water manometer for this purpose. Give IPPV rhythmically at 30 times per minute.
3. *Check heart rate*:

(a) if rising, then the asphyxia should be lessening.

(b) if the heart rate is less than 40 beats per minute or if cardiac arrest occurs then cardiac massage should be given, preferably by an assistant: depress the middle sternum sharply but gently with two fingers at a rate of 100–120 times per minute.

4. Drugs. The doctor may give:

(a) Sodium bicarbonate 8.4% solution intravenously once respiration is established to help correct metabolic acidosis. Some think this is associated with intraventricular haemorrhage in very preterm babies (Halliday et al., 1985).

(b) Dextrose 5 or 10% intravenously to prevent or treat hypoglycaemia.

(c) Dexamethasone either intramuscularly or intravenously to reduce the risk of cerebral oedema.

(d) Konakion to reduce the risk of haemorrhage.

(e) Calcium for hypocalcaemia.

The baby's condition is monitored constantly and observations and all treatment given are recorded. The midwife also supports the parents who will naturally be very anxious at this time.

As the condition improves, as indicated by the rising Apgar score, the baby will be extubated but requires careful observation for some time. The mother should be given her baby to cuddle as soon as it has recovered and, in cases of mild to moderate asphyxia, it may be transferred with her to the postnatal ward. Low-birth-weight babies and/or those who have been severely asphyxiated are transferred to the neonatal unit for skilled observation and care, but the parents are encouraged to visit frequently and are kept informed of progress.

Failure to improve with the measures described above needs full investigation by the paediatrician to exclude meconium aspiration, diaphragmatic hernia, pneumothorax or CHOANAL ATRESIA. Very rarely, it may be due to irreversible terminal apnoea resulting from prolonged intrauterine hypoxia or intracranial haemorrhage.

Reference

Halliday HL, McClure G & Reid M (1985) Handbook of Neonatal Intensive Care, p. 24. Baillière Tindall: London.

APPENDIX 17

Neonatal Problems

Low birth weight

A low-birth-weight baby is one which weighs 2500 g or less at birth, irrespective of the gestation period. About 6 per cent of the babies born in the United Kingdom are in the low-birth-weight group, but within this relatively small group occur more than 60 per cent of all the neonatal deaths.

Low-birth-weight babies may be subdivided into those which are genuinely preterm and those which are not. A premature or preterm baby is one which is born before the end of the 37th week of pregnancy. (A term baby is one born between the end of the 37th week and the end of the 41st week). A 'small for gestational age' or 'light-for-dates' baby is one having a birth weight below the tenth centile (some authorities say below the fifth centile) for the period of gestation. These babies constitute as many as one-third of all low-birth-weight babies, presenting problems in some respects different from those of the true preterm infants.

These groupings are, of course, approximate; obviously many preterm babies are, in addition, small for gestational age. All low-birth-weight babies need some special care, but it is convenient to note certain differences.

Preterm babies

The common known causes of preterm labour are pre-eclampsia, multiple pregnancy and antepartum haemorrhage. With good antenatal care, admission to hospital and rest, some pregnancies can safely be prolonged. Often, however, the background of preterm labour is more obscure. It occurs in women of poor socio-economic status, who may be anaemic, ill-nourished, tired or otherwise debilitated, and is much more difficult to assess, still more to prevent. It is also more likely to occur in a woman who has had a termination of pregnancy (TOP).

The mother should be delivered in a hospital with a neonatal intensive care unit. Her labour should be conducted with a minimum of respiratory-depressant drugs; the labour room must be well warmed with a heated portable incubator present. An episiotomy and, possibly a forceps delivery may make the birth safer, as less pressure is applied directly to the soft, vulnerable fetal skull. A paediatrician should be present for the delivery, ready to resuscitate if necessary. The baby should be transferred quickly to the neonatal unit to prevent hypothermia and for skilled care.

Preterm and small for gestational age babies present many similar features, with some clearly defined differences, which are set out in Table 7.

Both babies are of low birth weight, have a head large in proportion to the trunk and lack subcutaneous fat, though the small for gestational age baby is often the 'skinnier' looking one.

More precise clinical assessment may be made by the Dubowitz rating, which is based on such factors as oedema, colour, texture and opacity of the skin, lanugo, plantar creases, breast development, ear formation and genitalia, together with a wide range of neurological criteria.

Table 7. Features of preterm and small for gestational age babies.

	Preterm baby	Small for gestational age baby
Skin	Skin reddish pink; lanugo present	Skin grey or yellowish, from meconium, and dry, sometimes cracked
Length	Proportionate to weight	Proportionate to gestation, i.e. long for weight
Head	Cranial bones soft	Cranial bones hard and unyielding
Face	Eyes closed, peaceful expression	Eyes often open, expression may look anxious and worried
Pinna of ear	Soft, little cartilage allows it to remain folded	Resistant to folding unless also preterm
Breast size	No tissue palpable or less than 1 cm in diameter	Tissue palpable often more than 1 cm in diameter
Abdomen	May be prominent	Often scaphoid
Behaviour	Weak cry; no attempt to suck or swallow; often inactive. Lies in 'frog position' with limbs abducted due to a degree of flaccidity	Stronger, more 'mature' cry; sucks, often hungrily, and swallows; often active and lively with good muscle tone

Preterm infants—problems

These babies have many problems as all their organs are immature. The severity of the problems is related directly to the degree of immaturity. The main problems are as follows.

Respiratory. These are very likely to occur under 35 weeks' gestation, and the main condition is the RESPIRATORY DISTRESS SYNDROME (RDS) otherwise called HYALINE MEMBRANE DISEASE (HMD). The cause is a lack of SURFACTANT.

Signs. The onset of respiratory difficulty occurs within 4 hours of birth. The signs include:

1. Tachypnoea—where the respiratory rate is over 60 per minute.
2. 'Grunting' on expiration.
3. Recession of the sternum and rib cage.

Very-low-birth-weight (VLBW) babies (those <1500 g) may not show all these signs, but may simply not breathe at all or gasp, and be therefore deeply cyanosed. Oxygen therapy is needed urgently to maintain oxygen concentration in the arterial blood (Pao_2) at 7.0–12.0 kPa (50–90 mmHg) and the carbon dioxide ($Paco_2$) at 4.5–6.0 kPa (35–45 mmHg). These should be continuously monitored by umbilical arterial catheter containing an oxygen electrode or by a transcutaneous monitor. If the Pao_2 falls below 7.0 kPa then hypoxic brain damage can occur, and if they remain above these levels for prolonged periods, blindness from RETROLENTAL FIBROPLASIA can ensue. Concentration of oxygen above 30 per cent must be given in a head box in an incubator. About 30 per cent of babies will need to breathe against a CONTINUOUS INFLATING PRESSURE (CIP) to prevent collapse of the surfactant-deficient alveoli on expiration. Methods for CIP include continuous positive airways pressure (CPAP) with intranasal catheters, face mask and endotracheal tube, or CONTINUOUS NEGATIVE PRESSURE (CNP).

Babies with severe RDS may also need mechanical ventilation (intermittent positive pressure ventilation (IPPV)). This is used to prevent prolonged apnoea accompanied by bradycardia or frequent apnoeic attacks, and also where the Pao_2 is below the desired level in spite of 95 per cent oxygen.

IPPV is usually administered at a rate of somewhere between 20 and 60 breaths per minute. In between these inflations a background pressure is maintained in the chest to prevent alveolar collapse, i.e. a positive end expiratory pressure (PEEP).

The baby receiving IPPV requires constant care and observation to detect complications which may occur.

Feeding. A baby under 34 weeks' gestation is unlikely to be able to suck, swallow or cough efficiently. In the first days, therefore, feeds will be given by nasogastric or nasojejunal tube. All these babies need a high calorie intake of 120–150 cal/kg per day. Expressed breast milk (EBM) or a special artificial milk for preterm babies is usually given in a scheme similar to that below:

Day 1: 60 ml/kg per 24 hours
Day 2: 90 ml/kg per 24 hours
Day 3: 120 ml/kg per 24 hours
Day 4: 150 ml/kg per 24 hours

This should build up to at least 200 ml/kg in a day.

All babies being ventilated and most VLBW infants are given total intravenous feeding until their condition improves. Enteral feeding is then gradually introduced.

Jaundice. This is very common in preterm infants (*see* p. 447).

Hypothermia. Heat is rapidly lost, due to the large surface area, lack of brown fat and chilling at delivery when the baby is wet and naked. Oxygen and energy are used up rapidly unless the baby is kept in a neutral thermal environment. A special and intensive care nursery should be kept at between 26°C and 28°C (79–82.5°F) and an incubator between 32°C and 36°C (89.5–97°F). To maintain the skin temperature at 36.5°C various other aids may be needed, such as a Perspex shield, bubble plastic sheeting and clothes. Some servo-controlled incubators adjust automatically to control the baby's temperature.

Infection. A preterm baby lacks maternal antibodies, and has very little cellular immunity, so the infant is very vulnerable. Prevention of infection is essential, with meticulous frequent hand-washing on the part of the staff, and also the parents of the baby who will be taking part in the care.

Maternal/infant relationship. A baby receiving ventilation, in the midst of a battery of machinery, cannot be held close to its mother or carer. It lies in bright light and hears mechanical rather than human sounds. This lack of human contact may possibly adversely affect the baby. It is definitely known that it can affect the mother's relationship to her baby, and that she feels unlike a mother. The baby is more likely to be neglected or to suffer non-accidental injury when the mother has not been encouraged to make early physical contact. She should be encouraged to visit as soon as possible, and then be introduced to the baby with an explanation of the equipment, which may be very frightening. She should touch the baby inside the incubator, and as soon as the condition allows, cuddle, talk to, feed and change the baby. Midwives should be very careful to see that the mother feels comfortable about visiting the unit, and accompany her if possible or ensure that a member of the unit staff meets her until she feels more confident.

Small for gestational age (SGA) or light-for-dates (LFD) babies

A baby whose birth weight is below the tenth percentile for the period of gestation is termed small for gestational age. These babies are more likely to suffer from hypoxia *in utero* or birth asphyxia than are normal or preterm babies.

Management at birth

Hypoxia during labour must be detected at the soonest possible moment (*see* Appendix 16) and where possible the midwife will ensure that a paediatrician is present at delivery to resuscitate the baby.

When hypoxia occurs, meconium may be passed into the liquor, which in turn may be inhaled during delivery. Respiratory distress then may develop as the bronchioles get plugged and pneumonitis occurs. This can be prevented by intubating the baby, who has meconium in the pharynx and trachea, before the first breath is taken. It cannot then be sucked further down during inhalation.

Subsequent problems

Hypoglycaemia. This is a common problem, as the liver becomes depleted of glycogen stores *in utero*, and is not apparent until the levels of glucose have fallen below 1.4 mmol/l (25 mg/dl). Apnoeic attacks may then occur and brain damage can follow then. Other signs of hypoglycaemia are very unspecific: lack of muscle tone, poor feeding and jittering. All babies below the tenth percentile should be screened frequently for 72 hours or so after birth using Dextrostix or BM-Test-Glycemie. Early and frequent feeding is essential to prevent hypoglycaemia and these babies usually suck well. Treatment of hypoglycaemia is by continuous intragastric feeding or by intravenous infusion of 10% dextrose.

Hypothermia. This occurs for the same reasons as in the preterm infant.

Infection. Aspiration pneumonia is a particular problem of SGA babies. The baby's dry, cracked, often meconium-stained skin also predisposes to skin infections.

Poor growth. This may occur in babies whose growth *in utero* has been retarded from early pregnancy, thus neurological damage is more likely. The outlook is better for babies whose growth has only been retarded in the last trimester of pregnancy.

Babies of diabetic mothers

The baby of a diabetic mother, though himself or herself very unlikely to be a diabetic, is at risk in other ways. There is a greater than average chance of congenital defect, and the fetus may be 'large for dates' if the diabetes is not well controlled. There is then a risk of intrauterine death during the last 3–4 weeks of pregnancy, or alternatively of cephalopelvic disproportion.

With expert antenatal care shared between a specialist physician and an obstetrician, the diabetes is well controlled and the fetus healthier and less large. Labour may then be allowed to commence spontaneously at term. In cases of poor diabetic control or a deterioration in maternal or fetal condition, early induction of labour or a ceasarean section will be necessary. If the baby's condition at birth gives rise to anxiety, he or she will be transferred to a neonatal unit. The particular risks to this large but preterm baby are: respiratory distress syndrome, particularly if delivery has been by caesarean section; and severe hypoglycaemia, due to transient hyperinsulinaemia, which, being foreseen, can be promptly corrected. The blood glucose level will therefore be monitored soon after birth and thereafter initially 2 hourly because hypoglycaemia can cause brain damage. Early feeding is essential and the Dextrostix reading should not be allowed to drop below 1.4 mmol/l (25 mg/dl) as this hypoglycaemia can cause brain damage.

Jaundice

Jaundice is seen very commonly in young babies. It is usually slight in degree, sometimes moderate and, occasionally, severe.

Enzyme deficiency or 'physiological' jaundice. These conditions or jaundice due to immaturity of hepatic function and the breakdown of excess red blood cells which occurs soon after birth affects about 25 per cent of apparently mature and healthy babies. Characteristically it appears about the third day, is slight in degree, is not accompanied by anaemia and fades by the seventh or eighth day. The child remains in good condition and either behaves normally or is slightly lethargic. In these mild cases no treatment is required, though the serum bilirubin should be monitored and it is necessary to ensure that a sleepy baby is having sufficient food and fluid. Sometimes the jaundice may become serious, necessitating the use of phototherapy and even, occasionally, exchange transfusion.

When red blood cells are broken down or haemolysed (a process that continues throughout life), bilirubin is released. It is fat soluble and has to be changed to water-soluble bilirubin before it can be excreted. This process is called conjugation and takes place in the liver by the action of the liver enzyme glucuronyl transferase, after which it can be excreted. If this function is delayed for a few days, the bilirubin accumulates in the blood and leaks into the tissues, and the yellow tinge is seen in the skin and sclerae. In a fair-skinned baby, jaundice is apparent when the serum bilirubin has reached a level of approximately 51 μmol/l (3 mg/100 ml).

In preterm babies, as might be expected, jaundice is commoner and may be more severe. Phototherapy is often used successfully to reduce the level of the unconjugated bilirubin to avoid the danger of kernicterus.

Kernicterus or nuclear jaundice. This may occur where the levels of unconjugated bilirubin exceed the following levels, depending on gestation:

Under 27 weeks	250 μmol/l
28–30 weeks	280 μmol/l
31–34 weeks	310 μmol/l
35–38 weeks	350 μmol/l
39+ weeks	380 μmol/l

The bilirubin crosses the blood/brain barrier and stains the basal ganglia of the brain. Irreversible changes take place, leading to athetoid spasticity, mental retardation or death. Exchange transfusion is very occasionally needed to prevent the above levels being exceeded, but is not without risk.

Haemolytic jaundice
  Caused by blood incompatibility. The commonest type is due to Rhesus incompatibility where the mother is Rhesus-negative and the father Rhesus-positive, either HOMOZYGOUS or HETEROZYGOUS. Where the Rhesus-positive factor, usually D, is transmitted to the fetus who carries d from its mother, the fetal blood group will be Rhesus-positive because D is dominant to d. This always occurs when the father is homozygous, but may not do so when he is heterozygous. Isoimmunization can arise whenever Rhesus-positive blood, even as little as 0.25 ml, enters the circulation of the mother who is Rhesus-negative. Very rarely isoimmunization is caused by mismatched blood transfusion, but usually by a transplacental haemorrhage (TPH) at either abortion or delivery of the fetus or following premature separation of the placenta or trauma to it during procedures such as external cephalic version, chorionic villus biopsy or amniocentesis. Unless these Rhesus-positive cells are

identified by the KLEIHAUER TEST and eliminated by giving anti-D within 72 hours of delivery or abortion or the investigative procedures described above, *sensitization* will occur. In this process the body's own antibody production is initiated, and cannot be reversed once started, so that anti-D is now useless.

Prevention. All women who are Rhesus-negative and giving birth must have their blood tested for Rhesus-positive fetal cells and, if present, anti-D is given as soon as possible. This is now given routinely even if the Kleihauer test is negative. Even where the cord blood showed the fetus to have been Rhesus-positive, and no fetal cells were seen, some cases developed antibodies. Similarly, Anti-D is given in pregnancy when there is a risk of transplacental haemorrhage, as described above (Clarke *et al.*, 1985).

Antibodies are sought by testing the blood antenatally at booking and at 28 and 34 weeks' gestation; if antibodies are detected, antibody titres are estimated at more frequent intervals.

Treatment. In specialist units, amniocentesis, under the control of ultrasound scanning to avoid the placental site, is carried out to estimate the amount of bilirubin in the liquor amnii. This indicates whether the maternal antibodies have crossed the placenta to the fetus and caused haemolysis. Where this is severe, the fetus may receive intraperitoneal blood transfusions (IPT) of Rhesus-negative blood to keep it alive until it is mature enough to be delivered—usually at about 34 weeks' gestation.

Mild cases of incompatibility may need no treatment apart from induction of labour before full term.

Where the haemolysis is *severe* and hydrops fetalis is certain to occur before it is safe to deliver the fetus, a series of IPTs are attempted. After birth this baby will need exchange transfusions and will be nursed in the neonatal intensive care unit.

ABO incompatibility. This occurs in 1 in 200 pregnancies where the maternal blood group is O, the serum containing anti-a and anti-b. If the fetus is therefore group A or B or AB, an antibody differing immunologically from normal anti-a and b may cross the placenta and cause haemolysis in the neonate, even the first-born. Jaundice appears within 24 hours of birth, but is usually mild. The bilirubin level rises very rapidly but anaemia is less obvious. The COOMB'S TEST is usually negative, unlike Rhesus incompatibility. Treatment is as for any jaundice—by phototherapy or, rarely, by exchange transfusion.

Other causes of jaundice.

Infections. Those acquired *in utero* include CYTOMEGALOVIRUS, TOXO-PLASMOSIS and RUBELLA. After birth severe infections such as pyelonephritis and septicaemia may cause haemolysis and therefore jaundice.

Cephalhaematoma and severe bruising. These are due to excess breakdown of red blood cells.

Metabolic disorders. Those causing jaundice include glucose-6-phosphate dehydrogenase (G6PD) deficiency (see dictionary section), HYPOTHYROIDISM, GALACTOSAEMIA and CYSTIC FIBROSIS.

Breast milk jaundice. This is thought to be caused by the excretion of a steroid in the milk which interferes with liver function.

Obstructive jaundice. This is rare. The cause is biliary atresia, compression of the ducts or hepatitis.

The midwife should take note of any jaundice in a baby under her care, and if it appears in the first few hours, or deepens noticeably, the paediatrician should be called. Coloured babies, in whom skin change is not apparent, should have their sclera observed.

Infection in the neonate

Though less vulnerable than his preterm counterpart, the healthy newborn baby nevertheless needs careful protection from bacterial infection. Babies in hospital in particular are liable to cross-infection, and have little resistance to the strains of staphylococci and streptococci which cannot be completely eliminated from their environment.

Accordingly, various barrier-nursing procedures are common practice. Each baby has his own equipment in a cupboard attached to the cot and disposables are used wherever possible. Rooming-in is chosen in preference to overcrowded nurseries. Hand-washing is strict and frequent, and antiseptic hand creams are used. Staff are carefully screened and those having infections are, so far as is possible, excluded from contact with babies. Visitors having infections are asked not to visit. During influenza epidemics, for example, visitors are sometimes excluded.

Despite these and many other precautions, minor infections are quite common, whilst infection of a serious and disturbing kind occurs from time to time.

Ophthalmia neonatorum

A notifiable disease, ophthalmia neonatorum is caused by *Staphylococcus, Escherichia coli, Mycoplasma hominis, Chlamydia trachomatis* and the gonococcus. By definition, this is any purulent conjunctivitis occurring within 21 days of birth. Severe ophthalmia is quite a rarity, but 'sticky eye' is the commonest of all neonatal infections. The midwife should consult a doctor about the slightest stickiness. A conjunctival swab is sent to the laboratory to determine the infecting organism and the antibiotics to which it is sensitive. The eye may be very gently swabbed with sterile saline. In many mild cases the stickiness clears completely within 18–24 hours, and often the laboratory's report states that no pathogens were isolated. If the condition does not clear quickly, chloramphenicol or neomycin eye drops may be used, while in the occasional severe ophthalmia of gonococcal infection, a very vigorous regimen of frequent instillation of penicillin drops will be carried out. Where *Chlamydia* is the cause, tetracycline eye ointment is used and systemic erythromycin may also be prescribed to prevent the infection spreading to the respiratory tract.

Skin infections

The neonate's skin is very sensitive, and rashes are not uncommon—usually as a result of irritation without infection. Chafing (sometimes called intertrigo), sweat rash, napkin rash and sore buttocks are examples. Soreness of the axillae, groins and neck responds to careful washing and gently thorough drying and a light dusting of an antiseptic powder; the baby who is overheated may have a rash which soon disappears if excess clothing is removed. Napkin rash, if it is an ammoniacal dermatitis, will require very careful cleansing of the affected area and possibly protecting the skin with zinc and castor oil cream; strict attention is paid to the washing of the napkins, which should be either changed more frequently or temporarily discarded, the area being exposed to the air. The treatment of sore buttocks, not uncommon in artificially fed babies, is on similar lines.

Small crops of spots or pustules are usually staphylococcal in origin, as is paronychia (infection of the nail bed). The treatment of both is the same: dabbing with chlorhexidine in 1 per cent solution in spirit.

Signs of an umbilical infection include slight redness around the base of a moist, offensive cord and delay in separation. The infected cord requires frequent cleansing with antiseptic agents and close observation is essential, as severe omphalitis with septicaemia can occasionally develop with alarming rapidity.

Alimentary tract

Oral thrush is seen, not infrequently as greyish white patches in the mouth. It is caused by a fungus, *Candida albicans*, and occurs equally in breast-fed and artificially fed babies, and more often in the babies of mothers who have had candidal (monilial) vaginitis in pregnancy. The fungus tends to spread to the stomach and intestine and causes loose, offensive stools which may lead to sore buttocks. It is usually treated with nystatin suspension, 100 000 units in 1 ml, after feeds. The child should be isolated and, until the lesions clear, he/she should wear disposable napkins if they are not already in regular use. Nystatin cream may be applied to sore buttocks.

Gastroenteritis is not common, but it is so dangerous that the slightest suggestive symptoms create anxiety. With the onset of vomiting and frequent watery stools there is rapid dehydration and electrolyte imbalance, and the baby is soon in a state of collapse, whilst other babies are increasingly at risk. The affected baby should be rigidly isolated, given intravenous fluid replacement and oral feeding stopped. Contact cases should also be isolated. This may be due to rotavirus or to a particular strain of *Escherichia coli*, or to one of the *Salmonella* group. The appropriate antibiotics are prescribed and blood electrolyte balance restored.

Urinary tract

A baby does not have the characteristic signs and symptoms of an adult with a urinary tract infection. It is to be suspected if the baby is, first, not thriving, and soon, more positively ill—refusing feeds and becoming pallid or greyish, and limp or irritable. The diagnosis is made by finding pus cells and bacteria (usually *Escherichia coli*) in the baby's urine obtained by suprapubic aspiration. Treatment is by antibiotics; recovery is the rule, but remissions tend to occur, in which case there may be an underlying congenital defect of the urinary tract, and in any case adequate follow-up by X-ray is necessary. If diagnosis is delayed, there is a danger of septicaemia.

Respiratory tract

Infection may occur as an ascending or intrapartum infection or, after delivery, from air-borne organisms transmitted by parents or others in close contact with the baby. Initially the baby is snuffly and may develop a hoarse cry. If the infection spreads downwards and the baby develops pneumonia, the respirations will be rapid and the child may have cyanotic attacks. The temperature is not always raised and the diagnosis may be confused by diarrhoea and vomiting. A chest X-ray is taken to confirm the diagnosis and the organism identified where possible by nose and throat swabs. The appropriate antibiotic is given and the baby is nursed in an incubator with humidified oxygen. In severe cases treatment is similar to that given to babies with respiratory distress syndrome.

Septicaemia

This is growth of bacteria in the blood stream, usually following a localized infection. The baby's response to infection is typically non-specific, although the liver and spleen may be enlarged. Diagnosis is confirmed by blood culture. Treatment includes intravenous antibiotics, an intravenous infusion and drugs to combat shock and if necessary, a transfusion of white blood cells to help combat the infection, and ventilator therapy.

Meningitis

This may follow septicaemia. Initially the signs are non-specific but later vomiting, a high-pitched cry, raised anterior fontanelle, convulsions and neck rigidity occur. Diagnosis is confirmed by lumbar puncture and intravenous or intrathecal antibiotics are given. There is a high risk of brain damage or death.

It must be reiterated that this appendix deals very briefly with some, not all, of the commoner neonatal problems. In most cases, reference to a more detailed textbook account is necessary.

Reference

Clarke CA, Mollison PL & Whitfield AGW (1985) Deaths from rhesus haemolytic disease in England and Wales in 1982 and 1983. *British Medical Journal* 291: 17–19.

APPENDIX 18

Normal Blood and Urine Values and Tests

Adults

Blood

Normal volume	5 litres approx.
Red cells	4–5×10^{12}/l
Haemoglobin	8.1–9.9 mmol/l
Packed cell volume (PCV haematocrit)	0.42–0.50/l
Reticulocytes	0.005–0.015/l
Leucocytes	4.0–11.0×10^9/l
neutrophils	2.5–7.5×10^9/l
lymphocytes	1.8–3.5×10^9/l
monocytes	0.2–0.8×10^9/l
eosinophils	0.04–0.4×10^9/l
basophils	0.0–0.1×10^9/l
Platelets	200–300×10^9/l
Acid–base state:	
pH	7.35–7.45
$P\text{CO}_2$	4.7–6.0 kPa
Standard bicarbonate	24.0–32.0 mmol/l

Plasma	Non-pregnant	Pregnant
Calcium	2.1–2.6 mol/l	2.2–2.4 mmol/l
Chloride	95–105 mmol/l	
Creatinine	60–120 mmol/l	
Magnesium	0.8–1.0 mmol/l	
Osmolality	285–295 mOsm/kg	
Phosphate	0.8–1.4 mmol/l	0.8–1.5 mmol/l
Potassium	3.8–5.0 mmol/l	
Sodium	135–145 mmol/l	
Urea	2.5–5.8 mmol/l	2.3–5.0 mmol/l
Uric acid	0.09–0.36 mmol/l	0.15–0.52 mmol/l

	Non-pregnant	Pregnant
Serum		
Albumin	36–52 g/l	22–44 g/l
Bilirubin	<17 μmol/l	
Cholesterol	3.6–6.7 mmol/l	5.4–7.8 mmol/l
Protein (total)	62–75 g/l	50–70 g/l
Thyroid-binding globulin (TBG)	6–16 mg/l	6–32 mg/l
Thyroid-stimulating hormone (TSH)	1–3 mU/l	1.7–4.4 mU/l
Thyroxine (T4)	50–140 nmol/l	72–206 nmol/l
Triiodothyronine (T3)	0.9–3.0 nmol/l	
T4/TBG ratio	5–13	Lower
Blood		
Glucose (fasting)	3.3–5.3 mmol/l	3.3–6.1 mmol/l
Red cell		
Glucose-6-phosphate dehydrogenase	680–1095 IU/l	
Urine		
Calcium	2.5–7.5 mmol/24 h	
Creatinine	9–17 mmol/24 h	
Creatinine clearance	80–130 ml/min	80–140 ml/min
Osmolality	>600 mOsm/kg	
Potassium	26–123 mmol/24 h	
Protein	<0.05 g/l	
Reducing substances	<2.5 g/l	
Sodium	27–287 mmol/24 h	

Babies

Blood		
Erythrocytes		
Birth	6–6.5 × 10^{12}/l	
4 weeks	4.5 × 10^{12}/l	
Glucose	1.0–6.0 mmol/l	
Haemoglobin		
Birth	20 g/dl	
1 week	13.2 g/dl	
Glucose-6-phosphate	>1800 IU/l	

dehydrogenase

Packed cell volume	
Day 1	52–58%
2 weeks	46–54%
Leucocytes	
Day 1	8×10^9/l (8000/mm³)
Day 7	1.6×10^9/l (16 000/mm³)
pH	7.3–7.4
Phenylalanine	0.37 mmol/l

Plasma

Calcium	1.9–2.9 mmol/l
Chloride	96–106 mmol/l
Creatinine (day 2)	9–62 mmol/l
Magnesium	0.6–1.6 mmol/l
Osmolality	280–305 mOsm/kg
Phosphate	1.3–2.7 mmol/l
Potassium	4.0–6.0 mmol/l
Sodium	136–143 mmol/l
Urea	3.4–8.4 mmol/l

Serum

Albumin	28–40 g/l
Cholesterol	2.1–4.1 mmol/l
Protein (total)	50–65 g/l
Thyroid-stimulating hormone	<0.5–8.0 mU/l
Thyroxine (T4)	125–200 mmol/l

CSF

Glucose	2.5–3.8 mmol/l
Protein	0.4–1.2 g/l

Urine

Osmolality	40–1400 mOsm/kg
Potassium	26–125 mmol/l
Protein	<0.5 g/l
Reducing substances	<2.5 g/l
Sodium	43–211 mmol/l

Stool

Reducing substances	<2.5 g/l
Bilirubin (preterm)	
cord	68 μmol/l total

	9 μmol/l conj.
<24 h	137 μmol/l total
	10 μmol/l conj.
<48 h	205 μmol/l total
	10 μmol/l conj.
3–5 days	274 μmol/l total
	17 μmol/l conj.

Bilirubin (term)

cord	43 μmol/l total
	9 μmol/l conj.
<24 h	103 μmol/l total
	10 μmol/l conj.
<48 h	128 μmol/l total
	12 μmol/l conj.
3–5 days	205 μmol/l total
	17 μmol/l conj.

Changes in blood in pregnancy

Total volume: increased by 25–30 per cent; maximum at about 28th week and gradually declining.

Red cells: small increase in relation to total volume, therefore hydraemia or apparent anaemia, preventable by consumption of foods rich in iron.

White cells: increase to 15.0–20.0×10^9/l (15 000–20 000 mm³).

Plasma protein: Relatively small increase; concentration at term 5 g/dl (5 g/100 ml).

Blood urea: falls to 2.3–5.0 mmol/l (10–20 mg/100 ml).

Platelets: increase to about 500×10^9/l at term

Blood groups

There are two agglutinogens, named A and B, found in blood and other tissues. Any individual's blood may contain A, or B, or A and B or neither, and thus four blood groups are described: A, B, AB and O. The serum contains a natural antibody, or agglutinin, as seen below:

Red blood cell agglutinogen	Serum agglutinin or antibody
A	Anti-b
B	Anti-a
AB	—
O	Anti-a and b

When a blood transfusion is given, attention must be paid in order to avoid a fatal reaction. If the same group as the antibody or agglutinin in the serum is given (e.g. group B blood to a group A person, who contains anti-b in their serum) then agglutination of the donor cells will occur.

Universal recipient. Group AB has no agglutinin or antibody in the serum; this group can accept any other, and so is called the universal recipient.

Universal donor. Group O cells contain neither a nor b so can be safely given to any other group, and is kept for use in acute emergencies provided it is also Rhesus-negative. The proportions of the groups are summarized below:

Group	Proportion
A	40%
B	10%
AB	5%
O	45%

Rhesus types. People whose red cells contain Rhesus antigen (so called because it was first isolated in Rhesus monkeys) are described as Rhesus positive (RH+), and constitute about 85 per cent of the population of white people in Europe and North America. The remainder, who carry no such antigen, are termed Rhesus-negative (Rh−). Rhesus grouping differs from ABO grouping in that there are no natural antibodies or agglutinins in the serum. A Rhesus-negative person should never be given Rhesus-positive blood, as it stimulates the formation of antibodies (isoimmunization). This could cause a severe reaction to a subsequent transfusion. Similarly, a Rhesus-negative woman may develop antibodies to a Rhesus-positive fetus in her uterus (see Appendix 17).

Blood tests routinely carried out in pregnancy
1. *ABO grouping*.
2. *Rhesus typing*. In cases of antepartum or anticipated postpartum haemorrhage suitable blood can thus be cross-matched and set aside for the patient.
3. A serological test to detect *syphilis*.
4. The *haemoglobin* value is ascertained when the pregnancy is first diagnosed and repeated at least twice; more often if anaemia is suspected.
5. *Antibody* tests are carried out both early and late in pregnancy in Rhesus-negative women.
6. *Sickling* tests are made in patients of those races in which sickle cell disease occurs.

7. *Rubella*. Screening for antibody formation is carried out. If none is present, rubella vaccination is arranged in the puerperium.

Routine tests on babies' blood

1. The *Guthrie test* is performed on the 6th or 7th day of life to detect phenylketonuria and other inborn errors of protein metabolism.
2. *Dextrostix test*. The risks of hypoglycaemia are such that this simple test is undertaken at least every 6–8 hours, or more often if readings are low, on all babies in special care units and on all small for gestational age or large for gestational age babies.

Examination of the urine

The examination should be methodical, and all findings should be recorded at once.

All apparatus should be absolutely clean.

Most chemical tests require the urine to be acid. Alkaline specimens should therefore be acidified unless the reagent itself is acid.

The following features should be noted.

Amount. In an adult, about 1500 ml daily.

The output is increased (polyuria) by a greater fluid intake, in the normal early puerperium, in cold weather (when the skin is less active), in diabetes of all kinds, in chronic nephritis and following the administration of such drugs as caffeine and digitalis.

It is decreased (oliguria) following a diminished intake, in hot weather, in febrile conditions, in acute nephritis, in severe pre-eclampsia, in cardiac failure, in severe sweating, vomiting, diarrhoea and haemorrhage, and by drugs such as opium.

Suppression of urine (anuria) means that no urine is excreted by the kidney.

Retention of urine means that it is retained in the bladder.

Colour. Normally pale amber and clear. Dilution makes it paler, and concentration darker. It is smoky or even bright red if blood is present, and greenish-brown in the presence of bile.

Deposits. Urates form a pink 'brick-dust' deposit which dissolves on heating. Phosphates form a white precipitate in alkaline urine, which dissolves on the addition of acid. Pus cells make the specimen cloudy, and infected urine sometimes has a faintly greenish 'sheen'. Mucus shows as a flocculent deposit.

Smell. Ketones may be recognized by a sweetish smell. In *Escherichia coli* infection there is a disagreeable 'fishy' odour.

Reaction. Normally slightly acid, but not uncommonly neutral or slightly alkaline. Urine becomes alkaline on standing. It may be strongly acid in the presence of ketones or in *E. coli* infection.

Acid urine turns blue litmus paper red.

Alkaline urine turns red litmus paper blue.

If neither colour changes the reaction is neutral.

Specific gravity. This is a measure of the density compared with that of water, which is 1000. Normal urine is 1010–1020. The greater the amount passed, the more dilute the urine and the lower the specific gravity, as for example in chronic nephritis. In diabetes mellitus a large volume of pale urine is passed, but the specific gravity is high on account of the sugar content. The specific gravity is raised in concentrated urine, as for example in severe vomiting.

The urinometer should be floated clear of the glass for an accurate reading.

Urine tests
See Tables 8 *and* 9.

Interpretation of urine tests

During pregnancy
1. *Proteins* may signify:
   (a) Contamination—possibly from a vaginal infection or discharge, which is common in pregnancy, or from the container used for the specimen. A mid-stream specimen (MSU) should be tested to exclude contamination.
   (b) Infection. Protein in an uncontaminated specimen may be present as a constituent of pus in infected urine. This is revealed by microscopic examination.
   (c) Renal damage. If no pus is present, the protein is serum albumin or even serum globulin from the blood. This is true proteinuria; in early pregnancy it would suggest chronic renal disease, and in late pregnancy, pre-eclampsia.
2. *Sugar* may be:
   (a) Lactose, distinguished from glucose by Clinistix or chromatography. Requires no treatment.
   (b) Renal glycosuria. This is due to a lowering of the renal threshold for glucose, which is common in pregnancy. It is of no

significance but cannot be distinguished without testing the blood sugar.

(c) Alimentary glycosura. Here the glucose is absorbed normally, and reaches a higher concentration than usual, but falls to normal within 2 hours. The patient is well, and there is no ketosis.

(d) Diabetes mellitus. The urine contains more glucose and ketone, the patient probably has symptoms and her blood sugar is raised.

3. *Ketones* signify carbohydrate starvation and disordered fat metabolism. They are found:

(a) When 'morning sickness' is worsening to hyperemesis gravidarum.

(b) In conjunction with glucose in diabetes mellitus. The urine should always be tested for ketones if the woman complains of persistent vomiting, or if she should appear dehydrated.

4. *Pus*. Pus cells found in a mid-stream specimen of urine signify infection of some part of the urinary tract. This is relatively common in pregnancy.

5. *Chlorides*. A diminution of urinary chlorides is found in hyperemesis gravidarum, and in pre-eclampsia where there is marked oedema.

6. *Blood and bile pigments* are found only rarely during pregnancy.

During labour

1. *Protein*. This is usually due to contamination of the urine with liquor amnii, mucus or blood.

2. *Ketones*. These are found in abnormal and prolonged labour, especially if the woman is vomiting. This is serious, and indicates the necessity for intravenous dextrose.

During the puerperium

1. *Lactose*. This is commonly present.

2. *Protein*. This test would be carried out only in mothers who had had proteinuria during pregnancy. A mid-stream specimen is necessary, as the lochia contaminates the urine.

3. *Pus*. Urinary tract infection—in the puerperium, more often cystitis—is not uncommon. It is diagnosed by the finding of pus cells on microscopy.

Renal function tests
These include blood urea, plasma creatinine and uric acid estimations.

Table 8. Ames strip tests for urine. The Ames strip tests are so quick, easy and accurate that they have largely replaced the older tests carried out with Bunsen burners and bottles of (often poisonous) chemicals. (Tests for fluids other than urine are included below.)

Name of reagent	Nature of test	Procedure	Interpretation
Acetest	Ketones	Place tablet on a filter paper and put one drop of urine on tablet. Exactly 30 s later compare with colour chart	Shows presence of acetone and acetoacetic acid. Tablet lavender or purple = positive, the deeper the colour the greater the concentration. Tablet white or cream = negative
Albustix strips	Protein	Dip end of stick in urine, remove immediately and compare closely with colour chart at once	Test end turns to shade of green = positive, nearest shade on chart giving approximate amount. Test end remains yellow = negative
Clinistix strips	Glucose	Dip test end in fresh urine, remove at once and in 10 s compare with colour chart. Ignore changes after 10 s	Test end changes to purple = positive; 'light' generally 0.25% or less; 'dark' generally 2% or more. Test end remains red = negative
Clinitest tablets	Sugar	With dropper upright put 5 drops of urine in test-tube. Rinse dropper and add 10 drops of water. Add 1 tablet; 15 s after boiling stops, shake tube gently and read, comparing with colour chart	Change to green or orange = positive, nearest shade on chart giving amount. Transient bright orange, turning brown at any time = more than 2%. Blue = negative. Reduced by lactose and glucose
Hemastix	Blood	Dip test end in well-mixed urine; remove immediately. Read in exactly 30 s. Ignore changes after 30 s	Test end changes to blue = positive; test end remains off-white = negative

Table 8. Continued

Name of reagent	Nature of test	Procedure	Interpretation
Icotest tablets	Bilirubin	Place 5 drops of urine on special mat. Put tablet on moist area. Flow 2 drops of water over tablet. Note mat around tablet 30 s later	Mat turns bluish purple = positive; concentration roughly proportionate to depth of colour and speed of development. Mat unchanged or faintly red or orange at 30 s = negative
Ketostix strips	Ketones	May be used for serum, plasma and milk as well as urine. Dip test end in specimen; remove at once. In 15 s compare with colour chart	Test end changes to lavender or purple = positive, the deeper the colour, the greater the concentration. Shows acetone and acetoacetic acid. Test end remains off-white = negative

Two or more tests may be carried out simultaneously, using compound reagent strips

Name of reagent	Nature of test	Procedure	Interpretation
Hema-Combistix	pH Glucose Protein Blood	Dip test end in well-mixed urine, remove immediately and, keeping tip downwards, read: glucose exactly 10 s and blood exactly 30 s after dipping; pH and protein, time not critical	pH range from 5 to 9 shown by colour change of orange through green to blue Accurate to ±0.5. Glucose, protein and blood as Clinistix, Albustix and Hemastix, respectively, above
Labstix	pH Protein Glucose Ketones Blood	Similar to Hema-Combistix, above	With addition of Ketostix reagent strip. Useful in antenatal clinics since the tests for protein, glucose and ketones are those routinely required
Uristix	Protein Glucose	Dip test end of stick in urine and remove immediately. Read protein portion at once and glucose portion 10 s later	Interpret as Albustix and Clinistix above

Table 9. Chemical tests for abnormal constituents in urine. Before the introduction of reagent strips, urine testing was a time-consuming procedure, necessitating the use of bottles of chemicals, often poisonous or otherwise dangerous. Of these traditional tests, those set out below are still in occasional use

Test	Reagent	Method	Interpretation	Remarks
For protein Cold	Salicylic acid, 30% solution	Pour 2.5 cm of urine into each of two test tubes. To one add 3 drops of salicylic acid	A cloud indicates the presence of protein. In case of doubt compare with the control specimen	
Esbach's quantitative	Esbach's reagent of citric and picric acids	Into the graduated tube pour urine to the mark U and reagent to the mark R. Mix well. Leave for 24 h	The protein sinks as a sediment, the level of which is read, according to the figures on the tube, in g/l	The specific gravity should be 1010 or less, otherwise the precipitate may not sink. This test is only approximate

	Reagent	Method	Result
For sugar Benedict's	Benedict's copper sulphate solution	Pour 5 ml of reagent into a test-tube. Add 8–10 drops of urine. Boil for 2 min	A change of colour through green and yellow to deep red-orange indicates an increasing amount of sugar	Benedict's solution is reduced by both galactose and lactose. Differentiation may be necessary
For chlorides Fantus	Silver nitrate, 2.9% solution. Potassium dichromate, 20% solution	Into a clean dry test-tube put 10 drops of urine. Add 1 drop of potassium dichromate. Rinse pipette with distilled water, and add silver nitrate drop by drop, counting the drops until the colour changes from yellow to red	The number of drops of silver nitrate needed to accomplish the colour change indicates the number of grams of sodium chloride per litre of urine. Normal is about 5 g/l	In order to assess the chloride excretion accurately, it is necessary to know the total volume of urine passed

APPENDIX 19

Drugs Used in Midwifery, Including Controlled Drugs

Drugs of any description should be avoided in pregnancy if possible because of the risk of their harmful effect on the fetus. This is especially relevant during the first trimester, when the fetus is undergoing development. There are times, however, when the benefits of a drug outweigh the risks—for example, in epilepsy where there is little choice but to continue the anticonvulsant therapy.

Following the thalidomide tragedy, a Committee on the Safety of Drugs was set up in 1962 to ensure that every new drug is tested for toxicity on pregnant animals in a laboratory before it is considered safe to be prescribed to the pregnant woman.

The need for drugs in midwifery and paediatrics can be divided into five categories:

1. To relieve pain in labour—an effective analgesic which does not adversely affect the mother, the contractions or the fetus.
2. To induce labour.
3. To prevent/treat haemorrhage.
4. To resuscitate the neonate.
5. To treat medical conditions.

Legislation

1. Medicines Act, 1968 regulates use of all medicinal products.
2. Misuse of Drugs Act, 1971 is concerned with abuse of controlled drugs (formerly classified as 'dangerous drugs').
3. Misuse of Drugs Act, 1971, Modification Order, 1985.
4. Misuse of Drugs Regulations, 1985, and Misuse of Drugs Act, 1971 Modification Order, 1985 lay down conditions whereby controlled drugs may be used by medical practitioners and certain others such as midwives. The safe custody of controlled drugs and the procedure whereby midwives must surrender or destroy unwanted stock is also outlined.
5. Medicines (Prescription Only) Order, 1980. Medicines can be prescribed only by a doctor but midwives are authorized to obtain certain ones, e.g. oxytocic drugs, sedatives, analgesics, local anaesthetics and drugs for maternal and neonatal resuscitation.

Controlled drugs are stored in a locked compartment within a locked cupboard, the keys of which are held by the midwife in charge to prevent unauthorized access to them.

Controlled drugs

Five Controlled Drug Schedules were introduced in the 1985 Regulations:

Schedule 1: Cannabis, hallucinogens etc.

Schedule 2: Drugs which are strongly addictive such as diamorphine, morphine and pethidine.

Schedule 3: Drugs such as barbituates and pentazocine (Fortral).

Schedule 4: This includes benzodiazepine tranquillizers such as diazepam, nitrazepam and temazepam.

Schedule 5: Medicines which contain a limited amount of controlled drugs such as some cough mixtures.

Since 1951, practising midwives who have notified their intention to practise to the Local Supervising Authority have been allowed to use pethidine on their own responsibility, provided they abide by the UKCC Midwives' Rules and the relevant Acts of Parliament.

The possession and administration of controlled drugs of midwives is covered by the Misuse of Drugs Regulations, 1985 (S1 1985 No. 2066) the Misuse of Drugs (Northern Ireland) Regulations 1986 (SR 1985 No. 52), and the Medicines Act 1968 (UKCC, 1991). These Regulations are concerned with the control of narcotic drugs and other substances which can cause drug dependence. They also provide for the supply of pethidine to midwives (and any other controlled drug listed in Schedule 3 Parts I and III of the Medicines (Products Other Than Veterinary Drugs) (Prescription Only) Order 1983, S1 1983 No. 1212 and subsequent orders using the supply order procedure.

Pentazocine (Fortral) is a Schedule 3 drug which a midwife can use.

Supply of controlled drugs to midwives

When a midwife working in the community requires a supply of pethidine, she applies to her supervisor of midwives. Together they check the entries in the midwife's personal register and drug book. Provided they tally, the remaining stock is checked, and all being in order the supervisor issues a supply order form, signed by her. It is normal practice to issue the smallest practicable amount. The midwife takes the drug book and order form to the agreed chemist or hospital pharmacist, who issues the new stock. Both the pharmacist and the midwife make the appropriate entries. The midwife should have been introduced to the pharmacist, who should have a sample signature from the supervisor.

All controlled drugs held by the midwife must be stored in a fixed locked cupboard which is only accessible to her.

Midwives may *surrender* unwanted drugs to an 'authorized' person, such as the pharmacist from whom the drug was obtained, or to a medical officer, but not a supervisor of midwives. *Destruction* of controlled drugs obtained by a midwife through a supply order procedure is carried out by the midwife but only in the presence of an 'authorized' person who may be one of the following:

1. A supervisor of midwives in England, Wales and Northern Ireland.
2. A Regional Pharmaceutical Officer in England.
3. Pharmaceutical Adviser, Welsh Office.
4. Chief Administrative Pharmaceutical Officer of Health Boards in Scotland.
5. In Northern Ireland, an inspector appointed by the Department of Health under the Misuse of Drugs Act, 1971.
6. Medical officers of the Regional Medical Services in England, Scotland and Wales.
7. An inspector of the Pharmaceutical Society of Great Britain.
8. A police officer.
9. An inspector of the Home Office Drugs Branch (UKCC, 1991).

Controlled drugs obtained by a woman on a prescription from her general practitioner belong, in law, to the woman. The midwife should advise the mother to destroy any unused drugs and may be a witness to this action. Any advice given by the midwife and destruction of drugs by the mother should be fully recorded in the mother's notes.

Use of controlled drugs by midwives in hospital/institution

The midwife caring for a woman in hospital usually uses controlled drugs supplied by the hospital and must follow the locally agreed policies and procedures. These may include a standing order signed by a medical consultant and senior midwife authorizing the administration of controlled drugs and medicines for use by the midwife in her practice in the institution. In some hospitals/institutions it may be decided that midwives follow the same practice as midwives working in the community (UKCC, 1991).

'Topping-up' epidurals

Midwives are permitted by the UKCC to top up epidurals provided that:

1. The midwife has been fully instructed in the technique.
2. There are written instructions regarding the dose to be given.
3. The drug and the dose are checked by one other person.
4. The midwife has been instructed by the anaesthetist as to the

woman's position, blood pressure recordings and steps to take if
there are side effects.
5. The ultimate responsibility rests with the anaesthetist concerned.

Drugs commonly used
The drugs mentioned in Table 10 are those which are commonly used
in midwifery and paediatrics, and the doses given are those most
frequently employed. These may vary according to the purpose for
which a drug is administered.

The categories of drugs are listed in alphabetical order.

Reference
UKCC (1991) *A Midwive's Code of Practice*, UKCC: London.

Table 10. Drugs commonly used in midwifery and paediatrics.

Drug	Proprietary name	Dose	Mode of administration	Uses/remarks
Anaesthetics, general				
Halothane		0.5–3%	Inhalation	Postpartum haemorrhage may result due to relaxation of the uterus
Methohexitone sodium	Brietal sodium	1 mg/kg body weight	Intravenous	—
Thiopentone sodium	Intraval sodium	Up to 4 mg/kg body weight	Intravenous	2.5% solution only must be used
Anaesthetics, local				
Bupivacaine hydrochloride	Marcain	0.25%, 0.5% 0.75%	Epidural Intrathecal	Greater duration than lignocaine, so useful where prolonged analgesia is required, e.g. caesarean section
Lignocaine hydrochloride	Xylocaine	0.5% or 1% 2%	Infiltration Epidural	10 ml 0.5% solution or 5 ml 1% solution may be used by midwives for infiltration prior to episiotomy and prior to perineal repair
Prilocaine hydrochloride	Citanest	0.5 or 1% solutions	Infiltration	For nerve blocks
Analgesia, inhalational Nitrous oxide + oxygen	Entonox	50% of each gas (in a cylinder)	Entonox apparatus	Safe and effective. Excreted via the lungs

Trichloroethylene	Trilene	0.35% in air 0.5% in air	Tecota MK 6 or Emotril inhalers	Accumulative. Excreted via the kidneys. No longer to be administered by midwives in the UK, unless prescribed by a doctor
Analgesics				
Dextropropoxyphene hydrochloride	(Co-proxamol) Distalgesic	2 tabs t.d.s./q.d.s.	Oral	May be addictive, especially if taken with alcohol. Safety in pregnancy has not been established
Dihydrocodeine tartate	DF 118	30 mg q.d.s. 50 mg	Oral i.m.	Side effects: headache, nausea, vertigo. Avoid in asthmatics, as it causes histamine release
Fentanyl Mefenamic acid	Sublimaze Ponstan	0.05–0.1 mg 2 caps t.d.s. (250–500 mg t.d.s.)	i.v. Oral	For intra- and postoperative pain Anti-inflammatory as well as analgesic
Methadone hydrochloride	Physeptone	5–10 mg	Oral, subcutaneous or i.m.	May be prescribed to drug addicts in pregnancy as maintenance drug
Morphine sulphate		10–15 mg	s.c., i.m. or i.v.	Opioid analgesic to relieve severe pain, e.g. placental abruption. Causes respiratory depression
Morphine sulphate	Oramorph Sevredol	5–20 mg	Oral	
Paracetamol	Panadol	2 tabs q.d.s.	Oral	Mild. Also anti-pyretic.
Pentazocine hydrochloride	Fortral	25–100 mg 3–4 hourly 30–60 mg	Oral i.m./i.v.	Relief of moderate to severe pain. Relief is variable
Pethidine hydrochloride		25–150 mg 25–50 mg	i.m. i.v.	Short-acting but effective. May cause depression of respiratory centre of baby

Continued over

Table 10. (Continued) Drugs commonly used in midwifery and paediatrics.

Drug	Proprietary name	Dose	Mode of administration	Uses/remarks
Anticoagulants				
Heparin	—	Prophylaxis: 10 000 units b.d. Treatment: up to 40 000 units daily	s.c. i.v. infusion	Heparin is rapidly excreted. Protamine sulphate is used to counteract over dosage, but if used in excess it has an anticoagulant effect
Warfarin	—	Maintenance: 2–15 mg daily (dose depends on prothrombin time)	Oral	In general: contraindicated in pregnancy and labour but may be given at 16–36 weeks' gestation if heparin not available. Dose should control prothrombin time to 2.5–3.5 times above normal
Anticonvulsants Chlormethiazole edisylate	Heminevrin	0.8% solution, 15–60 d.p.m. until patient drowsy, then maintenance at 15 drops per minute	i.v. infusion	Hypnotic as well as anticonvulsant. Useful in eclampsia and status epilepticus
Phenobarbitone Phenytoin sodium	Gardenal Epanutin	60–300 mg daily 100 mg b.d./t.d.s. (max. 600 mg daily)	Oral Oral	Avoid in early pregnancy Avoid in early pregnancy if possible unless potential benefits outweigh risk of congenital abnormality

Sodium valproate	Epilim	2.5 g daily (maximum) in divided doses	Oral	Anti-epileptic. Plasma concentrations should be monitored in pregnancy. Breast feeding acceptable
		Initial dose up to 10 mg/kg followed by maximum of 2.5 g daily	i.v.	
Carbamazepine	Tegretol Retard	0.8–1.2 g daily Maximum 1.6 g daily	Oral	Benefit of treatment outweights risk to fetus. Breast feeding acceptable

NB. The use of barbiturates should be avoided, except when required as anticonvulsants, because dependence and tolerance occur readily.

Anti-emetics				
Perphenazine	Fentazin	4 mg t.d.s.	Oral	Avoid in 1st trimester
Promazine hydrochloride	Sparine	25–100 mg q.d.s.	Oral	May be given in conjunction with pethidine in labour
		25–50 mg	i.m.	
Promethazine hydrochloride	Phenergan	25–50 mg	im./i.v.	May be given in conjunction with pethidine in labour
Promethazine theoclate	Avomine	25 mg at bedtime, increased to maximum of 100 mg daily if necessary	Oral	Only prescribed if vomiting severe in early pregnancy

Continued over

Table 10. (Continued) Drugs commonly used in midwifery and paediatrics.

Drug	Proprietary name	Dose	Mode of administration	Uses/remarks
Thiethylperazine	Torecan	10 mg 2 to 3 times a day 6.5 mg	Oral i.m.	Only prescribed if vomiting severe in early pregnancy
Anti-hypertensives Hydralazine	Apresoline	25–50 mg 20–40 mg	oral i.v. (physiological saline)	Contraindicated in early pregnancy and in women with tachycardia
Methyldopa	Aldomet	250 mg t.d.s. (max. 3 g daily)	Oral	Crosses placenta but no evidence that it affects fetus
Labetalol hydrochloride		100–200 mg b.d. max 2.4 g daily 20 mg/h, doubled every 30 min; maximum 160 mg/h	Oral i.v. infusion	Combines alpha and beta receptor blocking activity. Used for pregnancy-induced hypertension

NB. Beta blockers have been used successfully in pregnancy to lower the blood pressure. When used during the third trimester of pregnancy may cause neonatal hypoglycaemia and bradycardia; risk greater in severe hypertension.

Antimicrobials		Route	Dose	Notes
Acyclovir	Zovirax	Oral i.v. infusion	200 mg 5 times daily 5 mg/kg over 1 h; repeat 8 hly	Antiviral drug. Active against herpes viruses but does not eradicate them
Amoxycillin	Amoxil	Oral	250 mg t.d.s.	Same action as ampicillin but better absorption
Ampicillin	Penbritin	Oral i.m./i.v.	250–500 mg q.d.s. 0.5–1 g	Broad-spectrum antibiotic
Cefotaxime	Claforam	i.m. or i.v.	1–2 g every 8–12 h	A cephalosporin; a broad-spectrum antibiotic, less active than other cephalosporins against Gram-positive bacteria, especially *Staphylococcus aureus*
Cefuroxime	Zinacef	i.m./i.v.	750 mg t.d.s.	Active against both Gram-positive and Gram-negative bacteria
Cephaloridine	Ceporin	Oral i.m./i.v.	125–250 b.d. 1–2 g daily in divided doses	
Chloramphenicol	Chloromycetin ophthalmic	Topically	2 drops to affected eye every 3 hours	For bacterial conjunctivitis
Ciprofloxacin	Ciproxin	Oral i.v.	250–750 mg twice daily. For gonorrhoea 250 mg as a single dose. 200 mg b.d	Active against Gram-negative organisms and Chlamydia in particular. Used with caution in pregnancy and breast feeding

Continued over

Table 10. (Continued) Drugs commonly used in midwifery and paediatrics.

Drug	Proprietary name	Dose	Mode of administration	Uses/remarks
Clotrimazole	Canesten	Vaginal cream 2%, 5 g p.v. twice daily for 3 days, or once nightly for 6 nights Vaginal tablets, 100 or 200 mg nightly for 3 or 6 nights	p.v.	Pessaries or cream inserted high into the vagina. Anti-fungal.
Doxycycline	Nordox	200 mg initially, then 100 mg daily	Oral	A tetracycline used for Chlamydia. Tetracyclines should not be prescribed in pregnancy because of the risk of dental staining and hypoplasia in the infant
Erythromycin	Erythrocin	1–2 g daily (divided doses) 100 mg q.d.s. (max 5–8 mg/kg per 24 h)	Oral Deep i.m.	Highly effective in the treatment of a wide variety of clinical infections
Flucloxacillin	Floxapen	250 mg q.d.s.	Oral i.v./i.m.	Active against most staphylococci and streptococci, including majority of penicillinase-producing staphylococci

Drug	Trade name	Dose	Route	Notes
Fluconazole	Diflucan	150 mg single dose, or 50 mg daily for 7–14 days	Oral	Anti-fungal drug for acute or recurrent candidiasis. Single dose of 150 mg given for vaginal candidiasis and 50 mg daily for 7–14 days given for oropharyngeal candidiasis
Gentamicin	Cidomycin Genticin Lugacin	2.5 mg/kg daily in divided doses 8 hly Paediatric dose: up to age 2 weeks 3 mg/kg every 12 hours; 2 weeks–12 years, 2 mg/kg every 8 hours	i.m., i.v. or i.v. infusion	Avoided in pregnancy because can cause fetal 8th nerve damage. Used for septicaemia, neonatal sepsis, including CNS infections
Metronidazole	Flagyl	400 mg t.d.s.	Oral	For anaerobic infections and *Trichomonas vaginalis*
Miconazole	Gyno-Daktarin	200 mg nightly	p.v.	For vulvovaginal candidiasis
Nitrofurantoin	Furadantin Macrodantin	50–100 mg 6 hly	Oral	Prescribed for urinary tract infections. May produce neonatal haemolysis if used at term
Nystatin	Nystan	500 000 units 6 hly 100 000 units q.d.s. 1–2 pessaries	Oral Oral p.v.	Prescribed for intestinal candidiasis Dose per child with oral candidiasis Vaginal candidiasis
Phenoxymethyl-penicillin	Penicillin V	250–500 mg 6 hly	Oral	Commonly used for mild streptococcal infections

Continued over

Table 10. (Continued) Drugs commonly used in midwifery and paediatrics.

Drug	Proprietary name	Dose	Mode of administration	Uses/remarks
Procaine penicillin	Bicillin	300 mg (procaine penicillin) 60 mg (Benzylpenicillin sodium) every 12–24 hours	i.m.	Commonly used for the treatment of syphilis and gonorrhoea
Sultrin		Cream or tablets. 1 pessary or applicator of cream b.d. for 10 days, then daily if required	p.v.	For bacterial vaginitis and cervicitis
Trimethoprim	Ipral Monotrim Syratrim Trimogel Trimopan	200 mg 12 hly, 150–250 mg 12 hly	Oral, i.v. or i.v. infusion	Used for urinary and respiratory tract infections. Contraindications include use in pregnancy and for neonates

NB. The sulphonamides have not been included here because—due to the large selection of relatively safe and effective antibiotics, and the many contraindications and side effects of the sulphonamides—they are rarely used in midwifery.

Antiseptics				
Benzalkonium chloride	Roccal	0.05% antiseptic 1% disinfectant		Skin antiseptic and general disinfectant. Not effective against viruses, fungi, spores

Cetrimide	Cetavlon Savlon	1% solution 1:100 solution 1:30 solution	Skin antiseptic Swabbing Disinfection of wounds
Chlorhexidine	Hibitane	1:2000 solution 1% obstetric cream	Potent antibacterial Vaginal examinations
Glutaraldehyde	Glutarol	10% solution	For viral warts
Anti-thyroid Carbimazole	Neo-Mercazole	5–60 mg daily	Oral	For thyrotoxicosis. May cause fetal hypothyroidism
Contraceptives (*see also* Appendix 12) Medroxyprogest- erone acetate	Depo-Provera	150 mg	i.m.	Effective for 12 weeks. A useful single-dose contraceptive to be given following rubella vaccination or to the woman whose husband has had vasectomy performed
Combined contraceptives Ethinyloestradiol 30 µg	Microgynon 30 Loestrin 30 Marvelon 30 Ovran 30 Conova 30 Eugynon 30 Femodene 30 Minulet Ovranette	1 tab. daily for 21 days starting 5th day of menstrual cycle, then 7 day pill-free interval	Oral	30 µg is the standard strength for oral contraceptives. 20 µg pills also available but may be less effective. 50 µg pills are associated with increased side effects. Can be commenced 3–4 weeks post-partum. Contraindicated if breast feeding

Continued over

Table 10. (Continued) Drugs commonly used in midwifery and paediatrics.

Drug	Proprietary name	Dose	Mode of administration	Uses/remarks
Progestogen-only contraceptives				
	Femulen Micronor Microval Neogest Norgeston Noriday	1 tab daily, no pill-free interval	Oral	Prescribed where oestrogens are contraindicated, e.g. breast feeding. Higher failure rate than combined pill
Medroxyprogest- erone acetate	Depo-Provera	150 mg	i.m.	Long-acting progestogen, which may be prescribed for women who are unable to use other methods. Can be administered in the puerperium without adverse effects. Risk of heavy bleeding if given before 5th postnatal week
Norethisterone	Noristerat		i.m.	Long-acting progestogen
Norethisterone	Micronor Noriday	1 tab. daily 350 µg	Oral	Examples of the progesterone-only pill. Not as reliable as combined pill but can be prescribed to postnatal mothers even if breast feeding

Phased formulations (combined)

BiNovum Logynon Logynon ED Synphase Triordiol TriNovum	1 tab. daily for 21 days then 7 day pill-free interval	Oral	Phased formulations are a little more complex to take but provide better control than the fixed-dose preparations

Postcoital contraceptives

Schering PC4	2 tabs as soon as possible after coitus (up to 72 h), then further 2 tabs. after 12 h	Oral	Used as an occasional emergency measure

Corticosteroids

Betamethasone sodium phosphate	Betnesol	24 mg in divided doses	i.m.	Thought to stimulate the production of surfactant in the immature fetal lungs

Diabetic

Chlorpropamide	—	250–500 mg daily	Oral	Contraindicated in pregnancy. Causes neonatal hypoglycaemia
Insulin	—	Determined by patient's requirements	s.c.	Requirements rise in 2nd and 3rd trimesters

Diuretics

Frusemide	Lasix	20–40 mg	i.m./i.v.	May inhibit lactation. Should be reserved for pulmonary oedema and selected oliguric patients

Continued over

Table 10. (Continued) Drugs commonly used in midwifery and paediatrics.

Drug	Proprietary name	Dose	Mode of administration	Uses/remarks
Mannitol		50–200 mg in 24 h	i.v. infusion	Not recommended in pregnancy. Used when acute tubular necrosis presents following postpartum haemorrhage. Never add mannitol to whole blood
Hypnotics/sedatives				
Diazepam	Valium	2 mg t.d.s. 5–10 mg nightly up to 40 mg	Oral Oral i.m. or i.v.	For mild anxiety For insomnia For treatment of eclampsia
Nitrazepam	Mogadon	5–10 mg	Oral	Side effect: morning sickness
Temazepam	Normison	10–30 mg	Oral	Should not be given in 1st trimester. Otherwise, effective hypnotic with no side effects
Iron Ferrous fumarate 304 mg + folic acid 0.35 mg	Pregaday	1 tab. daily	Oral	Treatment for iron deficiency and megaloblastic anaemia in pregnancy
Ferrous sulphate 150 mg + folic acid 0.5 mg	Fefol	1 spansule daily	Oral	Treatment for iron deficiency and megaloblastic anaemia in pregnancy
Ferrous sulphate 325 mg + folic acid 0.35 mg	Ferrograd-folic	1 tab. daily	Oral	Treatment for iron deficiency and megaloblastic anaemia in pregnancy

Ferrous sulphate Iron dextran	Imferon	200 mg b.d. or t.d.s. According to body weight and Hb level	i.v. infusion	For iron-deficiency anaemia Test dose must be given first at rate of not more than 5 drops/min for 10 min under supervision
Iron sorbitol	Jectofer	2 ml	i.m.	For severe iron-deficiency anaemia
Laxatives Ispaghula Lactulose Senna	Fybogel Duphalex Senokot	1 sachet b.d. 15 ml b.d. 2-4 tabs	Oral Oral Oral	Increases faecal mass May take up to 48 hours to act
Enema Sodium citrate	Micro-enema Microlette Micro-enema Microlax Micro-enema Relaxit Micro-enema	Single-dose disposable pack		For constipation
Suppositories Glycerol (or glycerine)		1-2 suppositories	Rectal	Act as rectal stimulant
	Anusol	Cream or suppositories	Rectal	Used to relieve pain associated with haemorrhoids

Continued over

Table 10. (Continued) Drugs commonly used in midwifery and paediatrics.

Drug	Proprietary name	Dose	Mode of administration	Uses/remarks
Myometrial relaxants				
Isoxsuprine hydrochloride	Duvadilan	100 mg in 500 ml saline	i.v. infusion	Start at 0.5 ml/min; increase every 10 min until labour arrested
Ritodrine hydrochloride	Yutopar	0.05 mg per minute	i.v. infusion and tablets	Increase by 0.05 mg every 10 min. Effective dose: 0.15–0.35 mg
Salbutamol	Ventolin	4 mg q.d.s. 5 ml/500 ml sodium chloride/dextrose	Oral i.v. infusion	Contraindicated in pre-eclampsia and antepartum haemorrhage
Myometrial stimulants				
Dinoprostone	Prostin E₂	In solution. 100 µg, then 100–200 µg 2 hly	Extra-amniotic instillation	For therapeutic abortion
	Prostin E₂	Gel. 1 mg, then after 6 h 1–2 mg if required (max. 3 mg)	Inserted high into posterior fornix of vagina	For induction of labour
	Prostin E₂	Vaginal tabs. 3 mg, then 6–8 h. Later repeat 3 mg if required	Inserted high into posterior fornix of vagina	For induction of labour

	Prostin E₂	Tabs. 500 µg followed by 0.5–1 mg at hly intervals (max. 1.5 mg)	Oral	For induction of labour
	Prepidil gel	Dose variable depending on reason for usage 500 µg	i.v.	Rarely used i.v. because of high incidence of side effects
			Inserted into cervical canal	For pre-induction cervical softening and dilatation
Ergometrine		0.5 mg	i.v.	Acts in 45 s, so is useful in prevention/treatment of postpartum haemorrhage
			i.m. Oral	Acts in 7 min and gives sustained contraction of uterus
Gemeprost	Cervagem	1 mg 3 h before surgery	Pessaries	To soften and dilate cervix to facilitate transcervical procedures in the 1st trimester. Second trimester abortion, 1 mg every 3 h for a maximum of 5 doses. Second course may begin 24 hours later

Continued over

Table 10. (Continued) Drugs commonly used in midwifery and paediatrics.

Drug	Proprietary name	Dose	Mode of administration	Uses/remarks
Oxytocin	Syntocinon	1 i.u. in 1 litre solution 1–3 milliunits per min, adjusted according to response.	i.v. infusion	Induction and augmentation of labour—stimulates contraction of uterine muscle.
		10–20 units/500 ml increased to max. of 100 units/500 ml, 10–30 drops/min.		Missed abortion.
		5–10 units/500 ml at 15 drops/min, adjusted according to response		Postpartum haemorrhage
Syntometrine		1 ml	i.m.	Consists of oxytocin 5 units + ergometrine maleate 0.5 mg, and so has rapid and sustained action. Active management of 3rd stage of labour

Thyroid				
Thyroxine sodium	Eltroxin	50–300 μg, adjusted monthly until normal metabolism is maintained	Oral	For hypothyroidism
Anti-oestrogens				
Clomiphene citrate	Clomid	50 mg daily for 5 days, starting on 5th day of cycle	Oral	Used for treatment of female infertility. Induces gonadotrophin release
Other endocrine drugs				
Bromocriptine	Parlodel	2.5 mg on 1st day, then 2.5 mg b.d. for 14 days	Oral	Used for suppression of lactation
Neonatal drugs				
Alprostadil	Prostin VR	50–100 ng/kg/min, then decreased	i.v. infusion	Maintains patency of ductus arteriosus in neonates with congenital heart defects prior to corrective surgery in centres where intensive care is immediately available
Ampicillin	Penbritin	62.5 mg q.d.s.	Oral/i.m./i.v.	For listeriosis
Cefotaxime	Claforan	50 mg/kg daily in 2–4 divided doses (can increase to 150–200 mg/kg)	i.m. or i.v.	Used to treat infections. Broad-spectrum antibiotic active against certain Gram-negative bacteria

Continued over

Table 10. (Continued) Drugs commonly used in midwifery and paediatrics.

Drug	Proprietary name	Dose	Mode of administration	Uses/remarks
Chloramphenicol	Chloromycetin	Infants under 2 weeks 25 mg/kg daily in divided doses. Under 1 year 50 mg/kg daily in divided doses	i.v. or i.v. infusion	Prescribed for treatment of meningitis. May cause 'grey syndrome' in neonate. Plasma concentration monitoring required in neonates
Chloramphenicol eye drops	Chloromycetin eye drops	2 drops to affected eye every 3 hours	Topical	For bacterial conjunctivitis
Erythromycin		Child up to 2 years 125 mg every 6 hours. 25–50 mg/kg daily in divided doses	Oral i.v. Infusion	Respiratory tract infections. Active against many penicillin-resistant staphylococci; also chlamydia
Flucloxacillin		250 mg q.d.s. 0.25–1 g q.d.s. Child under 2 years ¼ adult dose	Oral or i.m. i.v. or i.v. infusion	Effective in infections caused by penicillin-resistant staphylococci
Frusemide	Lasix	1–3 mg/kg daily, 0.5–1 mg/kg i.v. min	Oral	Oedema, oliguria due to renal failure

Gentamicin	Genticin	7.5 mg b.d.	i.m.	For urinary tract infection and respiratory tract infections. Blood levels need careful monitoring in neonatal use
Indomethacin	Indocid PDA	200 µg/kg t.d.s., then adjusted	i.v.	Patent ductus arteriosus in preterm babies
Naloxone	Narcan	0.01 mg/kg	i.v./i.m.	To counteract respiratory depression in neonate, resulting from pethidine given to mother in labour
Nystatin	Nystan	100 000 units q.d.s.	Oral	For *Candida albicans*
Paraldehyde	—	0.1 ml/kg	i.m. deep	To abort prolonged or recurrent fits
Penicillin G	—	100 000 units q.d.s.	Oral/i.m./i.v.	
Phenobarbitone	Gardenal	2 mg/kg	i.m./i.v.	Accumulation may occur
Phenobarbitone elixir (5 mg/ml)		1.25 mg/kg	Oral	Anticonvulsant
Phytomenadione	Konakion	1 mg	i.v./i.m.	Prevention and treatment of haemorrhage
Tetracycline hydrochloride		2–4 times daily. Ointment every 2 h	Eyedrops or ointment	Eye infections

APPENDIX 20

SI Units and Statistics

SI units
Metric measures of all kinds have now replaced those which have traditionally been in use in the United Kingdom. These had to be standardized precisely to meet the needs of modern science. Following international conferences, the metric unit system was revised and extended for use as an international system for scientific measurement as well as general use. This was agreed in 1960 and is known as the Système International d'Unités (SI).

Systeme International d'Unités—SI units
The SI unit of weight is the gram (g), of length the metre (m), and of capacity, the litre (l). These can be used with standard prefixes to make them into convenient sizes by multiplication or division. For example a patient can be weighed in kilograms (one thousand gram units) or drugs in milligrams (one thousand times smaller than a gram).

Measurements smaller than a unit

Prefix	Symbol	Meaning	Example
deci	d	one-tenth	dl, one-tenth of a litre—0.1 l
centi	c	one-hundredth	cm, one-hundredth of a metre—0.01 m
milli	m	one-thousandth	ml, one thousandth of a litre—0.001 l
micro	μ	one-millionth	μg, one-millionth of a gram—0.000 001 μg
nano	n	one-thousand-millionth	ng, one-thousand-millionth of a gram—0.000 000 001 g

Multiples of units

Prefix	Symbol	Meaning	Example
deca	da	ten	dal, ten litres—10 l
hecto	h	one hundred	hg, one hundred grams—100 g
kilo	k	one thousand	kg, one thousand grams—1000 g
mega	M	one million	MJ, one million joules—1 000 000 J

Mass

The most common SI fundamental unit that a midwife will use is that for measuring mass or weight.

Calculation of drug dosages is of vital importance. This is particularly so with paediatric drugs, which are given according to the weight of the baby. The following equivalents are helpful to start with:

$$
\begin{aligned}
1 \text{ kilogram (kg)} &= 1000 \text{ grams (g)} \\
1 \text{ gram (g)} &= 1000 \text{ milligrams (mg)} \\
1 \text{ milligram (mg)} &= 1000 \text{ micrograms } (\mu g) \\
1 \text{ microgram } (\mu g) &= 1000 \text{ nanograms (ng)} \\
1 \text{ nanogram (ng)} &= 1000 \text{ picograms}
\end{aligned}
$$

The following is an example of calculating drug dosage for a prescription of a baby weighing 4.0 kg:

$$
\begin{aligned}
&4 \text{ kg baby: dose } 0.1 \text{ mg prescribed} \\
&\text{The elixir contains } 0.05 \text{ mg/ml}
\end{aligned}
$$

Calculation:

$$
\frac{\text{Required dose}}{\text{Strength available}} = \frac{0.1 \text{ mg}}{0.05 \text{ mg}} = 2 \text{ ml}
$$

If it is prescribed in micrograms, decimals can be avoided:

$$
\begin{aligned}
0.1 \text{ mg} &= 100 \ \mu g \text{ dose} \\
0.05 \text{ mg/ml} &= 50 \ \mu g \text{ elixir}
\end{aligned}
$$

Calculation:

$$
\frac{\text{Required dose}}{\text{Strength available}} = \frac{100 \ \mu g}{50 \ \mu g} = 2 \text{ ml}
$$

The index notation

Since one unit is used for large or small quantities the numbers can involve many zeros and be very clumsy to read or write, and inaccuracies can occur. The 'index' is a small raised number to *multiply* the products of 10. For example:

$$
\begin{aligned}
100 &= 10 \times 10 &&= \text{index, } 10^2 \\
10\ 000 &= 10 \times 10 \times 10 \times 10 &&= \text{index, } 10^4
\end{aligned}
$$

Where fractions of a unit are used, the index has a minus sign to represent the number of times the unit should be *divided* by 10. For example:

$$
0.1 = \frac{1}{10} = \text{index, } 10^{-1}
$$

$$0.01 = \frac{1}{100} = \text{index}, 10^{-2}$$

Index notation is now used in pathology reports. For example:

	Old value	Index notation
Total white blood count (WBC)	5000–10 000/mm³	5–10.0×10⁹/l
Red cell count (RBC)	4.5 million/mm³	4.5×10¹²/l

SI units are now coming into general use and it is better to use only the one system. Older people, however, still use Imperial measurements so the following conversion charts (see Figures 20–22 and Table 11) are included for convenience. It should be noted that it is now illegal in the United Kingdom for drugs to be prescribed or dispensed in any other units other than SI units.

Thermometers

The CELSIUS scale is now used in most hospitals in preference to the Fahrenheit scale. The name 'Centigrade' should not now be used because it is not internationally recognized as a measurement of temperature; in some countries it is used to measure an angle.

To convert Fahrenheit to Celsius is a complicated calculation. It is safer to use a double scale (Figure 22) in the rare event of a conversion being required.

Records

Graphs, which have the advantage of showing a number of facts at a time, are now used extensively. If accurately compiled, they are valuable in saving time which would otherwise be spent searching case notes, and they can also help to overcome language barriers and show the relationships of different factors in a way which would not otherwise be possible. Deviations from the normal can be seen at a glance.

Vital statistics

The vital statistics for the United Kingdom used to be published in one book from the Registrar General. They are now produced in booklet and pamphlet form by the Office of Population Censuses and Surveys (OPCS). The majority of statistics which concern a midwife are contained in the biennial booklet, *Population Trends*, published in the Spring and Autumn each year and obtainable from the OPCS (see Appendix 25 for the address).

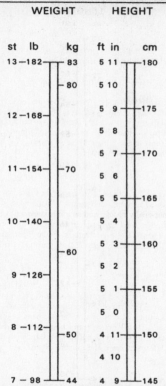

Figure 20. Weight and height conversion charts for antenatal women.

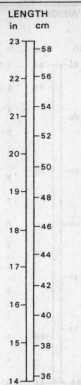

LENGTH

in   cm

Figure 21. Linear equivalents for lengths of babies.

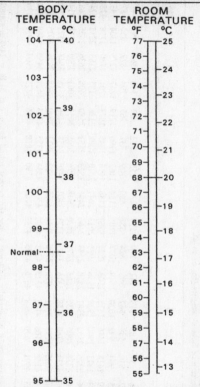

Figure 22. Celsius/Fahrenheit equivalents.

Table 11. Conversion of babies' weights (lb, oz to g).

oz	0	1	2	3	4	5	6	7	8	9	10	11	12	13	14	15
lb																
0		28	57	85	113	142	170	198	227	255	283	312	340	368	397	425
1	454	482	510	539	567	595	624	652	680	709	737	765	794	822	850	879
2	907	935	964	992	1020	1049	1077	1105	1134	1162	1190	1219	1247	1275	1304	1332
3	1360	1389	1418	1446	1475	1503	1531	1560	1588	1616	1645	1673	1701	1730	1758	1786
4	1815	1843	1871	1900	1928	1956	1985	2013	2041	2070	2098	2126	2155	2183	2211	2240
5	2268	2296	2325	2353	2381	2410	2438	2466	2495	2523	2551	2580	2608	2636	2655	2683
6	2721	2750	2778	2806	2835	2863	2891	2920	2948	2976	3005	3033	3061	3090	3118	3146
7	3175	3203	3231	3260	3288	3316	3345	3373	3401	3430	3458	3486	3515	3543	3571	3600
8	3628	3656	3685	3713	3741	3770	3798	3826	3855	3883	3911	3940	3968	3996	4025	4053
9	4081	4110	4138	4166	4195	4223	4251	4280	4308	4336	4355	4383	4421	4450	4468	4506
10	4535	4563	4591	4620	4648	4676	4705	4733	4761	4790	4818	4846	4875	4903	4931	4960

In making this conversion it is generally sufficient to use the nearest round figure, e.g. 5½ lb = 2495 g, rounded to 2.5 kg

Table 12. Comparison of Celsius and Fahrenheit recordings.

	Celsius	Fahrenheit
Boiling point of water at normal atmospheric pressure	100°	212°
Freezing point of water at normal atmospheric pressure	0°	32°
Normal body temperature	36.5°–37.0°	98.4°

Birth rates
See Table 13.

Death rates
Those relevant to midwifery are maternal mortality, stillbirth, neonatal and perinatal mortality, and infant death rates. These figures can be used to compare the efficiency of maternity and paediatric services in the United Kingdom with those of other countries, while at the same time they indicate where necessary improvements should be undertaken in order to reduce such deaths to an absolute minimum.

The most important death rates from the midwife's point of view are as follows:

Maternal mortality rate. This is defined as the number of maternal deaths

Table 13. Birth rates in the United Kingdom (per 1000 population, all ages) by year.

1961	17.9
1966	18.0
1971	16.2
1976	12.1
1980	13.5
1985	13.3
1990	13.9

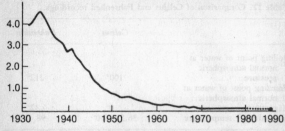

Figure 23. Maternal deaths (recorded per 1000 registered live and stillbirths for England and Wales).

(deaths due to pregnancy and childbearing) per 1000 registered births (live and still). From about 1900 to 1935 the rate remained approximately constant at about 4, but since the latter date it has fallen steadily (*see* Figure 23). During recent years it has been as shown in Table 14.

The improvement is due to improved social and medical/midwifery care and facilities. The NHS provides complete maternity care for all childbearing women. Women are healthier and better nourished, and education, housing and other social conditions are steadily improving. Medical factors which have helped to reduce maternal mortality include: higher standards of antenatal care; the use of antibiotics in treating sepsis; oxytocic drugs and blood transfusion in dealing with haemorrhage; improvements in anaesthetics; the prevention and better treatment of

Table 14. Maternal mortality rates in England and Wales (per 1000 registered births) per year.

1966	0.26
1971	0.17
1976	0.13
1980	0.11
1985	0.07
1990	0.08

anaemia; and the increased use and safety of operative measures such as caesarean section. In addition, the education and training of both midwives and doctors has improved, and they are supported by a range of other health care professionals such as radiographers, physiotherapists and haematologists.

The 1985–1987 Confidential Report on Maternal Deaths showed that the chief direct causes of maternal death were:

Thromboembolism	29
Hypertensive disorders	27
Early pregnancy deaths (including abortions)	22
Haemorrhage (ante and post partum)	10
Amniotic fluid embolism	9

Indirect deaths result from either a pre-existing disease or from a disease which developed in pregnancy and which was aggravated by pregnancy (Dept of Health, 1991). Of the 29 deaths due to *thromboembolism*, 16 occurred in the antenatal period and half of them were before 17 weeks' gestation. The majority of the antenatal deaths were caused by deep vein thrombosis which had not been recognized. It is therefore recommended that an otherwise healthy pregnant or postpartum woman who complains of pain in the leg or chest, or of dyspnoea should be treated for thrombosis or pulmonary embolism until proved otherwise.

Hypertensive disorders of pregnancy continue to be a major cause of maternal death. Of the 27 deaths, only in one case was there essential hypertension present before the onset of pregnancy. Maternal age, particularly over 35 years, increases the risk of the conditions. Severe pre-eclampsia was present in 15 cases and eclampsia in 12. Twenty-six women died after delivery. The major causes of death were pulmonary complications and intracerebral haemorrhage. Local specialized teams are strongly recommended to advise or care for these women.

Early pregnancy deaths includes deaths from both ectopic pregnancy and abortion. Of the 22 direct deaths, 16 were due to ectopic pregnancy. In seven of these cases there was a history of sub-standard care, often delay in making a correct diagnosis. Ultrasound scan is recommended to aid diagnosis and, in cases of doubt, a laparoscopy should be done.

Of the 10 deaths due to haemorrhage, four were caused by placental abruption and six by postpartum haemorrhage, and there was sub-standard care in seven cases. This includes anaemic women in labour, high-risk women booked for delivery in small units and unsatisfactory resuscitative measures.

Nine women died from amniotic fluid embolism. Risk factors include age over 35 years, high parity, excessive or strong uterine contractions, the use of oxytocic drugs for induction or augmentation of labour, overdistension of the uterus, rupture of the uterus and intravascular coagulation. The signs and symptoms are sudden dyspnoea, hypoxia and hypotension, and cardio-respiratory arrest may follow in minutes. Urgent resuscitative measures are necessary.

A significant fall in maternal deaths due to abortion and anaesthetics was noted.

Reference
Department of Health (1991) *Report on Confidential Enquiries into Maternal Deaths in England and Wales 1985–1987.* HMSO: London.

Stillbirth rate. This is defined as the number of stillbirths per 1000 registered births (live and still). The rate in 1931 was 41, after which it slowly declined in 1939 to 38, and then more rapidly until 1947 when it reached 24. There was then little change in the next 10 years. More recent stillbirth rates have been as shown in Table 15. The main causes of stillbirth are fetal anoxia and congenital abnormalities.

Duties imposed on midwives by statute regarding stillbirths
1. Notification of stillbirth.
2. Certification of stillbirth. It is usual for the doctor who was present at the birth or examined the body to give one of the parents the certificate but, failing this, a midwife who was present at the birth or examined the body should complete the certificate.
3. Registration of stillbirth. The midwife explains to the parents that they must take the Certificate of Stillbirth to the Registrar of Births and Deaths who will then issue them with a certificate for burial or cremation. The hospital or health authority will make arrangements for the burial or cremation, unless the parents prefer to do so.
4. The midwife notifies her supervisor of midwives.

Table 15. Stillbirth rates in the United Kingdom (per 1000 registered births) by year.

1965	15.8
1970	12.9
1975	10.5
1980	7.2
1985	5.5
1990	4.6

Neonatal mortality rate. This represents the number of infant deaths during the first 4 weeks of life per 1000 registered *live* births. Between 1928 and 1941 the rate was approximately constant at 30, but subsequently it has fallen, at first considerably, then more gradually.

During recent years the neonatal mortality rate has been as shown in Table 16.

The reduction in the neonatal death rate is largely due to the same factors that have led to the improvement in the stillbirth rate, the most important being the greater antenatal attention to the welfare of the fetus, avoidance and better treatment of low birth weight babies, and greater obstetric skill leading to fewer birth injuries; other factors are the improved treatment of asphyxia and sepsis.

Perinatal mortality rate. This is the number of stillbirths, and the number of neonatal deaths which occur during the first week of life per 1000 total births. It is often a matter of chance whether a fetus dies just before or just after birth, i.e. whether it is a stillbirth or a neonatal death. The perinatal mortality rate, by comprising all such deaths, is a more accurate index of the number of such deaths which are due to purely obstetric causes.

In 1931 the rate was 62.1, in 1941 it was 54.7 and in 1951 38.2. By 1958 it was 35 and this slow reduction in the 1950s focused such attention on the problem that in 1958 a National Survey of Perinatal Mortality was undertaken under the auspices of the National Birthday Trust. The findings were so revealing that an interim report was published in the hope that some avoidable deaths would be prevented. The report, published in 1963, is well known, and has clearly been instrumental in achieving better care of infants before, during and after birth. In particular, much more attention has been focused on 'antenatal paediatrics', namely, close observation of the growth and development

Table 16. Neonatal mortality rate in the United Kingdom (per 1000 registered *live* births) by year.

1966	12.9
1971	11.6
1976	9.7
1980	7.7
1985	5.4
1990	4.5

of the fetus. This close attention is clearly saving many lives. Some of the rates published since are shown in Table 17.

The main causes of perinated mortality are:

1. Low birthweight.
2. Intra- and extrauterine hypoxia.
3. Intracranial injury.
4. Congenital abnormality.

The Short Committee in 1984 welcomed the improvement but expressed concern that the highest fetal and infant mortalities were still mainly associated with the lower socio-economic groups.

Infant mortality rate. This is defined as the number of deaths of infants under 1 year per 1000 registered *live* births. This has been steadily dropping throughout the present century; in 1930 it was over 60, in 1940 56.8, in 1950 29.1 and in 1960 21.8 (*see* Figure 24). Recent figures are shown in Table 18.

The improvement is partly due to the lower neonatal mortality rate, whilst advances in paediatric medicine and better social conditions and health education constitute their share. The chief causes of infant mortality are infection, mainly acute respiratory and gastrointestinal infections, accidents, child abuse, sudden infant death and the causes of neonatal death described above.

Table 17. Perinatal mortality rates.

Year	England and Wales	United Kingdom
1966	26.3	26.7
1971	22.3	22.6
1976	17.7	18.0
1980	13.3	—
1985	9.8	9.9
1990	8.1	8.1

Table 18. Infant mortality rates.

Year	England and Wales	United Kingdom
1966	19.0	19.6
1971	17.5	17.9
1976	14.3	14.5
1980	12.0	12.1
1985	9.4	9.4
1990	7.9	7.9

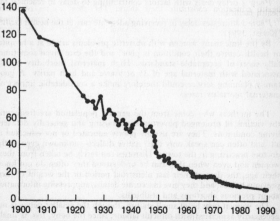

Figure 24. Infant mortality (deaths under 1 year recorded per 1000 registered births).

APPENDIX 21

Midwifery in the Developing Countries

Maternal mortality

Half a million women die in pregnancy and childbirth each year, 99% occurring in developing countries, especially in the rural areas. The main causes of death are haemorrhage, sepsis, pregnancy-induced hypertension, obstructed labour and illicitly induced abortion (Kwast, 1992). Morbidity rates are also high, many women suffering life-long ill-health following childbirth. Thaddeus & Maine (1990) describe factors contributing to maternal death in developing countries as 'the three phases of delay', in the book entitled *Too Far To Walk*:

Phase 1 delay deals with the woman's situation and her family setting and includes her status, her decision-making power, her financial opportunity and perceptions of health care and benefits.

Phase 2 delay deals with factors contributing to delay in reaching the health facilities.

Phase 3 addresses delay in receiving adequate care at the health facility (Kwast, 1991).

By the time many women with obstetric problems arrive at a hospital or health centre their condition is poor, and the care given sometimes falls short of acceptable standards. High maternal morbidity is also associated with maternal age of 35 or above and high parity. A good family planning service could therefore make a considerable impact on maternal mortality rates.

The mothers who come from the general population are frequently the victims of prolonged poverty, poor housing and generally deficient living conditions. They are usually poorly educated or not educated at all, and often can speak only their native dialect—unknown even to the doctors practising in the towns. Histories can rarely be taken from these women and even when they can be understood they often do not know their age, the date of their last menstrual period or the weight of their previous babies, and they give inaccurate details, suppressing information about previous abortions and stillbirths.

The women may be of small stature, though the smaller pelvis is not necessarily associated with difficult labour, since the baby, too, is small. Chronic anaemia, the result of prolonged dietary iron deficiency, is common. Many women are unable to eat protein every day, as they are too poor to afford it. In certain areas anaemia due to chronic malaria, schistosomiasis (bilharziasis), hookworm infestation and sickle cell disease may also occur.

All developing countries have some specialist obstetricians, doctors and trained midwives working in their health services, but in many areas they are seriously insufficient in number for the population they serve. In large towns will be found up-to-date and adequately staffed hospitals, but small towns may contain only medical attendants and locally trained midwives working on their own. In the developing parts of the world it is estimated that between 60 and 80 per cent of births are attended by traditional birth attendants (TBA). These are sometimes called 'indigenous midwife', 'hilot', 'dunken' or 'dai'. These traditional midwives are familiar figures in most villages and many urban areas of Africa, Asia and Latin America. There are varying attempts to educate and integrate them into health care services, but often financial constraints work against this. Those who are trained and become aware of better facilities are often unwilling to return to the needy areas from which they came.

Supervision and regulation of practice are often very difficult, as they require first-hand knowledge of beliefs, customs, economics, environmental and health conditions of the people living in remote rural areas. This will take both time and money. Evaluation of schemes presents difficulties, as in many areas maternal mortality rates are not known. In an enquiry in rural Bangladesh, one-third of maternal deaths were due to complications of pregnancy requiring anaesthesia, surgery or blood transfusion—which were not available.

Infant mortality, which is high, is no more easy to use as an indicator.

Clinical differences

In areas of poverty where poor nutrition is common, or where taboos exist on eating iron-rich food and protein, a very low level of haemoglobin is common. Many of the primigravida may be very young, in their early teens, whilst the number of women of high parity is likely to be large. Many of the emergency cases will be obstructed labour due to disproportion, transverse lie and brow presentation, neglected cases being admitted with the uterus ruptured. The midwife may expect to participate in the performance of caesarean sections and symphysiotomies, and she could be asked to assist with perforation or embryotomy. Some women will have permanent urinary fistulas, especially in countries such as the Sudan, where female circumcision is still practised, leading to delay in labour, necrosis of the bladder wall, and later, vesicovaginal fistula.

Some of the babies are born preterm and many are small. Teaching hospitals are likely to have well equipped and adequately staffed special care baby units, but for the most part these facilities are lacking. Outside hospital, and with simple and sometimes primitive equipment, a conscientious and painstaking attendant can rear small babies with remarkable success, but the neonatal death rate remains high, with gastroenteritis one of the major problems, particularly where babies are not breast-fed.

Most mothers breast feed their babies, simply accepting that it is natural to do so. Many prolong breast feeding for 2 years or more, possibly as part of a tribal taboo which forbids intercourse during the lactation period or perhaps as a contraceptive measure. But, as women become better educated, read, travel and make greater contact with other races, so they see more of artificial feeding and begin to accept it as something desirable, so that the feeding bottle is easily seen as a status symbol. This has been encouraged by commercial advertising, but is not a good idea, especially where standards of hygiene are poor.

This issue is of major concern in developing countries because infant mortality rates are greatly increased when babies are artificially fed. In 1981, the World Health Organisation (WHO) and the United Nations Children's Fund (UNICEF) produced the WHO International Code of Marketing of Breast Milk Substitutes which was accepted by the WHO later that year. Its purpose is to protect breast feeding and to help control the marketing of products for artificial feeding, especially in developing countries, where the risks of infection are greatly increased in babies who are artificially fed. Recommendations included in the Code are:

1. Advertising or promotion directly to the public is prohibited.
2. No free samples of breast-milk substitutes are to be given to mothers.
3. No free gifts are to be given to mothers, including special offers or discounts.
4. No financial or free gifts are to be given to health workers for the purpose of promoting artificial milk substitutes.
5. Information on artificial milks, provided by the manufacturers for health workers, should include only scientific and factual information, and should not suggest that artificial milks are equivalent or superior to breast milk.

The implementation of the Code depends on agreements between manufacturers and governments, backed by legislation if necessary. Some countries have adopted their own version of the Code, including the UK where the Food Manufacturing Federation (FMF) in conjunction with the Ministry of Agriculture, and the then Department of Health and Social Security drew up what appeared to be a modified version. Despite the well-publicized problems associated with artificial feeding, some manufacturers have continued to actively promote their products in developing countries.

In 1991 WHO and UNICEF launched an initiative aimed at promoting breast feeding through the creation of baby-friendly hospitals. It aims to promote adoption of 'ten steps to successful breastfeeding' by hospitals and maternity services. Many of these are included in the management of breast feeding in Appendix 14.

Pathological and radiological facilities, blood banks and an efficient blood transfusion service are often poor or non-existent away from the large towns. Of particular concern now is that adequate facilities should be available to screen all blood for the HIV virus because the disease is a major problem in some countries.

Lack of transport is another problem, and contributes to the delay in transferring women with complications to a hospital or health centre.

Education

The education of midwives and TBAs in developing countries is a key factor in reducing maternal mortality and morbidity. In some developing countries, midwifery training schemes are based on inappropriate and out-of-date curricula from developed nations, thus midwives are ill-equipped to practise competently in their own situations. There is also a shortage of trained midwives in most countries and little or no continuing education for those practising.

In 1990 the International Confederation of Midwives (ICM), WHO and UNICEF held a workshop on midwifery education prior to the 22nd ICM Congress in Japan. From this workshop recommendations were made regarding the initial and continuing education of midwives in clinical practice, education and supervisory positions. Emphasis is placed on providing a realistic community-based education and enhancing clinical skills with special emphasis on prevention and emergency management of obstructed labour, eclampsia, haemorrhage, sepsis and abortion. The educational framework devised for those obstetric emergencies, together with distance-learning packages being developed by WHO have started to be implemented in some developing countries, for example, Tanzania. Greater uptake of this educational framework is necessary if it is to make an impact on maternal mortality and morbidity over the next decade.

Commitment by government and non-governmental organizations is also required, not only for education, but also for resources to provide a sufficient number of midwives since at present there is no trained person present at 58% of all births in the world per annum. The shortage of midwives is compounded by inappropriate distribution since the majority practise in towns, yet most of the population live in rural areas where there are few trained midwives or doctors to attend them. Because of this situation, the midwife in rural areas often has to lead a team of partially or untrained helpers such as TBAs and/or maternal and child health workers (MCH) and/or auxiliary midwives. The midwife's training therefore needs to prepare him/her for a leadership role and include management and teaching skills.

Organizations such as the Overseas Development Association (ODA) are also involved in initiatives to improve maternal and child health in developing countries. Such initiatives included schemes to educate midwife teachers in Zimbabwe and provide a programme of continuing education for midwives in Bangladesh.

Whether working in a government hospital, a mission hospital, or as part of a World Health Organization or Voluntary Services Overseas scheme, the British midwife will find much that is different from home.

Certainly specialized knowledge and skill will be required since, on the one hand, the work will include infant care and health and family planning education, and on the other it may include endotracheal intubation, forceps or ventouse delivery or symphysiotomy; but as today there are increasing opportunities to gain this knowledge and experience, the midwife will not begin this work unprepared.

The midwife will gain a sense of fulfilment in realizing that he/she is playing a role in the development of midwifery services and using his/her skill and knowledge to improve the health and welfare of the mothers and babies in the developing countries.

References

Kwast BE (1991) Maternal mortality: the magnitude and causes. *Midwifery* 7(1): 4–7.

Kwast BE & Bentley J (1991) Introducing confident midwives: midwifery education—action for safe motherhood. *Midwifery* 7(1): 8–19.

Thaddeus S & Maine D (1990) *Too Far to Walk. Maternal mortality in context.* Center for Population and Family Health, Columbia University.

APPENDIX 22

The Statutory Framework for Midwifery

The Central Midwives Board

The Central Midwives Board (CMB) was set up in 1902, and governed the education and practice of midwives until 1983 when the Nurses, Midwives and Health Visitors Act of 1979 was implemented. The functions of the CMB were to:

- regulate midwifery training and practice;
- conduct examinations;
- issue certificates;
- frame rules and directives;
- deal with complaints and panel cases

Throughout its existence it was medically dominated, although in its final decade before dissolution in 1983, the chairman was a midwife.

Nurses, Midwives and Health Visitors Act, 1979

The Nurses, Midwives and Health Visitors Act, 1979 was implemented in 1983 with a new statutory framework (*see* Figure 25). Since 1983, therefore, midwives have no longer had their own statutory body.

An outline of the Nurses, Midwives and Health Visitors Act 1979 follows, but when the new Nurses, Midwives and Health Visitors Act 1992 is implemented in 1993, the membership, committee structure and functions of the statutory bodies as described below, will change. An outline of the proposed changes is included at the end of this Appendix.

UKCC

Membership totals 45 and is made up as follows:

twenty members from the four National Boards, five from each board:
  two nurses;
  one midwife;
  one health visitor;
  one teacher (a nurse midwife or health visitor); and
twenty-five members appointed by the Secretary of State from nominations received from appropriate organizations.

The minimum number of midwives on the Council is four, one from each of the four National Boards, although this number is increased

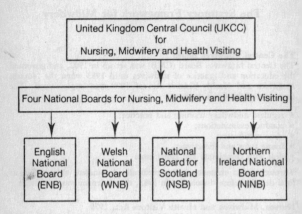

Figure 25. Statutory bodies for nursing, midwifery and health visiting.

due to those appointed by the Secretary of State. Nevertheless, midwives are in a minority on the UKCC.

Functions of the UKCC
1. To establish and improve standards of training.
2. To make rules for entry to training, and for the kind and standard of training to qualify for registration; to make rules for recording additional qualifications.
3. To maintain a professional register.
4. To establish and improve standards of professional conduct.
5. To make rules for practice of midwives.
6. To deal with international matters, including compliance with relevant European community Directives.

Committee Structure of the UKCC
To enable the UKCC to carry out its functions, the following committees have been established:

Midwifery Committee;
Education Policy Advisory Committee (EPAC);
Research Committee;
Finance Committee;
Registration Committee.

Midwifery Committee
This comprises 11–14 members, the majority of whom are midwives. Two medical practitioner members are required. The functions of the Midwifery Committee are defined in the Act: the Council (UKCC) shall consult the (Midwifery) Committee on all matters relating to midwifery and the Committee shall, on behalf of the Council, discharge such of Council's functions as are assigned to them either by the Council or the Secretary of State' (Section 4(2)). The same functions are designated to the Midwifery Committees of the Boards.

National Boards
The National Boards for

England   ⎫
Wales   ⎬   maximum of 45 members
Scotland   ⎭
Northern Ireland   maximum of 35 members

Two-thirds of the members of the National Boards are elected and one-third appointed by the Secretary of State. The English National Board (ENB) has 30 elected members, five of whom are midwives and the other three Boards have 24 elected members, four of whom are midwives. Despite the fact that the Secretary of State may appoint some midwives to each Board, they are in the minority, as is the case on the UKCC.

Functions of the National Boards
1. To collaborate with the UKCC in the promotion of improved training.
2. To approve training institutions and ensure courses meet UKCC requirements for registration, both initial and for additional qualifications.
3. To award qualifications.
4. To investigate cases of alleged professional misconduct and refer to UKCC as appropriate.

5. To be consulted by the UKCC.
6. To be consulted on midwives' rules and give guidance to local supervising authorities on supervision of midwives.

Committee structure of National Boards
All boards are required to have a *midwifery* and *finance* committee. Apart from this there is considerable variation in the committee structure of the National Boards. The *midwifery committee* of the Boards have the same number of members and functions as described for the UKCC Midwifery Committee.

Proposed changes to statutory bodies
In 1988 the government commissioned a firm of management consultants, Peat Marwick McLintock, to review the UKCC and four National Boards as part of the regular programme of reviews of non-Departmental public bodies, and their Report was published in 1989. As a result of the Report (Peat, Marwick McLintock Report), the government has agreed that the following changes should be made:

1. The UKCC should be the body elected by the professionals.
2. The Boards should cease to be elected bodies and become small, appointed, executive bodies.
3. The whole of the professional conduct function should be centralized at the UKCC.

The changes proposed required legislation.

Nurses, Midwives and Health Visitors Act 1992
The Nurses, Midwives and Health Visitors Act 1992 amends the Nurses, Midwives and Health Visitors Act of 1979. The new Act fundamentally changes the membership, powers and responsibilities of the United Kingdom Central Council (UKCC) and the national boards. It allows nurses, midwives and health visitors to directly elect the majority of members to the UKCC and gives the Council greater jurisdiction over the management of its professional affairs.

Changes to the UKCC

Membership
Membership should not exceed 60

Two thirds of the members of Council are to be elected by the professions (40).

One third will be appointed by the Secretary of State (20).

At the time of writing the UKCC is consulting the professions about the election process. Agreement is expected to be reached by July 1992 and elections will then take place in October 1992. The new Council takes over in April, 1993.

The titles President and Vice-President of the UKCC will replace the existing titles of Chairman and Vice-Chairman.

Committee Structure of the UKCC

The UKCC has been given greater freedom in the creation of its committee structure, and is required by the Act to pay proper attention to minority interests. The only two committees which the Council is obliged to establish under the new Act are the *finance* and *midwifery committees*.

Midwifery Committee

There will be a UKCC Midwifery Committee, but no national board midwifery committees under the new Act. The UKCC no longer has to consult the national boards before acting on the recommendations of its midwifery committee.

Professional Conduct

1. All professional conduct matters will become the sole function of the UKCC.
2. Members of conduct committees need not be exclusively from members of the UKCC, although a majority of the committee is required to consist of UKCC members.
3. Professional conduct committees will have two new powers:
   1. The power to caution a nurse, midwife or health visitor about his/her future conduct. A record of a caution will be kept.
   2. The power to suspend from practice for a specified period.

These powers are in addition to the existing options of removal from the register, taking no action or referral to the health committee.

Supervision of Midwifery

1. The UKCC is given new powers to prescribe standards for the supervision of midwifery.
2. The local supervising authorities (LSA's) are required to inform the UKCC and not the national boards of receipt of notice of intention to practice. The national boards will retain the responsibility to give advice and guidance to the LSA's on the supervision of midwives, but will be required to take account of the Council's policy and guidelines.

Discussions between the UKCC and the midwifery profession are taking place to determine the detailed nature and implementation of these changes.

Changes to the National Boards

The national boards will become smaller executive bodies, perhaps with only 9 or 10 members who will be appointed by the Secretary of State. Their main function will be to approve institutions and validate education programmes in relation to the provision of training for nurses, midwives and health visitors. They will no longer have responsibility for:

- funding education;
- Standing Committees, Joint Committees and Local Training Committees;
- initial investigation into illegal cases of misconduct;
- supervision of midwifery, although they will retain the responsibility to give advice and guidance to LSA's.

The Nurses, Midwives and Health Visitors Act 1992 will be implemented in April 1993.

APPENDIX 23

Publications of Current Interest

Of the many publications of particular topical interest to the midwife, a few are listed below.

Books for Midwives 1992 (Haigh and Hochland). This includes over 1000 titles. The titles in this catalogue have been selected for both students and practising midwives, and can be obtained by a postal service from Haigh and Hochland, Manchester M13 9QA.

The Common Market and the Common Man. European Community: The Facts. London: European Communities Press. These two small booklets set out, in outline only, a great deal of factual information about the European Economic Community, which midwives (and others) could learn with advantage.

Current Awareness Service (Royal College of Midwives). This is a bimonthly publication which contains a very full list of recent literature on midwifery and allied subjects.

Direct Entry: A Preparation for Midwifery Practice. N Radford & A Thompson, 1986 (University of Surrey). A study funded by the Department of Health and Social Security to investigate the current situation of direct entry midwifery training, to consider the implications of such programmes, and recommend ways of promoting their development.

Domiciliary Midwifery and Maternity Bed Needs (HMSO). Better known as the Peel Report, after its chairman, Sir John Peel, this report of the Subcommittee of the Standing Maternity and Midwifery Advisory Committee of the Central Health Services Council was published in 1970 and is well known to many midwives. The title is self-explanatory and, although the committee's recommendations were widely publicised some time ago, they remain the subject of much discussion.

Effective Care in Pregnancy and Childbirth. I Chalmers, M Enkin & M Keirse, 1989 (Oxford University Press). These two large volumes provide systematic analysis of evidence which is relevant in assessing the effects of care in pregnancy and childbirth.

ENB Framework and Higher Award for Continuing Professional Education for Nurses, Midwives and Health Visitors, 1991 (ENB). The aim of the framework is to provide a flexible system for continuing professional education and a structure leading to the ENB Higher Award.

Health and Personal Social Services Statistics for England (HMSO). This is an annual publication presenting health statistics and related social services data. As well as vital statistics, finance, manpower and administration, a range of services are included with hospital and community maternity services, and other data of interest to a midwife.

Journal of the Office of Population Censuses and Surveys [OPCS]. *Population Trends.* This is published quarterly and regularly contains tables of statistics as well as articles of medical interest. The OPCS library produces many other publications, and details are obtainable from St Catherine's House, 10 Kingsway, London WC2B 6TP.

Law and Professional Conduct in Nursing. AP Young, 1991 (Scutari Press). Again an important area for practising nurses and midwives study.

Legal Aspects of Nursing. B Dimond, 1990 (Prentice Hall). In view of the litigation problems of the present day, its importance to nurses and midwives cannot be gainsaid.

Local Government Reform. Short Version of the Report of the Royal Commission on Local Government in England (HMSO). Lord Redcliffe-Maud and his committee published in 1969 a ponderous volume, an admirable précis of which is presented in this 22-page booklet. It should be read with frequent reference to its accompanying map. It is of immediate interest, not only to nurses and midwives, but to all English citizens.

Maternity Services Advisory Committee: Maternity Care in Action; 1982 Part I, Antenatal Care; 1984 Part II, Care during Childbirth; 1985 Part III, Care of the Mother and Baby. These are guides for good practice and include checklists that are designed to aid professionals and users to review current practice, and raise standards of care.

MIDIRS Midwifery Digest. A midwifery information and research service which includes all topics of current interest to midwives. Four issues are published each year to enable midwives to keep up to date with current issues and research. (*See* Appendix 25.)

The Midwife: Her Legal Status and Her Accountability (Royal College of Midwives). This booklet clearly explains the practising midwife's legal status and accountability.

Midwifery Index 1980–1986, with selective coverage of 1976–1979 (Royal College of Midwives). An accumulation of journal articles which have been indexed in the RCM Current Awareness Service since 1980. It includes over 12 000 entries. A new *Midwifery Index*, 1986–1991, will be published in 1992 with a further 12–13 000 entries.

MIRIAD Midwifery Research Database. This is a national register of all completed and ongoing research in midwifery in the United Kingdom. An annual report is published. MIRIAD is based at the National Perinatal Epidemiology Unit in Oxford. (*See* Appendix 25.)

The National Council for Vocational Qualifications (NCVQ) in England, Wales and Northern Ireland. Its aims and purposes. A useful booklet explaining that the NCVQ has been set up by the government to enhance a coherent national framework for vocational qualifications in England, Wales and Northern Ireland for Health Care Assistants.

Offical Journal of the European Communities, L33, volume 23, 1980 (HMSO). This publication contains the midwifery directives, which concern freedom of movement in the Community and the training programme. (The requirements for the latter are included in the changes made in the United Kingdom 18-month training which came into effect in September 1981.)

On the State of the Public Health (HMSO). This is the annual report of the Chief Medical Officer of the Department of Health, a sizeable document which can usually be borrowed from a hospital library. Every aspect of public and community health is reviewed, including vital statistics, sexually transmitted diseases, all aspects of maternal and child health, and many other, wider, health issues.

Patients First—a consultative paper on the structure of the National Health Service in England and Wales, December 1979 (HMSO). This is a booklet produced after the Royal Commission on the National Health Service made certain criticisms of the health service: too many tiers, too many administrators, slow decision-making and money wasted. This consultative document formed the basis of the 1981 reorganization outlined in Appendix 1.

Present-day Practice in Infant Feeding (HMSO). A short report submitted by a panel of experts on child nutrition set up by the DHSS Committee on Medical Aspects of Food Policy. These reports give unequivocal support to the value of breast feeding, supply much succinct information about problems related to artificial feeding and obesity, and underline the need for improved education, both of mothers and of all professional personnel. Since the first publication in 1974, breast feeding has greatly increased in popularity. The most recent edition is due to be published in 1992.

Project 2000: A New Preparation for Practice. 1986 (UKCC for Nursing, Midwifery and Health Visiting). This important document recommended fundamental changes in nurse education which were accepted by the government and are now being implemented.

Report of the Committee on Child Health Service (HMSO). This report was produced by an eminent committee of professionals concerned with children, under the chairmanship of Emeritus Professor S. D. M. Court. Regrettably there was no midwife representative, although evidence was taken from the Royal College of Midwives. It examined issues concerning children and their families, their state of health and the quality of services provided for them, in the context of those offered in other industrialized countries. The range of maternity services was assessed, and areas of concern were highlighted. The inadequacy of preparation for parenthood, deprivation of choice in some areas of institutionalized maternity care were particularly noted. Early contact between the mother and her baby was advocated, as was the provision of regional neonatal intensive care centres to reduce the sequelae of neonatal illness. Many major recommendations were made, a number of which have yet to receive attention. These are contained in volume 1, volume 2 being the statistical appendix.

Report on the Committee on Nursing (HMSO). In October 1972 this committee, under the chairmanship of Professor Asa Briggs, published a lengthy but very readable report, which makes a number of recommendations which are creating radical changes in the careers of nurses and midwives. While much of the report had a very favourable reception, there remain a number of controversial issues. The report might well be borrowed from a hospital or public library. The Nurses, Midwives and Health Visitors Act, 1979, was based on this report.

Report on Confidential Enquiries into Maternal Deaths in England and Wales (HMSO). Each edition of this report covers three years, the most recent, the 12th, dealing with 1985, 1986 and 1987, having been published in 1991. Every maternal death in each three-year period is studied confidentially, individually and impartially by an expert committee, all the circumstances being closely reviewed, in an attempt to assess possible avoidable factors. These widely read reports are greatly respected and the adoption of their various recommendations has undoubtedly led to a steady decrease in the maternal mortality rate.

Report of the Expert Group on Special Care for Babies (HMSO) 1971. This expert committee reviewed the history and the facilities at present available for the nursing of special care babies and considered in detail how the needs of the future might best be met. Their important recommendations are of interest to midwives whether or not they are wanting to work in special care baby units.

Review of the UKCC and Four National Boards for Nursing, Midwifery and Health Visiting 1989 (Peat Marwick McLintock). This review was commissioned by the government as part of the regular programme of reviews of non-departmental public bodies. Some of the recommendations altering the roles of the statutory bodies have been included in the Nurses, Midwifery and Health Visitors' Act, 1992.

Report of the Post-registration Education and Practice Project. 1990 (UKCC). This document proposes a framework for continuing education in order to maintain and enhance the standards of nurses, midwives and health visitors.

Research and the Midwife Conference Proceedings (Department of Nursing, University of Manchester). Published annually following the Research and the Midwife Conferences.

The Role and Preparation of Support Workers to Nurses, Midwives and

Health Visitors and the Implications for Manpower and Service Planning 1987 (Department of Health and Social Security).

Second Report from the Social Services Committee, Session 1979–80, Perinatal and Neonatal Mortality, volume 1 (HMSO). An enquiry resulting from public concern over the differences in the mortality rates between different socio-economic groups and different areas in England and Wales. Other developed countries' rates were falling more quickly, and a large number of conclusions were reached by the Committee, under the chairmanship of Renee Short. Recommendations were made for improving antenatal clinics, redrafting the criteria for admission to the Obstetric List of General Practitioners, and making better use of the skills of the midwife.

Select Committee Report on the Maternity Services. 1992. The all-party House of Commons maternity services enquiry lasted 1 year and the report recommends a major shift in the provision of NHS care for healthy women and their babies. It is recommended that midwives should be the main care providers, giving continuity of care, that shared antenatal care should be largely abandoned in favour of care based in the community, midwife-led units should be established, and that women should be given sufficient information to make an informal choice about where they wish to have their baby. All midwives should read this important publication.

Social Trends (Central Statistical Office [SCO] London). Published annually and contains much valuable information about British Society, for example, births and deaths, population, households and families, education, crime, employment, health and social services are some of the areas covered.

Strategy for Nursing 1989 (HMSO). A document which takes nursing, midwifery and health visiting into the health service of the next century. It includes targets for action for practice, manpower, education and management.

Successful Breastfeeding. Royal College of Midwives, 2nd edn, 1991 (Churchill Livingstone). This book provides clear and effective guidelines to ensure successful breast feeding.

Towards a Healthy Nation. 2nd edn, 1991 (Royal College of Midwives). A statement on the Maternity Services by the RCM, setting out its review of the issues and its policies for the future. A document to stimulate discussion and lead to constructive attempts to meet the real needs of the women of the 21st century.

When a Baby Dies, N Kohner & A Henley, 1991 (Stillbirth and Neonatal Death Society Pandora Press). The experience of late miscarriage, stillbirth and neonatal death, based on letters from and interviews with many bereaved parents.

Women's Experience of Maternity Care—A Survey Manual. V Marson,

1989 (HMSO). A manual produced by Social Survey Division of OPCS on behalf of the Department of Health.

Working for Patients, Working Paper 10, Education and Training 1989 (HMSO). This paper was published soon after the Peat Marwick McLintock's Report was released by the government and put forward alternative proposals for the funding of non-medical education and training in the NHS. One of the proposals, namely that Regional Health Authorities should have the main responsibility for funding pre-registration nursing and midwifery education, was accepted by the government.

Writing a Research Proposal and Applying for Funding 1989 (Royal College of Midwives). A booklet providing useful information for those seeking help to get started on a research project.

UKCC Publications:

Midwives Rules, 1991.
A Midwife's Code of Practice, 1991.
Code of Professional Conduct for the Nurse, Midwife and Health Visitor, 1992.
Administration of Medicines, 1986.
Exercising Accountability, 1989.
Confidentiality, 1987.
Advertising by Registered Nurses, Midwives and Health Visitors, 1985.

APPENDIX 24

Abbreviations

Much controversy still exists over the use of abbreviations. In years gone by it was accepted that in oral and written reports, in examinations and in similar fairly formal statements, abbreviations were entirely inappropriate. Though this time is long past, the tradition remains. But, in the quickened tempo of life today and with an increasing multiplicity of committees and councils, of titles and designations and, indeed, of drugs, equipment and procedures, many having long and complex names, it is small wonder that conversation and reports appear often to be reduced to lists of initial letters.

In a hospital which has evolved its own code, describing its own particular treatments and procedures, the message is perfectly clear; elsewhere it is incomprehensible. In other words, though some abbreviations are nationally or even internationally recognized, others most certainly are not.

The midwife, trying to negotiate this maze of initial letters and short words, less obvious than NATO and UNO, for example, which evolved from those initials, may wonder when an abbreviation is or is not acceptable. There is no absolute answer, but these guidelines may help:

1. The more formal the occasion, the more abbreviations should be avoided. Those which may pass in casual conversation may well be unsuitable for a written statement.
2. Nationally recognized abbreviations are often acceptable where those coined locally are undesirable.
3. Above all, the communication must be clear to the recipient, who may be British or foreign, intelligent or slow-witted. If the abbreviated message is not clear or if there is any doubt as to its clarity, then it should be presented in full. Failure to observe this fundamental fact has led to many serious errors in communication.

There follows a list, necessarily incomplete, of some of the abbreviations in common use in the health service in the United Kingdom.

Titles, diplomas, organizations

ABPN	Association of British Paediatric Nurses
ADM	Advanced Diploma in Midwifery
ADMS	Assistant Director of Medical Services
AIDS	Advice and Information for the Deaf

AIMS	Association for the Improvement of the Maternity Services
AMS	Army Medical Service
ANA	Association of Nurse Administrators
ARRC	Associate of the Royal Red Cross
ARSH	Associate of the Royal Society of Health
ASH	Action on Smoking and Health
BA	Bachelor of Arts
BAO	Bachelor of the Art of Obstetrics
BAON	British Association of Orthopaedic Nurses
BC, BCh	Bachelor of Surgery
BChD	Bachelor of Dental Surgery
BDA	British Dental Association
BDS	Bachelor of Dental Surgery
BDSc	Bachelor of Dental Science
BEd	Batchelor of Education
BHyg	Bachelor of Hygiene
BM	Bachelor of Medicine
BMA	British Medical Association
BP	British Pharmacopoeia
BPC	British Pharmaceutical Codex
BPharm	Bachelor of Pharmacy
BRC	British Red Cross
BRCS	British Red Cross Society
BS	Bachelor of Surgery
BSc	Bachelor of Science
BSI	British Standards Institute
BTA	British Thoracic Association
BVP	British Volunteer Programme
CAMO	Chief Administrative Medical Officer
ChB	Bachelor of Surgery
CHC	Community Health Council
ChD	Doctor of Surgery
ChM	Master of Surgery
CHSC	Central Health Services Council
CM	Master of Surgery
CNF	Commonwealth Nurses Federation
CNN	Certified Nursery Nurse
CNO	Chief Nursing Officer
CSP	Chartered Society of Physiotherapy
CStJ	Commander of the Order of St John of Jerusalem

DA	Diploma in Anaesthetics
DA	District Administrator
DCh	Doctor of Surgery
DCH	Diploma in Child Health
DCP	Diploma in Clinical Pathology
DFO	District Finance Officer
DGH	District General Hospital
DGM	District General Manager
DGO	Diploma in Gynaecology and Obstetrics
DHA	District Health Authority
DH	Department of Health
DMC	District Medical Committee
DMU	Directly managed unit
DN	Diploma in Nursing
DNS	Director of Nursing Services
DObst	Diploma in Obstetrics
DPH	Diploma in Public Health
DPM	Diploma in Psychological Medicine
DPSM	Diploma in Professional Studies in Midwifery
DRCOG	Diploma of the Royal College of Obstetricians and Gynaecologists
DT	District Treasurer
EEC	European Economic Community
ENB	English National Board for Nursing, Midwifery and Health Visiting
ENT	Ear, nose and throat
FFA	Fellow of the Faculty of Anaesthetists
FHSA	Family Health Services Authority
FICS	Fellow of the International College of Surgeons
FIGO	International Federation of Gynaecology and Obstetrics
FPA	Family Planning Association
FRCOG	Fellow of the Royal College of Obstetricians and Gynaecologists
FRCP	Fellow of the Royal College of Physicians
FRCS	Fellow of the Royal College of Surgeons
FRS	Fellow of the Royal Society
GMC	General Medical Council
GP	General practitioner
HAS	Health Advisory Service

HASAW	Health and Safety at Work Act
HCPT	Health Care Planning Team
HMSO	Her Majesty's Stationery Office
HSA	Hospital Savings Association
HSC	Health and Safety Commission
HSE	Health and Safety Executive
HV	Health Visitor
HVA	Health Visitor's Association
HVCert	Health Visitor Certificate
ICM	International Confederation of Midwives
ICN	International Council of Nurses
ICRC	International Committee of the Red Cross
INR	Index of Nursing Research
ISD	Information Services Division
ITU	Intensive therapy unit
IVS	International Voluntary Service
JCC	Joint Consultative Committee
JCPT	Joint Care Planning Team
JLC	Joint Liaison Committee
KFC	King's Fund Centre
KFC	King's Fund College
LA	Local authority
LSA	Local supervising authority
MA	Master of Arts
MAO	Master of the Art of Obstetrics
MB	Bachelor of Medicine
MC, MCh	Master of Surgery
MD	Doctor of Medicine
MO	Medical Officer
MRC	Medical Research Council
MRCOG	Member of the Royal College of Obstetricians and Gynaecologists
MRCS	Member of the Royal College of Surgeons
MS	Master of Surgery
MTD	Midwife Teacher's Diploma (no longer awarded)
NAHA	National Association of Health Authorities
NAMCW	National Association for Maternal and Child Welfare
NB	National Board

NBS	National Board for Scotland for Nursing, Midwifery and Health Visiting
NCT	National Childbirth Trust
NCW	National Council of Women
NCUMC	National Council for the Unmarried Mother and her Child
NERU	Nursing Education Research Unit
NHS	National Health Service
NINB	Northern Ireland National Board for Nursing, Midwifery and Health Visiting
NO	Nursing Officer
NSC	National Staff Committee (Nurses and Midwives)
OHNC	Occupational Health Nursing Certificate
ONC	Orthopaedic Nursing Certificate
OPCS	Office of Population Censuses and Surveys
OStJ	Officer of the Order of St John of Jerusalem
PGCE(A)	Postgraduate certificate in education (adults)
PHI	Public Health Inspector
PMRAFNS	Princess Mary's Royal Air Force Nursing Service
PNO	Principal Nursing Officer
PSW	Psychiatric Social Worker
QARANC	Queen Alexandra's Royal Army Nursing Corps
QARNS	Queen Alexandra's Royal Naval Nursing Service
QIDN	Queen's Institute of District Nursing
QNI	Queen's Nursing Institute
RA	Regional Administrator
RCGP	Royal College of General Practitioners
RCM	Royal College of Midwives
RCN	Royal College of Nursing and National Council of Nurses of the United Kingdom
RGM	Regional General Manager
RGN	Registered General Nurse
RHA	Regional Health Authority
RM	Registered Midwife
RMN	Registered Mental Nurse
RMO	Regional Medical Officer
RMO	Resident Medical Officer
RNMS	Registered Nurse for the Mentally Subnormal
RNO	Regional Nursing Officer
RNT	Registered Nurse Tutor

RoSPA	Royal Society for the Prevention of Accidents
RSCN	Registered Sick Children's Nurse
RT	Regional Treasurer
RWO	Regional Works Officer
SCBU	Special care baby unit
SCM	State Certified Midwife
SEN	State Enrolled Nurse
SGT	Self-governing trust
SHHD	Scottish Home and Health Department
SHO	Senior House Officer
SNO	Senior Nursing Officer
SRN	State Registered Nurse
UGM	Unit General Manager
UKCC	United Kingdom Central Council (for Nursing, Midwifery and Health Visiting)
UN	United Nations
UNDP	United Nations Development Programme
UNICEF	United Nations International Children's Emergency Fund
WHO	World Health Organization
WNB	Welsh National Board for Nursing, Midwifery and Health Visiting
WRVS	Women's Royal Voluntary Service

Medical, Midwivery and Nursing Terms

ACH	After-coming head (in breech presentation)
ACTH	Adrenocorticotrophic hormone
AF	Artificially fed
AFP	Alpha-fetoprotein
AID	Artificial insemination (donor)
AIDS	Acquired immune deficiency syndrome
AIH	Artificial insemination (husband)
AN	Antenatal
ANC	Antenatal care; antenatal clinic
AP	Anteroposterior
APH	Antepartum haemorrhage
ARM	Artificial rupture of membranes
ASD	Atrial septal defect
AV, A/V	Anteverted

BBA	Born before arrival
BCG	Bacille Calmette–Guérin
b.d.	*bis in die* (twice a day)
BF	Breast-fed
BMR	Basal metabolic rate
BPD	Biparietal diameter
C	Celsius
CAT	Computerized axial tomography
CCT	Controlled cord traction
CDH	Congenital dislocation of the hip
CIP	Continuous inflating pressure
CNP	Continuous negative pressure
CPAP	Continuous positive airways pressure
CPD	Cephalopelvic disproportion
CRL	Crown–rump length
CS	Caesarean section
CSF	Cerebro-spinal fluid
CSU	Catheter specimen of urine
CTG	Cardiotocograph
Cx	Cervix
D&C	Dilatation and curettage
D&V	Diarrhoea and vomiting
DIC	Disseminated intravascular coagulation
DTA	Deep transverse arrest
DVT	Deep vein thrombosis
E_1	Oestrone
E_2	Oestradiol 17β
E_3	Oestriol
EBM	Expressed breast milk
ECV	External cephalic version
EDC	Expected date of confinement
EDD	Expected date of delivery
EUA	Examination under anaesthesia
F	Fahrenheit
FACH	Forceps to the after-coming head
FBS	Fetal blood sample
FD	Forceps delivery
FH(H)	Fetal heart (heard)
FHR	Fetal heart rate
FHS	Fetal heart sounds

FSH	Follicle-stimulating hormone
GIFT	Gamete intrafallopian transfer
GTT	Glucose tolerance test
Hb	Haemoglobin
HCG	Human chorionic gonadotrophin
HPL	Human placental lactogen
HVS	High vaginal swab
ICD	International classification of disease
IMV	Intermittent mandatory ventilation
INAH	Isonicotinic acid hydrazide
IPPV	Intermittent positive pressure ventilation
IUCD	Intrauterine contraceptive device
IUD	Intrauterine death
IUFD	Intrauterine fetal death
IUGR	Intrauterine growth retardation
IUT	Intrauterine transfusion
IVF	*In vitro* fertilization
IVP	Intravenous pyelogram
LBW	Low birth weight
LFD	Light-for-dates
LFT	Liver function test
LH	Luteinizing hormone
LMA	Left mentoanterior
LML	Left mentolateral
LMP	Left mentoposterior
LMP	Last menstrual period
LOA	Left occipitoanterior
LOL	Left occipitolateral
LOP	Left occipitoposterior
L/S ratio	Lecithin/sphingomyelin ratio
LSA	Left sacroanterior
LSCS	Lower segment caesarean section
LSL	Left sacrolateral
LSP	Left sacroposterior
MSU	Midstream specimen of urine
NAD	No abnormality detected
NBS	National Board for Scotland for Nursing, Midwifery

	and Health Visiting
ND	Normal delivery
NINB	Northern Ireland National Board for Nursing, Midwifery and Health Visiting
NND	Neonatal death
NNU	Neonatal unit
NTD	Neural tube defect
OA	Occipitoanterior
OCT	Oxytocin challenge test
OP	Occipitoposterior
OPD	Outpatient department
OT	Occipitotransverse
PA	*per abdomen*
P_{CO_2}	Partial pressure of carbon dioxide
PE	Pre-eclampsia
PKU	Phenylketonuria
PM	Post mortem
PMR	Perinatal mortality rate
PNC	Postnatal clinic
P_{O_2}	Partial pressure of oxygen
POP	Persistent occipitoposterior
PPH	Postpartum haemorrhage
PR	*per rectum*
p.r.n.	*pro re nata* (when necessary)
PUO	Pyrexia of unknown origin
PV	*per vaginam*
RDS	Respiratory distress syndrome
Rh	Rhesus
RMA	Right mentoanterior
RML	Right mentolateral
RMP	Right mentoposterior
ROA	Right occipitoanterior
ROL	Right occipitolateral
ROP	Right occipitoposterior
RSA	Right sacroanterior
RSL	Right sacrolateral
RSP	Right sacroposterior
RV, R/V	Retroverted
SB	Stillborn
SID	Sudden infant death syndrome

s.o.s.	*si opus sit* (if necessary)
stat.	*statim* (immediately)
SVD	Spontaneous vaginal delivery
t.d.s.	*ter die sumendus* (three times a day)
URTI	Upper respiratory tract infection
US	Ultrasound, ultrasonic
USS	Ultrasound scan
UTI	Urinary tract infection
VD	Venereal disease
Δ	Diagnosis
♂	Male (symbol of Mars)
♀	Female (symbol of Venus)
<	less than
>	more than
+ve	positive
−ve	negative

APPENDIX 25

Useful Addresses

Active Birth Centre (ABC), 55 Dartmouth Park Road, London NW5 1SL
  Tel. 071-267 3006

Association for Improvements in the Maternity Services (AIMS), 40 Kingswood Avenue, London NW6 6LS
  Tel. 081-969 5585

Association for Post-Natal Illness, 7 Gowan Avenue, London SW6 6RH
  Tel. 071-731 4867

Association for Spina Bifida and Hydrocephalus, ASBAH House, 42 Park Road, Peterborough PE1 2UQ
  Tel. 0733 555988

Association of Breast Feeding Mothers, Order Department, Sydenham Green Health Centre, Holmshaw Close, London SE26 4TH
  Tel. 081-774 4769

Association of Community Health Councils for England and Wales, 22 Columbo Street, London SE1 8DP
  Tel. 071-609 8405

Association of Radical Midwives (ARM), 62 Greetby Hill, Ormskirk, Lancashire L39 2DT
  Tel. 0695 572776

(This is a support and skill-sharing group—not a private midwifery service)

Baby Life Support Systems (BLISS), 17–21 Emerald Street, London WC1N 3QL
  Tel. 071-831 9393

Birthright, 27 Sussex Place, Regents Park, London NW1 4SP
  Tel. 071-262 5337

Breast Care and Mastectomy Association of Great Britain (BCMA), 15–19 Britten Street, London SW3 3TZ
  Tel. 071-351 7811

British Agencies for Adoption and Fostering, 11 Southwark Street, London SE1 1RQ
  Tel. 071-407 8800

British Association for Counselling, 37a Sheep Street, Rugby, Warwickshire CV21 3BX
  Tel. 0788 78328/9

British Council of Organisations of Disabled People (BCODP), St Mary's Church, Greenlaw Street, London SE18 5AR
    Tel. 081-316 4184

British Deaf Association, 38 Victoria Place, Carlisle CA1 1HU
    Tel. 0228 48844

British Diabetic Association, 10 Queen Anne Street, London W1M 0BD
    Tel. 071-323 1531

British Epilepsy Association, Anstey House, 40 Hanover Square, Leeds LS3 1BE
    Tel. 0532 439393

British Heart Foundation, 102 Gloucester Place, London W1H 4DH
    Tel. 071-935 0185

British Holistic Medical Association, 179 Gloucester Place, London NW1 6DX
    Tel. 071-262 5299

British Homeopathic Association (BHA), 27a Devonshire Street, London W1N 1RJ
    Tel. 071-935 2163

British Medical Association (BMA), BMA House, Tavistock Square, London WC1H 9JP
    Tel. 071-383 6101

British Organ Donor Society (BODY), Balsham, Cambridge CB1 6DL
    Tel. 0223 893636

British Pregnancy Advisory Service (BPAS), Austry Manor, Wootton Wawen, Solihull, West Midlands B95 6DA
    Tel. 05642 3225

British Red Cross Society (BRCS), 9 Grosvenor Crescent, London SW1X 7EJ
    Tel. 071-235 5454

British United Provident Association (BUPA), 24/27 Essex Street, London WC2
    Tel. 081-466 6531

Brittle Bone Society, 112 City Road, Dundee DD2 2PW
    Tel. 0382 817771

Brook Advisory Centres, 153a East Street, London SE17 2SD
    Tel. 071-708 1390

Bureau for Overseas Medical Service, Africa Centre, 38 King Street, London WC2E 8JT
    Tel. 071-836 5833

Childline, 50 Studd Street, London N1 0QJ
    Tel. 071-239 1000

Cleft Lip and Palate Association (CLAPA), 1 Eastwood Gardens, Kenton, Newcastle-upon-Tyne NE3 3DQ
    Tel. 091-285 9396

Coeliac Society of the United Kingdom, PO Box 220, High Wycombe, Buckinghamshire HP11 2HY
    Tel. 0494 437278

Commission for Racial Equality, Elliott House, 10–12 Allington House, London SW1E 5EH
    Tel. 071-828 7022

Confederation of Healing Organizations (CHO), 113 High Street, Berkhamsted, Hertfordshire HP4 2DJ
    Tel. 0442 870660

Committee on Safety of Medicines, Market Towers, 1 Nine Elms Lane, London SW8 5NQ
    Tel. 071-720 2188

Compassionate Friends, 6 Denmark Street, Bristol BS1 5DQ
    Tel. 0272 292778

Cruse (National Organization for the Widowed and their Children), Cruse House, 126 Sheen Road, Richmond, Surrey TW9 1UR
    Tel. 081-940 4818

Cystic Fibrosis Research Trust, Alexandra House, 5 Blythe Road, Bromley, Kent BR1 3RS
    Tel. 081-464 7211/2

Department of Health, Richmond House, 79 Whitehall, London SW1A 2NS
    Tel. 071-210 3000

Welsh Office

Crown Buildings, Cathays Park, Cardiff CF1 3NQ
    Tel. 0222 825111

Scottish Office

Dover House, Whitehall, London SW1A 2AU
    Tel. 071-270 3000

Scottish Home and Health Department

St Andrew's House, Regent Road, Edinburgh EH1 3DE
    Tel. 031 566 8400

Department of Health and Social Services, Northern Ireland

Dundonald House, Upper Newtownards Road, Belfast BT4 2SB
    Tel. 0232 650111

Department of Social Security, Richmond House, 79 Whitehall, London SW1A 2NS
    Tel. 071-210 3000

Disabled Living Foundation, 380–384 Harrow Road, London W9 2HU
    Tel. 071-289 6111

Down's Syndrome Association, 153–155 Mitcham Road, London SW17 9PG
    Tel. 081-682 4001

ENB Career's Advisory Office, PO Box 356, Sheffield S8 0SJ

English National Board for Nursing, Midwifery and Health Visiting (ENB), Victory House, 170 Tottenham Court Road, London W1P 0HA
    Tel. 071-388 3131

Equal Opportunities Commission, Overseas House, Quay Street, Manchester M3 3HN
    Tel. 061-833 9244

Family Planning Association (FPA), Margaret Pyke House, 27–35 Mortimer Street, London W1N 7RJ
    Tel. 071-636 7866

Family Welfare Association, 501–505 Kingsland Road, London E8 4AU
    Tel. 071-254 6251

Foresight Charity for Preconceptual Care, The Old Vicarage, Church Lane, Witley, Goldalming, Surrey GG8 5PN
    Tel. 0428 684500

The Foundation for the Study of Infant Deaths (Cot Death Research and Support), 3–5 Belgrave Square, London SW1X 8BQ
    Tel. 071-235 1721

Gingerbread, 35 Wellington Street, London WC2E 7BN
    Tel. 071-240 0953

Haemophilia Society, 123 Westminster Bridge Road, London SE1 7HR
    Tel. 071-928 2020

Health and Safety Executive, Baynards House, 1–13 Chepstow Place, Westbourne Grove, London W2 4TF
    Tel. 071-229 3456

Health Education Authority, Hamilton House, Mabledon Place, London WC1H 9TX
    Tel. 071-631 0930

Health Service Commissioner, Church House, Great Smith Street, London SW1P 3BW
    Tel. 071-276 3000

Health Services Superannuation Division, Hesketh House, 200–220 Broadway, Fleetwood, Lancashire FL7 8LG
    Tel. 0253 856123

Health Visitors' Association (HVA), 50 Southwark Street, London SE1 1UN
    Tel. 071-378 7255

Hospital Saving Association, Hambledon House, Andover, Hampshire SP10 1LQ
    Tel. 0264 53211

Institute for Complementary Medicine, 21 Portland Place, London W1N 3AF
    Tel. 071-636 9543

Institution of Environmental Health Officers (IEHO), Chadwick House, 7 Rushworth Street, London SE1 0QT
  Tel. 071-928 6006

International Confederation of Midwives, 10 Barley Mow Passage, London W4 4PH
  Tel. 081-994 6477

International Council for Nurses, 3 Place Jean-Marteau, 1201 Geneva, Switzerland
  Tel. 010 41(22)7312960

International Voluntary Service (IVS), (British Branch of Service Civil International), 162 Upper New Walk, Leicester LE1 7QA
  Tel. 0533 549430

King's Fund Centre (KFC), 126 Albert Street, London NW1 7NF
  Tel. 071-267 6111

Leukaemia Research Fund, 43 Great Ormond Street, London WC1N 3JT
  Tel. 071-405 0101

Listeria Support Group, 2 Wessex Close, Faringdon, Oxfordshire SN7 7YY

Margaret Pyke Centre, 15 Bateman's Building, Soho Square, London W1V 5TW
  Tel. 071-734 9351

Marie Stopes Clinic, Well Woman Centre, 108 Whitfield Street, London W1P 6BE
  Tel. 071-388 0662

Maternity Alliance, 15 Brittania Street, London WC1X 9JP
  Tel. 071-837 1265

Midwives Information and Resource Services, Institute of Child Health, Royal Hospital for Sick Children, St Michael's Hill, Bristol BS2 8BJ
  Tel. 0272 251791

MIND (National Association for Mental Health), 22 Harley Street, London W1N 2ED
  Tel. 071-637 0741

Miscarriage Association, PO Box 24, Ossett, West Yorkshire WF5 9KG
  Tel. 0924 830515

Multiple Births Foundation (MBFI), Queen Charlotte's and Chelsea Hospital, Goldhawk Road, London W6 0XG
  Tel. 081-748 4666

National Association for Maternal and Child Welfare, 1 South Audley Street, London W1Y 6JS
  Tel. 071-491 2772 and 1315

National Association of Bereavement Services (NABS), 122 Whitechapel High Street, London E1 7PT

Tel. 071-247 1080 (24-hour answerphone for referral requests); 071-247 0617 (admin.)

National Association of Citizens' Advice Bureaux, 115–123 Pentonville Road, London N1 9LZ
Tel. 071-833 2181

National Board for Nursing, Midwifery and Health Visiting for Northern Ireland, RAC House, 79 Chicester Street, Belfast BT1 4JE
Tel. 0232 238152

National Board for Nursing, Midwifery and Health Visiting for Scotland, 22 Queen Street, Edinburgh EH2 1JX
Tel. 031-226 7371

National Childbirth Trust, 9 Queensborough Terrace, London W2 3TB
Tel. 071-221 3833

National Council for One Parent Families, 255 Kentish Town Road, London NW5 2LX
Tel. 071-267 1361

National Council for Vocational Qualifications, 222 Euston Road, London NW1 2BZ
Tel. 071-387 9898

National Marriage Guidance Council, Herbert Gray College, Little Church Street, Rugby, Warwickshire CV21 3AP

National Perinatal Epidemiology Unit, Radcliffe Infirmary, Oxford OX2 6HE
Tel. 0865 224876

National Rubella Council, Bray Business Centre, Weir Bank, Monkey Island Lane, Bray-on-Thames, Berkshire SL6 2EP
Tel. 0628 770011

National Society for Phenylketonuria and Allied Disorders, Worth Cottage, Lower Scholes, Keighley, West Yorkshire BD22 0RR
Tel. 0535 44865

National Society for the Prevention of Cruelty to Children (NSPCC), 67 Saffron Hill, London EC1N 8RS
Tel. 071-242 1626

NSPCC National Advisory Centre on the Battered Child, Denves House, The Drive, Bounds Green Road, London N11
Tel. 081-361 1181

Office of Population Censuses & Surveys, St Catherine's House, 10 Kingsway, London WC2B 6TP
Tel. 071-242 0262

Pregnancy Advisory Service, 13 Charlotte Street, London W1P 1HD
Tel. 071-637 8962

Princess Mary's Royal Air Force Nursing Service (PMRAFNS), Ministry of Defence, First Avenue House, High Holborn, London WC1V 6HD

Tel. 071-430 5555

Queen Alexandra's Royal Army Nursing Corps (QARANC), Ministry of Defence, First Avenue House, High Holborn, London WC1V 6HD
Tel. 071-430 5555

Queen Alexandra's Royal Naval Nursing Service (QARNNS), Ministry of Defence, First Avenue House, High Holborn, London WC1V 6HD
Tel. 071-430 5555

Royal Association in Aid of Deaf People, 27 Old Oak Road, London W3 7HN
Tel. 081-743 6187

Royal British Nurses Association Club, 94 Upper Tollington Park, London N4 4NB
Tel. 071-272 6821

Royal College of General Practitioners, 14 Princes Gate, Hyde Park, London SW7 1PU
Tel. 071-581 3232

Royal College of Midwives (RCM), 15 Mansfield Street, London W1M 0BE
Tel. 071-580 6523

Royal College of Midwives, Scottish Board, 37 Frederick Street, Edinburgh EH2 1EP
Tel. 031-225 1633

Royal College of Midwives, Welsh Board, Suite 4, Floor 3, Alexandra House, 1 Alexandra Road, Swansea SA1 5ED
Tel. 0792 650082

Royal College of Midwives, Northern Ireland Board, Friends Provident Building, 58 Howard Street, Belfast BT1 6PU
Tel. 0232 241531

Royal College of Midwives, North of England Office, 18th Floor, Royal Exchange House, Boar Lane, Leeds LS1 5NY
Tel. 0532 444310

Royal College of Nursing of the United Kingdom (RCN), 20 Cavendish Square, London W1M 0AB
Tel. 071-409 3333

Royal College of Nursing and Council of Nurses of the United Kingdom (RCN) Scotland, 44 Heriot Row, Edinburgh EH3 6EY
Tel. 031-556 7231

Royal College of Nursing and National Council of Nurses of the United Kingdom (RCN) Welsh Board, Tŷ Maeth, King George V Drive, East Cardiff CF4 4XZ
Tel. 0222 751374/5

Royal College of Obstetricians and Gynaecologists (RCOG), 27 Sussex Place, Regent's Park, London NW1 4RG
    Tel. 071-262 5425

Royal Institute of Public Health and Hygiene, 28 Portland Place, London W1N 4DE
    Tel. 071-580 2731

Royal National Institute for the Blind (RNIB), 224 Great Portland Street, London W1N 6AA
    Tel. 071-388 1266

Royal National Institute for the Deaf (RNID), 105 Gower Street, London WC1E 6AH
    Tel. 071-387 8033

Royal National Pension Fund for Nurses, Burdett House, 15 Buckingham Street, Strand, London WC2N 6ED
    Tel. 071-839 6785

Royal Society of Health, 38a St George's Drive, London SW1V 4BH
    Tel. 071-630 0121

Royal Society of Medicine (RSM), 1 Wimpole Street, London W1M 8AE
    Tel. 071-408 2119

Royal Society for the Prevention of Accidents (RoSPA), Cannon House, The Priory, Queensway, Birmingham B4 6BS
    Tel. 021-200 2461

Samaritans, 17 Uxbridge Road, Slough, Berkshire SL1 1SN
    Tel. 0753 32713

Scottish Council for Single Parents, 13 Gayfield Square, Edinburgh EH1 3NX
    Tel. 031-556 3899

Sickle Cell Society (SCS), 54 Station Road, Harlesden, London NW10 4BO
    Tel. 081-961 7795

Spastics Society, 840 Brighton Road, Purley, Surrey CR8 2BH
    Tel. 081-660 8552

St John Ambulance Association (StJAA), 1 Grosvenor Crescent, London SW1X 7EF
    Tel. 071-235 5231

Stillbirth and Neonatal Death Society (SANDS), 28 Portland Place, London W1
    Tel. 071-436 5881

Tavistock Institute of Human Relations, Tavistock Centre, Belsize Lane, London NW3 5BA
    Tel. 071-435 7111 ext 2383

Tay-Sachs and Allied Diseases Association, 17 Sydney Road, Barkingside, Ilford, Essex IG6 2ED

Tel. 081-550 8989

Terence Higgins Trust, 52–54 Gray's Inn Road, London WC1X 8JU
Tel. 071-242 1010

Travellers Rights Organization, S. Crawley, 4 Toneborough Estate, Abbey Road, London NW6

Twins and Multiple Births Association (TAMBA), PO Box 30, Little Sutton, South Wirral L66 1TH
Tel. 051 348 0020

United Kingdom Central Council for Nursing, Midwifery and Health Visiting (UKCC), 23 Portland Place, London W1N 3AF
Tel. 071-637 7181 .

United Kingdom Thalassaemia Society, 107 Nightingale Lane, London N8 7QY
Tel. 081-348 0437

Vegan Society, 7 Battle Road, St Leonards-on-Sea, East Sussex TN37 7AA
Tel. 0424 427393

Vegetarian Society of the UK Ltd, Parkdale, Dunham Road, Altrincham, Cheshire WA14 4QE
Tel. 061-928 0793

Welsh Board for Nursing, Midwifery and Health Visiting, 13th Floor, Pearl Assurance House, Greyfriars Road, Cardiff CF1 3AG
Tel. 0222 395535

Women's Health Concern, PO Box 1629, London W8 6AU
Tel. 071-938 3932

Women's Natural Health Centre, 1 Hillside, Highgate Road, London NW5 1QT
Tel. 071-482 3293 (9.30 a.m.–1 p.m.)

Women's Therapy Centre, 6–9 Manor Gardens, London N7 6LA
Tel. 071-263 6200

Womens Royal Voluntary Service (WRVS), 234–244 Stockwell Road, London SW9 9SP
Tel. 071-733 3388

World Health Organization (WHO), Geneva, Switzerland

International Confederation of Midwives
Australia
Australian College of Midwives Inc., 260 Albert Road, East Melbourne, Victoria 3002

Austria
Verbindungsstelle der Hebammen, Österreichs, Heinrich Oschlgasse 19/6/8, A 3430 Tulln

Belgium
Comité de concertation des Accoucheuses Belges/Overlegcomite, van de Belgische Vroedvrouwen Square Vergote 43, 1040 Brussels

Brazil
Associacao Brasileira de Obstetrizes, Rua Roberto Dias Lopez 80/302, Rio de Janeiro

Burkina Faso
Association Burkinabé des Sages Femmes, BP 4686, Ouagadougou

Canada
The Alberta Association of Midwives, PO Box 1177, Station G, Calgary, Alberta, T3A 3G3
Midwives Association of British Columbia, International Section, 244–810 West Broadway, Vancouver, V4Z 5C9
Association of Ontario Midwives International Section, PO Box 85, Postal Station G, Toronto, Ontario M6J 3M7
Association des Sages-Femmes de Quebec, 675 av. Marguerite-Bourgeois, Quebec G1S 3V8

Chile
Colegio de Matronas de Chile A.G., Phillips 15, Depto L, 6 Piso, Santiago

Czechoslovakia
Czechoslovak Midwives' Association, c/o Mrs Olga Kubeckova, Pollitova 849/5, CS 120 00 Prague 10

Denmark
Den almindelige Dankse Jordemoderforening, Norre Voldgade 90, DK-1358 Copenhagen K

Ethiopia
Midwives' Section, EHPU, PO Box 7123, Addis Ababa

Finland
Suomen Katiloliitto, Asemamiehenkatu 4, 00520 Helsinki

Germany
Bund Deutscher Hebammen e.V., Reinhold-Frankstrasse 18, PO Box 1724, 7500 Karlsruhe 1
Bund freiberuflicher Hebammen Deutschlands e.V., Ludwig-Uhland-Str. 28, 6903 Neckargemund

Ghana
Ghana Registered Midwives' Association, PO Box 147, Accra

Greece
The Greek Midwives' Association, 2 Arist. Pappa. Ampelokipi, 115 21 Athens

Hong Kong
Hong Kong Midwives' Association, D1, 13th Floor, Hyde Centre, 221–226 Gloucester Road, Wanchai

Iceland
Icelandic Midwives' Association, Ljosmaedrafelag Islands, Grettisgata 89, 105 Reykjavik

Indonesia
Indonesian Midwives' Association, Jalan Johar Baru, V/13D Kayu Awet, Jakarta 10560, Pusat

Iran
Iranian Midwives' Association, PO Box 15878—1936, Tehran

Ireland
Ms H. Marchant, Midwives' Section, Irish Nurses' Organization, 11 Fitzwilliam Place, Dublin 2

Israel
Israel Midwives' Association, PO Box 7079, Tel-Aviv 61070

Italy
AIORCE, Piazza Tarquinia 5/D, 00183 Rome

Jamaica
Jamaican Midwives' Association, Victoria Jubilee Hospital, North Street, Kingston

Japan
Japan Academy of Midwifery, 1–12 Kata-machi, Shinjuku-ku, Tokyo 160
Japanese Midwives' Association, 1-8-21 Fujimi, Chiyoda-ku, Tokyo 102
Midwives' Division, Japanese Nursing Association, 8-2, 5-chome Jingumae, Shibuya-ku, Tokyo 150

Korea
Korean Midwives' Association, 35-5, 1-Ga, Chang Choong-Dong, Choong-gu, Seoul

France
Soeur Marie Leonard Mazraani, Présidente, Association des Sages-Femmes du Liban, 101 rue de Reuilly, Paris 75012

Liberia
Liberian Midwives' Association, c/o Mrs E. Ayomanor, JFK Maternity Centre, PO Box 1973, Monrovia

Luxembourg
Association des Sages-Femmes Luxembourgeoises, 22 rue Theodore Gillen, L-1625 Howald

Malta
The Midwives' Association, 167 Marina Street, Pieta, MSD 08

Morocco
Association morocaine des Sages-Femmes, Collège de Santé publique, Route de Casa KM4, Rabat

The Netherlands
Nederlandse Organisatie van Verloskundigen, p/Medisch Centrum Berg en Bosch, Prof. Bronkhorstlaan 10, 3723 MB Bilthoven

New Zealand
New Zealand College of Midwives, PO Box 7063, Wellington South, Wellington

Nigeria
Professional Ass. of Midwives, c/o Mrs G. E. Delano, Obstetrical & Gynaecology Dept., University College Hospital, Ibadan, Ogun State

Norway
Den Norske Jordmorforening, Tollbugaten 35, 0157 Oslo
Norsk Sykepleierforbunds Landsgruppe av Jordmodre, c/o Jorunn Wik Tunestweit, Våkleivskogen 130, 5062 Bones

Paraguay
Federacion Paraguaya de Obstetras, Gral. Colman No. 1852 y Panambireta, Casilla del Correo 2733, Asuncion

Philippines
Integrated Midwives' Association of the Philippines, IMAP Building, Corner Pinaglabanan & Ejercito Sts. San Juan, Metro Manila

Malaysia
Sarawak Midwives' Association, c/o School of Paramedical Personnel, Jalan Tun Abang Haji Openg, 93590 Kuching, Sarawak

Sierra Leone
Sierra Leone Midwives' Association, PO Box 1394, Freetown

Spain
Associacio Catalana de Llevadores, Tapineria, 10, 2o. 08002 Barcelona
Consejo General de Enfermeria, Seccion Matronas, Buen Suceso No. 6, Madrid 28008
Asociacion Nacional de Matronas, Espanolas, c/Menendez Pelayo 93, 28007 Madrid

Sudan
The Sudanese Midwives' Union, c/o Mrs N. Imam, Department of Midwifery, Khartoum Nursing College, PO Box 1063, Khartoum, Sudan

Sweden
Svenska Barnmorskeforbundet, Ostermalmsgatan 19, 114 26 Stockholm

Switzerland
Schweizerischer Hebammenverband, Flurstrasse 26, 3000 Bern 22

Taiwan
Midwifery Association of the Republic of China, Taoyan County Health Bureau, 55 Hsien Fu Road, Taoyan City

Uganda
Uganda Private Midwives' Association, PO Box 30962, Nakivubo, Kampala

UK
Royal College of Midwives, 15 Mansfield Street, London W1M 0BE
Association of Supervisors of Midwives, Maternity Unit, James Paget Hospital, Lowestoft Road, Gorleston, Great Yarmouth, Norfolk NR31 6LA
Association of Radical Midwives, 62 Greetby Hill, Ormskirk, Lancashire L39 2DT

USA
Midwives' Alliance of North America, c/o Karen Moran, PO Box 1121, Bristol, Virginia 24203-1121
American College of Nurse Midwives, 1522 K St NW, Suite 1000, Washington DC 20005

Kelnar & Harvey
The Sick Newborn Baby 2/e

This successful book is centred around the
team approach to neonatal care by nurses,
midwives and doctors. It includes information
on care of bereaved parents, AIDS and
management of the pregnant diabetic and her
baby.

CONTENTS:
The Challenge for Perinatal Care - Prenatal
Influences on the Baby - Resuscitation and
Care of the Baby at Delivery - Care of Normal
Newborn Babies - Care of Low Birth Weight
Babies - Respiratory Problems - Nutrition -
Congenital Disorders: General Principles -
Congenital Disorders: Specific Conditions -
Congenital Heart Disease - Birth Trauma -
Jaundice - Bleeding Disorders - Neurological
Disorders - The-Large-for-Dates Baby -
Infection - Sudden or Gradual Deterioration -
The Mother and Baby in Hospital - Perinatal
Care in Developing Countries - Appendix

0 7020 1185 1   384pp   118 ills   Pb   1986
Baillière Tindall   £10.00

Weller
Baillière's Encyclopaedic Dictionary of Nursing & Health Care

"...It contains a wealth of information and is much more than just a dictionary."
Nursing Standard

The first encyclopaedic dictionary of its kind to be published in Britain specifically for UK nurses and other health care professionals. In addition to defining the 24,000 entries included, for all of the more important nursing topics, comprehensive information on aetiology, complications and patient care is given.

Together with many figures and tables, an excellent pronunciation guide, and three Appendices, this dictionary is an invaluable companion as a comprehensive reference source for all in the nursing and related health care professions.

0 7020 1196 7   1312pp   158 ills   30 tables
Hb   1989   Baillière Tindall   £12.95

Ethics: A Primer for Nurses

Verena Tschudin

How do we know what is right? Or good or fair or honest? Who decides?

This beautifully designed **Workbook** allows you to explore your own ideas and opinions through imaginative and challenging exercises. Used as part of a workshop with the accompanying **Workshop Guide**, or for independent study, it aims to help you understand and evaluate the choices and decisions you need to make.

The **Workshop Guide** is designed to facilitate group learning about ethics in a workshop setting, and contains handouts, suggestions for role-play, and background material.

Workshop Guide 0 7020 1650 0 £55.00
Workbook 0 7020 1749 7 £9.95
Workshop Pack 0 7020 1679 9 £150.00
Oct 1992 Baillière Tindall

Halliday, McClure & Reid
Handbook of Neonatal Intensive Care (3/e)

A pocket-sized handbook that provides details of
how to manage very ill and premature babies.
Includes information on respiratory distress
syndrome, AIDS and improved non-invasive
imaging techniques. An indispensable reference
for all who work in the field.

Contents

Prenatal Diagnosis - Examination of the Normal
Newborn - High-risk Pregnancy - Asphyxia and
Resuscitation - Transitional Care and Transport -
The Low Birth Weight Infant - The Big Baby -
Basic Principles of Neonatal Intensive Care -
Procedures in Neonatal Intensive Care -
Respiratory Problems - Fluids and Nutrition -
Glucose, Calcium and Electrolyte Disturbances -
Jaundice - Fetal and Neonatal Infection -
Apnoeic Attacks - Neurological Problems -
Cardiovascular Problems - Gastrointestinal
Problems - Genitourinary Problems - Metabolic
and Endocrine Problems - Haematological
Problems - The Very Low Birth Weight Infant -
Congenital Malformations - Parental Attachment
- Infant Follow Up

0 7020 1399 4   414pp Pb 1989
Baillière Tindall £10.50

Hinchliff & Montague
Physiology for Nursing Practice

"The entire approach in this excellent book confirms the importance of a 'bionursing' view of the relation between the life sciences and the practice of nursing"
Nursing Times

This exciting and imaginative text enables the reader to understand the principles and mechanisms of normal body function and how these mechanisms alter in illness. The reader is provided with a rational basis for assessing patients' health problems and the planning, delivery and evaluation of care.

The book is divided into sections which logically illustrate the functions of the body as a complex homeostatic system. Multi-choice format review questions, suggestions for practical work and references of particular relevance enable readers to test and develop their knowledge.

0 7020 1194 0   695pp   384 ills   Pb   1988
Baillière Tindall £15.95

Education and Counselling for Childbirth

Kitzinger

This book is about the normal life crisis of having a baby and how those involved, whether doctor, nurse, midwife, physiotherapist, childbirth educator, psychotherapist, social worker or other, can help a woman, and often the prospective father too, meet the challenge arising from new emotional and social stresses which confront the couple when a baby is on the way.

0 7020 0642 4   317pp
Baillière Tindall Pbk   1977   £11.50

Before We Are Born: Basic
Embryology and Birth Defects
3rd Edition

KEITH L. MOORE

This concise embryology book is especially
designed as a convenient reference.

Coverage includes
- Reproduction
- Specific weeks of development
- Causes of congenital malformations
- *In vitro* fertilization
- Embryonic transfer
- Induction
- The embryonic period.

Features an increased use of full-colour
illustrations throughout.

0 7216 2207 0   280pp   210 ills   Pb   1989
W. B. Saunders   £19.00

Exhaustively Referenced

Blackburn & Loper
Maternal, Fetal, and Neonatal Physiology: A Clinical Perspective

This book provides a reference synthesising the latest research from physiology and the clinical sciences to present a detailed picture of the normal physiology of pregnancy, fetal and neonatal development. Comprehensive, detailed and well-illustrated, it consistently identifies clinical implications.

0 7216 2936 9   726pp   178 ills   1992
W. B. Saunders   £50.00

W. B. Saunders
24-28 Oval Road London NW1 7DX
071-267-4466

Concise and Logical Text

Cohen et al
Maternal, Neonatal and Women's Health Nursing

The first concise, logically organized maternal-neonatal textbook that takes the women's health focus beyond gynaecological care. It provides the basic components of physiology, clinical obstetrics, family-centred care, new-born care, and the Nursing Process along with a special section on women's health care. Also addresses the technological advances in maternal and new-born care and how it is being used by nurses.

0 87434 258 9   1296pp   Hb   1991
Springhouse Publishing Co.   £35.50

MATERNITY NURSING

Arlene Burroughs

Concise and easy to read, the new edition of this classic reference provides readers with essential knowledge for delivering quality maternity care.

Covers such topics as

- Health care during pregnancy
- Labour and delivery
- Parent-infant attachment,
- Assessment of fetal health
- Care of the newborn.

Also includes the latest on AIDS, infection control, sexually transmitted diseases, plus substance abuse, including cocaine.

0 7216 3313 7   544pp   200 ills   Hb
1992   W.B. Saunders   £16.50

Solomon & Davis
Human Anatomy & Physiology (2nd Edition)

This introductory text takes an integrated approach as it examines each body system's relationship to the organism as a whole. Basic concepts of human anatomy and physiology are explored in depth while emphasising the body as a homeostatic unit.

Key features of this edition include 130 new four colour photographs, and transparency acetate overlays for the human body and the human cell which facilitate a three-dimensional understanding of both. The immunology chapter has been revised to reflect the latest concepts in immunology.

0 03 053798 3 864pp Hb 1990 £41.50
International Edition 0 03 032389 4
£17.50
Study Guide 0 03 011918 9 £12.00